Molecular Mechanisms of Sensorineural Hearing Loss and Development of Inner Ear Therapeutics

Molecular Mechanisms of Sensorineural Hearing Loss and Development of Inner Ear Therapeutics

Editor

Srdjan M Vlajkovic

MDPI • Basel • Beijing • Wuhan • Barcelona • Belgrade • Manchester • Tokyo • Cluj • Tianjin

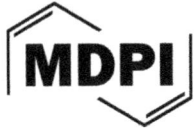

Editor
Srdjan M Vlajkovic
Department of Physiology
The University of Auckland
Auckland
New Zealand

Editorial Office
MDPI
St. Alban-Anlage 66
4052 Basel, Switzerland

This is a reprint of articles from the Special Issue published online in the open access journal *International Journal of Molecular Sciences* (ISSN 1422-0067) (available at: www.mdpi.com/journal/ijms/special_issues/Molecular_Hearing_Loss).

For citation purposes, cite each article independently as indicated on the article page online and as indicated below:

LastName, A.A.; LastName, B.B.; LastName, C.C. Article Title. *Journal Name* **Year**, *Volume Number*, Page Range.

ISBN 978-3-0365-1506-9 (Hbk)
ISBN 978-3-0365-1505-2 (PDF)

© 2021 by the authors. Articles in this book are Open Access and distributed under the Creative Commons Attribution (CC BY) license, which allows users to download, copy and build upon published articles, as long as the author and publisher are properly credited, which ensures maximum dissemination and a wider impact of our publications.

The book as a whole is distributed by MDPI under the terms and conditions of the Creative Commons license CC BY-NC-ND.

Contents

About the Editor vii

Preface to "Molecular Mechanisms of Sensorineural Hearing Loss and Development of Inner Ear Therapeutics" ix

Srdjan M. Vlajkovic and Peter R. Thorne
Molecular Mechanisms of Sensorineural Hearing Loss and Development of Inner Ear Therapeutics
Reprinted from: *Int. J. Mol. Sci.* **2021**, *22*, 5647, doi:10.3390/ijms22115647 1

Dong Jun Park, Sunmok Ha, Jin Sil Choi, Su Hoon Lee, Jeong-Eun Park and Young Joon Seo
Induced Short-Term Hearing Loss due to Stimulation of Age-Related Factors by Intermittent Hypoxia, High-Fat Diet, and Galactose Injection
Reprinted from: *Int. J. Mol. Sci.* **2020**, *21*, 7068, doi:10.3390/ijms21197068 5

Judit Szepesy, Viktória Humli, János Farkas, Ildikó Miklya, Júlia Tímár, Tamás Tábi, Anita Gáborján, Gábor Polony, Ágnes Szirmai, László Tamás, László Köles, Elek Sylvester Vizi and Tibor Zelles
Chronic Oral Selegiline Treatment Mitigates Age-Related Hearing Loss in BALB/c Mice
Reprinted from: *Int. J. Mol. Sci.* **2021**, *22*, 2853, doi:10.3390/ijms22062853 23

Chao-Hui Yang, Chung-Feng Hwang, Jiin-Haur Chuang, Wei-Shiung Lian, Feng-Sheng Wang, Ethan I. Huang and Ming-Yu Yang
Constant Light Dysregulates Cochlear Circadian Clock and Exacerbates Noise-Induced Hearing Loss
Reprinted from: *Int. J. Mol. Sci.* **2020**, *21*, 7535, doi:10.3390/ijms21207535 41

Sohyeon Park, Seung Hee Han, Byeong-Gon Kim, Myung-Whan Suh, Jun Ho Lee, Seung Ha Oh and Moo Kyun Park
Changes in microRNA Expression in the Cochlear Nucleus and Inferior Colliculus after Acute Noise-Induced Hearing Loss
Reprinted from: *Int. J. Mol. Sci.* **2020**, *21*, 8792, doi:10.3390/ijms21228792 57

Christine Fok, Milan Bogosanovic, Madhavi Pandya, Ravindra Telang, Peter R. Thorne and Srdjan M. Vlajkovic
Regulator of G Protein Signalling 4 (RGS4) as a Novel Target for the Treatment of Sensorineural Hearing Loss
Reprinted from: *Int. J. Mol. Sci.* **2020**, *22*, 3, doi:10.3390/ijms22010003 77

Sara Eitelmann, Laura Petersilie, Christine R. Rose and Jonathan Stephan
Altered Gap Junction Network Topography in Mouse Models for Human Hereditary Deafness
Reprinted from: *Int. J. Mol. Sci.* **2020**, *21*, 7376, doi:10.3390/ijms21197376 97

Antonino Germanà, Maria Cristina Guerrera, Rosaria Laurà, Maria Levanti, Marialuisa Aragona, Kamel Mhalhel, Germana Germanà, Giuseppe Montalbano and Francesco Abbate
Expression and Localization of BDNF/TrkB System in the Zebrafish Inner Ear
Reprinted from: *Int. J. Mol. Sci.* **2020**, *21*, 5787, doi:10.3390/ijms21165787 115

John Hoon Rim, Jae Young Choi, Jinsei Jung and Heon Yung Gee
Activation of KCNQ4 as a Therapeutic Strategy to Treat Hearing Loss
Reprinted from: *Int. J. Mol. Sci.* **2021**, *22*, 2510, doi:10.3390/ijms22052510 129

Dorota Olex-Zarychta
Hyperbaric Oxygenation as Adjunctive Therapy in the Treatment of Sudden Sensorineural Hearing Loss
Reprinted from: *Int. J. Mol. Sci.* **2020**, *21*, 8588, doi:10.3390/ijms21228588 . . . . **143**

About the Editor

Srdjan M Vlajkovic

Associate Professor Srdjan Vlajkovic holds an academic appointment in the Department of Physiology at the University of Auckland, New Zealand. His research focus is on molecular mechanisms of sensorineural hearing loss and the development of inner ear therapeutics. His research has contributed to the current understanding of the role of adenosine receptors in the repair of cochlear injury and restoration of hearing. His translational research in this area has implications for the treatment of several forms of sensorineural hearing loss, such as those induced by exposure to noise, ototoxic drugs and ageing.

Preface to "Molecular Mechanisms of Sensorineural Hearing Loss and Development of Inner Ear Therapeutics"

The scope of this book is to advance our understanding of the causes and mechanisms of hearing loss and propose novel strategies to protect and restore hearing.

The book contains original research articles and state-of-the-art reviews that address the mechanisms of sensorineural hearing loss caused by cochlear injury or gene mutations, propose new strategies to promote hearing rescue after cochlear injury, and identify novel biomarkers of hearing loss. This book can serve as a useful resource for auditory neuroscientists, audiologists, otolaryngologists, and all those who have a keen interest in this research field. We greatly appreciate the contributions of all authors and anonymous reviewers.

Srdjan M Vlajkovic
Editor

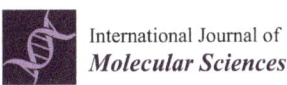

Editorial

Molecular Mechanisms of Sensorineural Hearing Loss and Development of Inner Ear Therapeutics

Srdjan M. Vlajkovic *[ ] and Peter R. Thorne

Department of Physiology and The Eisdell Moore Centre, Faculty of Medical and Health Sciences, The University of Auckland, Private Bag 92019, Auckland 1142, New Zealand; pr.thorne@auckland.ac.nz
* Correspondence: s.vlajkovic@auckland.ac.nz; Tel.: +64-9-923-9782

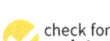

Citation: Vlajkovic, S.M.; Thorne, P.R. Molecular Mechanisms of Sensorineural Hearing Loss and Development of Inner Ear Therapeutics. *Int. J. Mol. Sci.* **2021**, *22*, 5647. https://doi.org/10.3390/ijms22115647

Received: 28 April 2021
Accepted: 24 May 2021
Published: 26 May 2021

Publisher's Note: MDPI stays neutral with regard to jurisdictional claims in published maps and institutional affiliations.

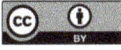

Copyright: © 2021 by the authors. Licensee MDPI, Basel, Switzerland. This article is an open access article distributed under the terms and conditions of the Creative Commons Attribution (CC BY) license (https://creativecommons.org/licenses/by/4.0/).

The sense of hearing enables us to enjoy sounds and music and engage with other people. The sense of hearing is, however, vulnerable to environmental challenges, such as exposure to noise. Indeed, more than 1.5 billion people experience some decline in hearing ability during their lifetime, of whom at least 430 million will be affected by disabling hearing loss. If not identified and addressed in a timely way, hearing loss can severely reduce the quality of life at various stages, for example by delaying language development, reducing social engagement, compromising economic independence and educational opportunities [1]. The cost of hearing loss has been estimated at more than USD 980 billion annually at a global level [1].

Some causes of hearing loss can be prevented, for example from occupational or leisure noise. The World Health Organization (WHO, Geneva, Switzerland) estimates that more than 1 billion young people put themselves at risk of permanent hearing loss by listening to loud music over long periods of time. Mitigating such risks through public health action is essential to addressing hearing loss in the community (WHO, World Report on Hearing, March 2021).

Hearing impairment often results from loss of the sensory hair cells and primary auditory neurons due to disease or trauma to the cochlea of the inner ear. The etiology of sensorineural hearing loss (SNHL) is complex and multifactorial, arising from congenital and acquired causes. Congenital hearing loss commonly manifests as hearing deficits at birth or during early development, while acquired hearing loss is usually sustained in later life from infection, exposure to excessive noise, ototoxic drugs, or the ageing process.

Substantial progress has been made in recent years towards understanding the underlying mechanisms of SNHL and the discovery of novel therapeutic targets to prevent and mitigate the hearing loss. In addition, the link between hearing loss and dementia has been established, with the view that hearing loss prevention may also protect cognitive function.

The aim of this special issue was to advance our understanding of the causes and mechanisms of hearing loss and propose novel strategies to protect and restore hearing. We invited investigators to contribute original research articles and state-of-the-art reviews to address the mechanisms of SNHL caused by cochlear injury or gene mutations, propose new strategies to promote hearing rescue after cochlear injury, and identify novel biomarkers of hearing loss. The collection includes seven original research papers and two reviews from the international groups investigating different aspects of SNHL.

Two articles focused on age-related hearing loss (ARHL). ARHL is the most common sensory disorder among the elderly, characterized by a decline in hearing sensitivity and speech discrimination, delayed central processing of acoustic information, and impaired localization of sound sources [2]. Multiple mechanisms have been proposed for age-related cochlear degeneration, and it appears that both genetic and environmental factors play a role [3]. There are currently no ARHL animal models induced by environmental challenges. Park and colleagues [4] presented a new model of ARHL established by exposing animals to continuous oxidative stress to promote cell ageing. Oxidative stress was induced in mice by intermittent hypoxic conditions, high-fat diet (HFD), or D-galactose injections. Hypoxia had the greatest effect on hearing loss induction, whilst HFD and D-galactose injections induced metabolic changes that promote cell ageing and apoptosis without significant changes in auditory thresholds. When two or more oxidative stress stimuli were combined, hearing loss occurred over a shorter period. The incidence of hearing loss was the highest in triple-exposure conditions than in any single factor model. The authors suggest that this novel animal model can aid in the development of preventative and treatment strategies for ARHL.

Even though approximately one in three people over the age of 65 years suffer from hearing loss, pharmacological therapies for ARHL are still lacking. Previous animal studies have shown that some antioxidants, apoptosis inhibitors, and neuroprotective compounds can delay the onset of ARHL, but none of these compounds successfully completed clinical trials. Szepesy and co-workers [5] propose selegiline, the FDA-approved anti-Parkinsonian drug, as a promising candidate for the treatment of ARHL due to its complex neuroprotective, antioxidant, antiapoptotic, and dopamine release-enhancing effects. In BALB/c mice, selegiline administered in drinking water mitigated the progression of ARHL at frequencies 8–16 kHz. The lack of otoprotective effect in DBA/2J mice indicated strain differences in response to selegiline, and the authors recognize that the otoprotective effect of selegiline depends on the host's genetic background.

Noise-induced hearing loss (NIHL) has become a leading occupational health risk in developed countries. NIHL may also result from unsafe recreational, social, and residential noise exposures. People with excessive exposure to noise are frequently the population with a lifestyle of irregular circadian rhythms, which may affect auditory function. The study by Yang and co-workers [6] provides evidence that the disturbed circadian clock induced by exposure to constant light leads to the suppression of circadian clock rhythmicity genes in the cochlea of CBA/CaJ mice without affecting auditory brainstem (ABR) thresholds. However, exposure to high intensity noise in those mice enhanced ABR threshold shifts and increased the loss of outer hair cells and synaptic ribbons relative to the control mice on normal circadian rhythm. This suggests that the dysregulation of the cochlear circadian clock can affect auditory function in the cochlea exposed to acoustic trauma. The study also underlines the importance of the normal circadian clock in the inner ear as a possible mitigation factor in noise-induced cochlear injury.

MicroRNAs are small non-coding single-stranded RNAs that regulate posttranscriptional gene expression. Acute exposure to traumatic noise induces microRNA expression changes not only in the cochlea, but also in central auditory pathways. Park and collaborators [7] demonstrated expression changes of several microRNAs involved in neural plasticity in the cochlear nucleus and inferior colliculus of the rat. Preliminary evidence suggests that these microRNAs may be involved in regulating the MAPK signaling pathway, axon guidance, and the TGF-β signaling pathway. Since miRNAs are stable and can be detected in the blood, they may represent biomarkers for early diagnosis of NIHL. The authors also suggest that the gene therapy involving the transfer of miRNAs to target cells could be used to promote neural plasticity in the central auditory pathways and thus reduce the impact of acoustic injury.

There is a significant need for the development of effective therapies to prevent permanent cochlear damage and hearing loss after acoustic overexposure. Fok and colleagues [8] identified a novel pharmacological target for the treatment of noise-induced cochlear injury in the post-exposure period. The Regulator of G protein Signaling 4 (RGS4) regulates the activity of G protein-coupled A_1 adenosine receptors, which confer considerable otoprotection against acoustic trauma and other forms of SNHL such as from cisplatin and aminoglycoside antibiotics. Intratympanic administration of a small molecule RGS4 inhibitor 48 h after exposure to traumatic noise attenuated noise-induced PTS in rats by up to 19 dB, whilst the earlier drug administration (24 h) led to even better preservation of auditory thresholds (up to 32 dB). This was linked to improved survival of sensorineural tissues and afferent synapses in the cochlea. This study demonstrates that intratympanic administration of an RGS4 inhibitor can rescue cochlear injury and hearing loss induced by acoustic overexposure. The authors postulate that the study presents a novel paradigm for the treatment of various forms of SNHL based on regulation of A_1 receptor signaling.

On a different note, the paper by Eitelmann and co-workers [9] reported the altered gap junction network topography in mouse models of human hereditary deafness. Mutations in various genes, such as those coding for the voltage-gated calcium channel CaV1.3 or the calcium sensor otoferlin in the inner hair cells of the cochlea, cause hereditary deafness. In genetically modified mouse models lacking these genes, auditory brainstem nuclei are deprived of spontaneous neuronal activity originating in the cochlea, which results in altered neuronal circuitry in auditory brainstem nuclei. This study demonstrates that the altered neuronal circuitry is linked to impaired topography of astrocyte networks in the brainstem. The immunoexpression of astrocytic connexin hemichannels Cx30 and Cx43 increased in the lateral superior olive (LSO) of CaV1.3 and otoferlin knockout mice, respectively. The authors conclude that the spontaneous neuronal activity in the cochlea is crucial for the proper formation of gap junction networks in LSO and point at a critical role of neuron-glia interactions in the auditory brainstem during early postnatal development.

An interesting contribution by Germana and colleagues [10] focused on the development of zebrafish inner ear. The zebrafish is recognized as an important experimental animal model for studying developmental biology and genetics, as well as modelling human disorders including SNHL. The hair cells of the zebrafish inner ear show structural similarity with the sensory hair cells of the mammalian inner ear, but they also have an extraordinary ability to regenerate. This study was undertaken to analyze the cellular localization of brain-derived neurotrophic factor (BDNF) and its receptor TrkB in the inner ear of the zebrafish. BDNF is essential for the development and neuronal plasticity in the brain, but also plays a key role in the regulation and development of the auditory system in mammals. The results of this study demonstrate that the BDNF/TrkB system is present in the sensory cells of the inner ear during the entire life of zebrafish, suggesting that the zebrafish inner ear represents a good model to study the role of neurotrophins in the biology of sensory hair cells. The similarity of the cellular localization of the BDNF/TrkB system in zebrafish and mammals suggests a similar role of this complex in the development and functional maintenance of the inner ear, but may also have implications for the regenerative processes.

The voltage-gated potassium channel KCNQ4 has an essential role in regulating auditory function in the inner ear, by contributing to potassium recycling and maintenance of cochlear homeostasis. Reduced activity of the KCNQ4 channel has been associated with a genetic form of hearing loss, noise-induced hearing loss, and age-related hearing loss [11]. Rim and colleagues presented a comprehensive review of 90 publications looking at the KCNQ4 as a potential therapeutic target for the treatment of hearing loss [11]. In this review, the authors updated the current concepts of the physiological and pathophysiological roles of KCNQ4 in the inner ear and focused on the role of KCNQ4 activators in therapeutic management of different forms of hearing loss. They propose that the simultaneous application of two activators with distinct modes of action may result in synergistic effects and reduced off-target effects. It was also suggested that drug repurposing may be an attractive option for clinical development of KCNQ4 activators as therapies for hearing loss.

Sudden sensorineural hearing loss (SSHL), also known as sudden deafness, is an unexplained, rapid loss of hearing which often affects only one ear and is considered a medical emergency [12]. SSHL can happen to people at any age, but most often affects adults in their late 40s and early 50s. Although about half of people with SSHL recover some or all their hearing spontaneously, usually within one to two weeks from onset, delaying SSHL diagnosis can decrease treatment effectiveness. The comprehensive review by Olex-Zarychta [12] presents hyperbaric oxygen therapy (HBOT) as a medical procedure used as an adjunct therapy for SSHL in addition to oral/intratympanic administration of steroids. In the treatment of SSHL, HBOT is used to reverse the lack of oxygen in the inner ear, which affects the viability of sensorineural tissues. This review focuses on the molecular mechanisms and clinical effectiveness of HBOT in the treatment of SSHL, carefully weighing the risks and benefits of its implementation.

In conclusion, this Special Issue highlights the diverse range of approaches to SNHL, from designing new animal models of ARHL, to the use of microRNAs as biomarkers of cochlear injury and drug repurposing for the therapy of age-related and noise-induced hearing loss. Further investigation into the underlying molecular mechanisms of SNHL and the integration of the novel drug, cell, and gene therapy strategies into controlled clinical studies will permit significant advances in a field where there are currently many unmet needs.

Author Contributions: Original draft preparation, S.M.V.; review and editing, P.R.T. All authors have read and agreed to the published version of the manuscript.

Funding: This research received no external funding.

Institutional Review Board Statement: Not applicable.

Informed Consent Statement: Not applicable.

Data Availability Statement: Not applicable.

Conflicts of Interest: The authors declare no conflict of interest.

References

1. McMahon, C.M.; Nieman, C.L.; Thorne, P.R.; Emmett, S.D.; Bhutta, M.F. The inaugural World Report on Hearing: From barriers to a platform for change. *Clin. Otolaryngol.* **2021**, *46*, 459–463. [CrossRef] [PubMed]
2. Gates, G.A.; Mills, J.H. Presbyacusis. *Lancet* **2005**, *366*, 1111–1120.
3. Van Eyken, E.; Van Camp, G.; Van Laer, L. The complexity of age-related hearing impairment: Contributing environmental and genetic factors. *Audiol. Neurootol.* **2007**, *12*, 345–358. [CrossRef] [PubMed]
4. Park, D.J.; Ha, S.; Choi, J.S.; Lee, S.H.; Park, J.-E.; Seo, Y.J. Induced short-term hearing loss due to stimulation of age-related factors by intermittent hypoxia, high-fat diet, and galactose injection. *Int. J. Mol. Sci.* **2020**, *21*, 7068. [CrossRef] [PubMed]
5. Szepesy, J.; Humli, V.; Farkas, J.; Miklya, I.; Tímár, J.; Tábi, T.; Gáborján, A.; Polony, G.; Szirmai, A.; Tamás, L.; et al. Chronic oral selegiline treatment mitigates age-related hearing loss in BALB/c mice. *Int. J. Mol. Sci.* **2021**, *22*, 2853. [CrossRef] [PubMed]
6. Yang, C.-H.; Hwang, C.-F.; Chuang, J.-H.; Lian, W.-S.; Wang, F.-S.; Huang, E.I.; Yang, M.-Y. Constant light dysregulates cochlear circadian clock and exacerbates noise-induced hearing loss. *Int. J. Mol. Sci.* **2020**, *21*, 7535. [CrossRef]
7. Park, S.; Han, S.H.; Kim, B.-G.; Suh, M.-W.; Lee, J.H.; Oh, S.H.; Park, M.K. Changes in microRNA expression in the cochlear nucleus and inferior colliculus after acute noise-induced hearing loss. *Int. J. Mol. Sci.* **2020**, *21*, 8792. [CrossRef]
8. Fok, C.; Bogosanovic, M.; Pandya, M.; Telang, R.; Thorne, P.R.; Vlajkovic, S.M. Regulator of G Protein Signalling 4 (RGS4) as a novel target for the treatment of sensorineural hearing loss. *Int. J. Mol. Sci.* **2021**, *22*, 3. [CrossRef] [PubMed]
9. Eitelmann, S.; Petersilie, L.; Rose, C.R.; Stephan, J. Altered gap junction network topography in mouse models for human hereditary deafness. *Int. J. Mol. Sci.* **2020**, *21*, 7376. [CrossRef]
10. Germanà, A.; Guerrera, M.C.; Laurà, R.; Levanti, M.; Aragona, M.; Mhalhel, K.; Germanà, G.; Montalbano, G.; Abbate, F. Expression and localization of BDNF/TrkB system in the zebrafish inner ear. *Int. J. Mol. Sci.* **2020**, *21*, 5787. [CrossRef]
11. Rim, J.H.; Choi, J.Y.; Jung, J.; Gee, H.Y. Activation of KCNQ4 as a therapeutic strategy to treat hearing loss. *Int. J. Mol. Sci.* **2021**, *22*, 2510. [CrossRef]
12. Olex-Zarychta, D. Hyperbaric oxygenation as adjunctive therapy in the treatment of sudden sensorineural hearing loss. *Int. J. Mol. Sci.* **2020**, *21*, 8588. [CrossRef] [PubMed]

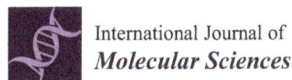

Article

Induced Short-Term Hearing Loss Due to Stimulation of Age-Related Factors by Intermittent Hypoxia, High-Fat Diet, and Galactose Injection

Dong Jun Park [1], Sunmok Ha [2], Jin Sil Choi [1], Su Hoon Lee [1], Jeong-Eun Park [3] and Young Joon Seo [1,*]

[1] Department of Otorhinolaryngology, Yonsei University Wonju College of Medicine, 20 Ilsan-ro, Wonju, Gangwon-do 26426, Korea; papapdj@gmail.com (D.J.P.); true_choi@yonsei.ac.kr (J.S.C.); tngns6049@daum.net (S.H.L.)
[2] Department of Biomedical Laboratory Science, College of Health Sciences, Yonsei University, wonju 26493, Korea; sunmok159@naver.com
[3] Department of Otorhinolaryngology Head and Neck Surgery, Hallym University College of Medicine, Dongtan Sacred Heart Hospital, Hwaseong 18530, Korea; omicsomics@naver.com
* Correspondence: okas2000@hanmail.net; Tel.: +82-33-741-0644

Received: 27 August 2020; Accepted: 23 September 2020; Published: 25 September 2020

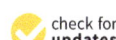

Abstract: Age-related hearing loss (ARHL) is the most common sensory disorder among the elderly, associated with aging and auditory hair cell death due to oxidative-stress-induced mitochondrial dysfunction. Although transgenic mice and long-term aging induction cultures have been used to study ARHL, there are currently no ARHL animal models that can be stimulated by intermittent environmental changes. In this study, an ARHL animal model was established by inducing continuous oxidative stress to promote short-term aging of cells, determined on the basis of expression of hearing-loss-induced phenotypes and aging-related factors. The incidence of hearing loss was significantly higher in dual- and triple-exposure conditions than in intermittent hypoxic conditions, high-fat diet (HFD), or D-galactose injection alone. Continuous oxidative stress and HFD accelerated cellular aging. An increase in *Ucp2*, usually expressed during mitochondrial dysfunction, was observed. Expression of *Cdh23*, *Slc26a4*, *Kcnq4*, *Myo7a*, and *Myo6*, which are ARHL-related factors, were modified by oxidative stress in the cells of the hearing organ. We found that intermittent hypoxia, HFD, and galactose injection accelerated cellular aging in the short term. Thus, we anticipate that the development of this hearing loss animal model, which reflects the effects of intermittent environmental changes, will benefit future research on ARHL.

Keywords: mitochondria dysfunction; reactive oxygen species; hypoxic; D-galactose; high-fat diet; aging; hearing loss

1. Introduction

Age-related hearing loss (ARHL), also known as presbycusis, is an emerging complication in the aging population worldwide. A gradual decrease of hearing function with increasing age is often perceived as an inevitable part of the human aging process. The overall contribution of ARHL to hearing impairment and decreased quality of life is underestimated. Since the average life expectancy of the population is increasing, hearing loss has significant implications on general health and quality of life [1,2]. Various clinical reports have investigated ARHL. According to the 2015 National Health and Nutrition Examination Survey conducted in the USA, 15% of individuals aged between 40 and 49 years were bilaterally deaf, while 19% of those aged between 50–69 and 43.2% of those aged over 70 years had the same condition [3].

Most studies on ARHL are aimed at its prevention and treatment and require long periods of aging for preclinical evaluation [1]. Factors and causes of ageing have been studied using genetically engineered mice, which have proven useful to uncover the mechanisms of aging and help in the discovery of therapeutic drugs [4]. It has been confirmed that oxidative stress caused by reactive oxygen species (ROS) is involved in cochlear cell death in transgenic mice, with an inhibited expression of the apoptosis-related *bax* gene [4]. In fact, mitochondrial DNA damage caused by aging was observed to induce cell death in the hearing organ. [4]. Similarly, increased expression of superoxide dismutase 1 (*Sod1*) and Cadherin 23 (*Cdh23*) have been reported to be associated with aging [5,6]. It has been shown that mouse strains susceptible to early-onset ARHL carry a specific mutation in the *Cdh23* gene, which encodes a component of the hair cell stereocilia tip-link associated with the mechanoelectrical transduction channels. [5,6]. As for *Sod1*, it has been reported that as the amount of oxidative stress in the cells of the auditory organ increases, the amount of *Sod1* also increases [7,8]. In addition, numerous reports have suggested that in these models, abnormal potassium channels resulting from mass transfer errors cause cell death [9,10]. However, these animal models have certain limitations since they do not reflect the lifestyle of the animals [4,11]. Cumulative damage caused by the surrounding environment contributes to ARHL. Oxidative stress accelerates the aging of auditory cells, ultimately causing hearing loss [12]. Therefore, in order to study the short-term effect of pharmaceutical targets, it is essential to develop a preclinical animal model in which oxidative stress can be induced by environmental changes [13].

We have previously conducted studies related to hearing loss caused by hypoxia. Moreover, an association between decreased oxygen saturation and hearing loss has been reported in the literature [14,15]. Therefore, in this study, we used a method based on the induction model of obstructive sleep apnoea syndrome (OSAS), wherein cell aging is promoted by temporarily blocking the supply of oxygen [16]. This model was designed so that the increase in ROS in the blood rapidly damages the auditory organs. We hypothesized that ARHL would be detected, among other aging phenotype changes, after intermittent exposure to a hypoxic environment.

Mitochondrial damage has been considered responsible for the death of auditory hair cells due to aging [6,17]. Therefore, based on relevant factors identified in the literature, we designed an aging animal model resulting from the exposure to a combination of three different lifestyles [9,18]. It has been reported that mitochondrial dysfunction can be induced by diet modification [19]. A high-fat diet (HFD) results in increased intracellular lipid content, diabetes-induced symptoms, and impairment of mitochondrial function due to oxidative stress. Caloric regulation associated with deafness has been reported to suppress cell aging through the inhibition of *Foxo3* and Sirt1 expression, as well as through the activity of apoptosis-related proteins [20]. In addition, clinical studies have reported that over 50% of diabetes patients suffer from hearing loss and that if diabetes persists for more than 5 years, the hearing loss rate doubles [21]. D-galactose (D-gal) injection animal models, established by administering successive subcutaneous D-gal injections to animals for approximately 6 to 8 weeks, have been frequently used in aging studies. In a study by Guo et al., an increase in aging factors was observed in rodents administered D-gal [22]. In addition, accelerated aging of the brain, kidney, liver, and blood cells has been proven in animal models using the galactose injection technique [23–25].

Therefore, we developed an ARHL animal model by changing various aspects of the lifestyle of mice, exposing them to intermittent oxidative stress for a short period of time in order to induce the death of auditory hair cells in the organ of Corti (OC) by stimulating the expression of aging-related factors. This study provides a realistic animal model that can be used to accelerate the development of therapeutic strategies for ARHL in the future.

2. Results

2.1. Phenotypic Analysis of the Different Groups for Ageing

The expected phenotype and hearing loss were observed at approximately 12 weeks. The mice were compared according to the three oxidative stress conditions: HFD, galactose injection (GI), and hypoxia. The exposure to the conditions was combinatory, which lead to the formation of 8 groups through a combination of three oxidative stresses. The physical characteristics of the mice in each group were also recorded. In the group under any of the oxidative stress conditions, it was confirmed that the shine of the hair had disappeared, and it became slightly grey in color (Figure S1). The body weight of mice was significantly increased in the normoxic (Figure 1a) and hypoxic HFD groups (Figure 1b) compared to the control group at 3 months. In terms of the different feeding conditions, the control group showed a minor change in body weight of less than 3 g, but the body weight in the HFD group increased by approximately 20 g after 3 months from baseline (0 months; Figure 1a). Under hypoxia, the control group showed a change in body weight of 4 g, and the HFD group showed an increase of over 20 g at 3 months from baseline (Figure 1b). In the group injected with galactose, a change of 8 to 10 g in body weight under normoxic conditions was observed; however, under hypoxic conditions, a change of 3 to 6 g in body weight was observed. Since we cannot determine aging based on changes in body weight alone, skin tissue from mice in each group was obtained to observe the changes in skin phenotype with aging. Interestingly, following an increase in body weight due to dietary conditions, a change in skin thickness was also observed (Figure 1c).

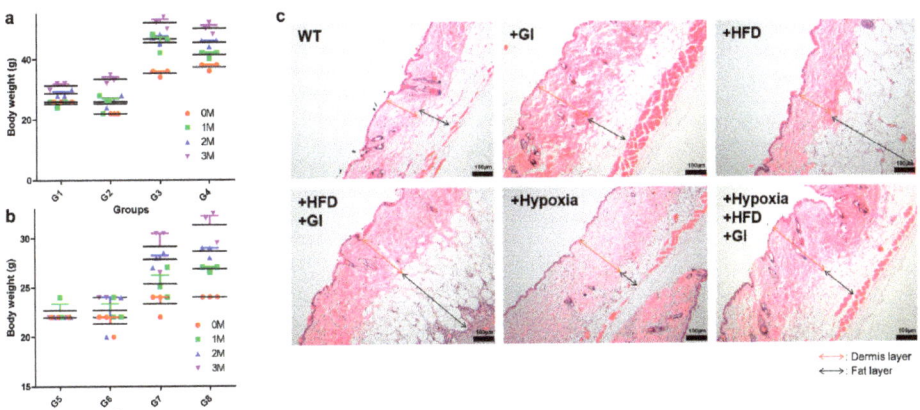

Figure 1. Phenotypic analysis of aging mice under oxidative conditions (**a**) Measured body weight of the normoxic groups. (**b**) Measured body weight of the hypoxic groups. HFD increased body weight regardless of the hypoxic environment. (**c**) The thickness of the dermis skin layer and the thickness of the fat layer were different. Interestingly, the fat layer was significantly thickened in the HFD groups, but it did not increase in size under hypoxic conditions, although the body weight increased. Rather, the dermis layer became thicker and a lot of wrinkles were observed on the skin surface. Abbreviations: HFD, high-fat diet; WT, wild-type.

The thicknesses of the dermis skin layer and of the fat layer were measured microscopically, and HFD was confirmed to produce the most notable effect on the fat layer [26–28]. The fat layer of mice in the HFD groups was the thickest (Table S1). In addition, hypoxia was confirmed to be the condition that affected the dermis the most. An increase in thickness of about 100 μm was observed under hypoxic conditions, and many deep wrinkles were observed on the skin surface in the GI group.

2.2. Oxidative Stress in Serum

Oxidative stress has been demonstrated to be the most important factor in causing aging [14,15]. Therefore, an increase in the levels of ROS and superoxide dismutase (SOD) in serum could be a major indicator of aging induction. In this study, we collected serum from mice in each of the groups throughout each month. SOD activity was measured to elucidate the amount of oxidative stress in each group (Figure 2). Interestingly, oxidative stress increased in the hypoxic group at 2 months from baseline. The normoxic group was associated with a tendency of decreased oxidative stress for 3 months (Table 1).

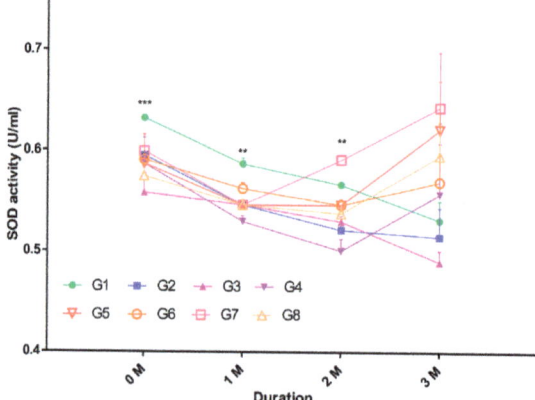

Figure 2. Monthly analysis of SOD activity in the serum from all groups. Serum was collected from mice in each group, and the amount of SOD in serum was measured. Significant values are shown for each month, with ** $p < 0.005$, *** $p < 0.0005$; Abbreviation: SOD, superoxide dismutase.

Table 1. Monthly measurement of SOD activity in serum.

Groups	0 Month	1 Month	2 Months	3 Months
1	0.6325 ± 0.000	0.5873 ± 0.005	0.5667 ± 0.000	0.5311 ± 0.019
2	0.5955 ± 0.017	0.5463 ± 0.005	0.5216 ± 0.005	0.5148 ± 0.028
3	0.5586 ± 0.011	0.5463 ± 0.005	0.5298 ± 0.005	0.4901 ± 0.011
4	0.5873 ± 0.005	0.5298 ± 0.005	0.5011 ± 0.011	0.5572 ± 0.050
5	0.5873 ± 0.029	0.5463 ± 0.005	0.5463 ± 0.005	0.6215 ± 0.048
6	0.5914 ± 0.000	0.5627 ± 0.005	0.5463 ± 0.005	0.5695 ± 0.059
7	0.5996 ± 0.000	0.5463 ± 0.005	0.5914 ± 0.000	0.6435 ± 0.055
8	0.5750 ± 0.011	0.5463 ± 0.005	0.5380 ± 0.005	0.5955 ± 0.022

Abbreviation: SOD, superoxide dismutase.

First, the hypoxic control returned a SOD value of 0.6215 ± 0.048, while the SOD value for the normoxic control was 0.5311 ± 0.019. The SOD values for the GI in hypoxic and normoxic groups were 0.5695 ± 0.059 and 0.5148 ± 0.028, respectively. The SOD values for the hypoxic and normoxic groups under HFD were 0.6435 ± 0.055 and 0.4901 ± 0.011, respectively. Finally, when the hypoxic and normoxic groups were exposed to both HFD and GI, the SOD values were 0.5955 ± 0.022 and 0.5572 ± 0.050, respectively. A 0.04 difference in SOD value is a significant error value and can be regarded as a positive trend. In other words, it was confirmed that the amount of SOD in the body increased with longer exposure to oxidative stress, and the difference in SOD values between hypoxic and normoxic groups was between 0.05 and 0.1534. Thus, we confirmed that hypoxia is the main factor for overall SOD activity increase, based on the significant increase in SOD values in G7, G5, and G8 after 3 months.

2.3. Comparison of the Hearing Threshold

Hearing loss due to aging occurs from the highest to the lowest frequencies [4,29]. Hearing thresholds in the mice groups were measured in the frequency range of 4 to 32 kHz by tone-burst auditory brainstem response (ABR; Figure 3). In the control group, the alteration of the hearing threshold was minimal during the 3 months (Figure 3a). We evaluated hearing loss in mice under all three conditions (hypoxia, HFD, and GI) and observed that there was a significant effect on the hearing threshold and that the value of the hearing threshold significantly decreased after 3 months from 35 to 67 dB at 8 kHz and from 31 to 70 dB at 16 kHz (Figure 3b). In the GI- and HFD-only groups, there was no change in the hearing threshold at any frequency (Figure 3c,d). Conversely, there was a significant elevation in the hearing threshold from 25 to 58 dB at 8 kHz and from 35 to 56 dB at 16 kHz in the hypoxic group (Figure 3e). Finally, the last three groups, characterized by exposure to two conditions each, HFD and GI (Figure 3f), hypoxia and GI (Figure 3g), and hypoxia and HFD (Figure 3h), confirmed the dual-exposure effect. The hearing threshold was significantly increased, from 34 ± 3.76 to 67 ± 10.13 dB at 8 kHz and from 38 ± 4.08 to 60 ± 7.33 dB at 16 kHz, in the hypoxic condition. The *p*-value was analyzed by a two-way analysis of variance (ANOVA), and it addressed the significance of hearing loss from 0 to 3 M.

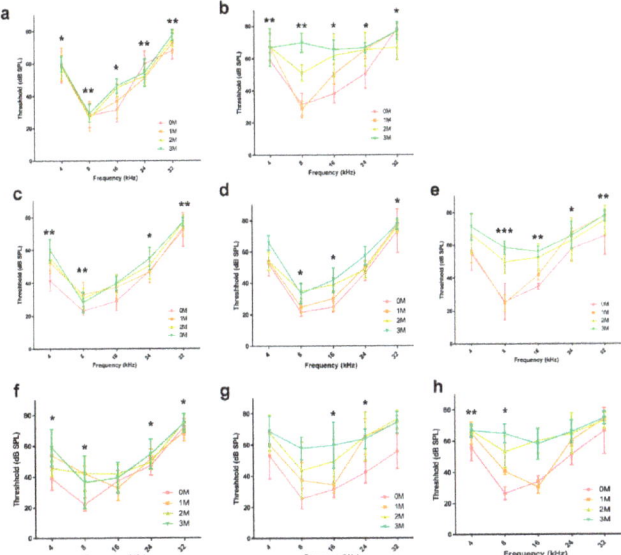

Figure 3. Comparison of the hearing threshold among all groups at various frequencies for each period using the auditory brainstem response (ABR) test. The hearing threshold was found to be greatly decreased under the hypoxic condition. Galactose did not affect hearing loss alone but led to hearing loss in combination with HFD and hypoxic conditions. (**a**) Control group (G1), (**b**) Hypoxia, HFD, GI group (G8), (**c**) GI group (G2), (**d**) HFD group (G3), (**e**) Hypoxia group (G5), (**f**) HFD, GI group (G4), (**g**) Hypoxia, GI group (G6), and (**h**) Hypoxia, HFD group (G7). Significant values are shown, with * $p < 0.05$, ** $p < 0.005$, *** $p < 0.0005$. Abbreviations: HFD, high-fat diet; GI, galactose injection.

The hearing threshold of mice in each group was compared and analyzed among the three conditions through a two-way ANOVA. The analysis was performed by selecting the three frequencies that changed the most: 8, 16, and 24 kHz. The hearing threshold values of the mice in groups G2, G3, and G5 were compared with the control group to analyze the effect of the independent conditions. The results of G2 and G3 showed that the hearing threshold did not decrease significantly compared to that of the control group (Figure S2). In contrast, in the case of G5, hearing loss due to hypoxia showed a significant tendency to appear from the second month onwards (Figure 4a–c). In the group G4, which was the dual-condition group of HFD and GI, hearing did not decrease at any of the frequencies (Figure 4d–f). Interestingly, in the dual-condition groups in which one of the conditions was hypoxia, G6 (plus GI; Figure 4g–i) and G7 (plus HFD; Figure 4j–l), the hearing threshold was significantly reduced from the first month onwards, from about 30 to 60 dB. The triple-condition group, which was characterized by HFD with GI in a low-oxygen environment (G8), showed a tendency of significant decrease in the hearing threshold over a short period of time (Figure 4m–o). Therefore, the hypoxic condition was the one that exerted the maximum effect on hearing loss, while HFD and GI had the least effect.

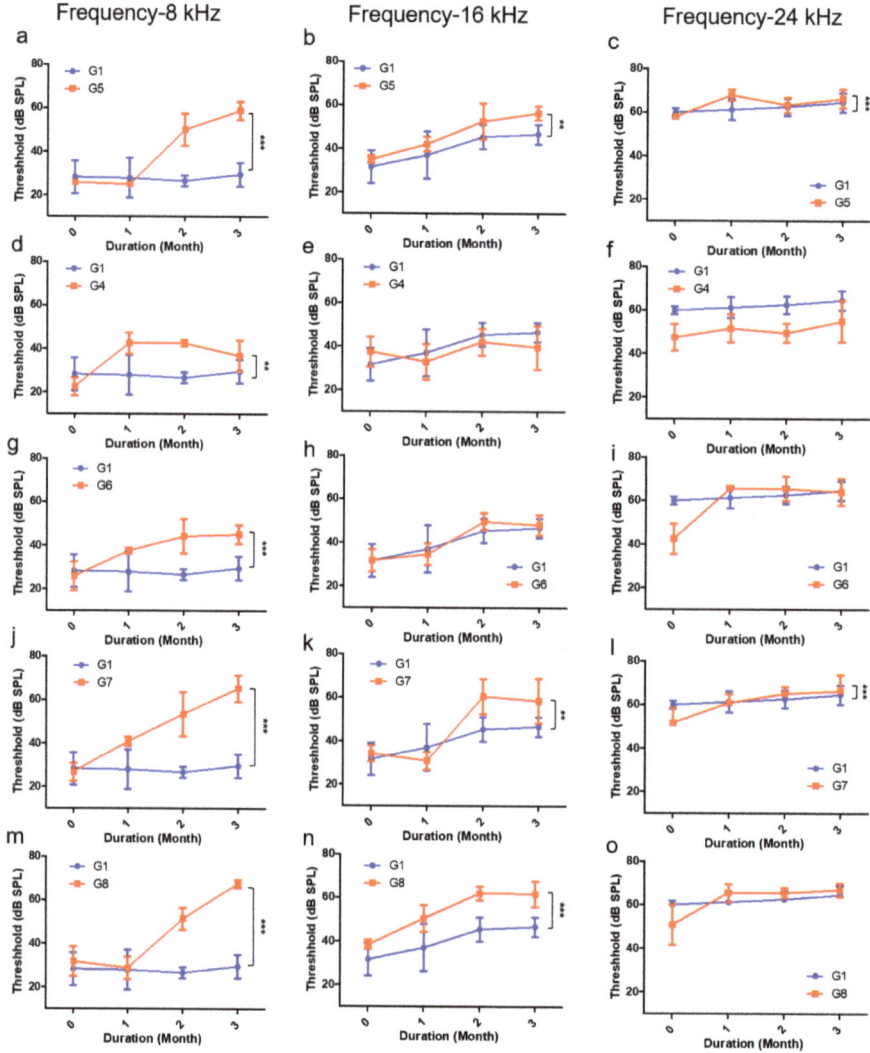

Figure 4. Detailed monthly comparison of hearing thresholds between all the groups and controls for three different frequencies (8, 16, and 24 kHz) by using two-way ANOVA. The analysis of 8 kHz is shown in (**a,d,g,j,m**); that of 16 kHz is shown in (**b,e,h,k,n**); that of 24 kHz is shown in (**c,f,I,l,o**). (**a–c**) G1 and G5, (**d–f**) G1 and G4, (**g–i**) G1 and G6, (**j–l**) G1 and G7, and (**m–o**) G1 and G8. ** $p < 0.005$, *** $p < 0.0001$. Abbreviation: ANOVA, analysis of variance.

For a more specific comparison of the groups, we selected the 8 kHz frequency to assess the determining factors in single-, dual-, and triple-condition exposures. When the results for GI were analyzed, no effective decrease in the hearing threshold was observed, even after including HFD and hypoxia as second exposure conditions (Figure 5a). Analyzing the results of HFD confirmed that hearing loss did not occur with HFD alone, but the hearing threshold did decrease within 2 months when hypoxic conditions were added as a second effect (Figure 5b). In addition, when analyzing the results of hypoxic conditions, it was confirmed that the hearing threshold decreased after 2 months if the hypoxic condition was included (Figure 5c). Therefore, based on the results, it was confirmed that the hypoxic condition and HFD have the greatest effect on hearing loss.

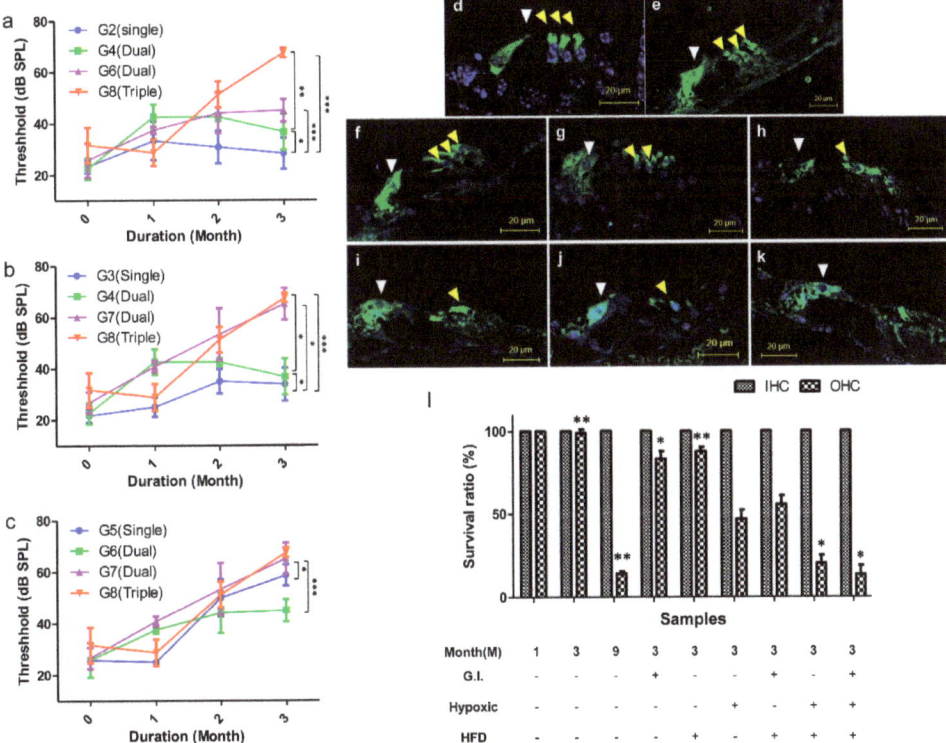

Figure 5. The threshold comparison of single, dual, and triple exposure to three factors (hypoxic condition, HFD, and GI) by two-way ANOVA. (**a**) Hearing threshold analysis of GI between single, double, and triple conditions for 3 months. (**b**) Hearing threshold analysis of HFD between single, double, and triple conditions for 3 months. (**c**) Hearing threshold analysis of the hypoxic condition between single, double, and triple exposure for 3 months. Observation of the damaged OHC and IHC exposed to various conditions. The yellow arrow indicates OHC, and the white arrow indicates IHC in all images (**d–k**). Microscope magnification ×20, scale bar = 20 µM. (**d**) Young mouse, 4 weeks, (**e**) 3 months, (**f**) 3 months + GI, (**g**) 3 months + HFD, (**h**) 3 months + hypoxia, (**i**) 3 months + HFD, GI, (**j**) 3 months + hypoxia, HFD, (**k**) 3 months + hypoxia, HFD, GI, and (**l**) the survival ratio of OHC and IHC in the different groups. Significant values are shown for each month, with * $p < 0.05$, ** $p < 0.005$, *** $p < 0.0001$. Abbreviations: HFD, high-fat diet; GI, galactose injection; ANOVA, analysis of variance; OHC, outer hair cells; IHC, inner hair cells.

2.4. Histological Observations of Hair Cells

We next evaluated the survival rates of auditory hair cells under the different conditions by histological analysis. The survival rate was evaluated by analyzing a major protein, *Myo7a*, present in the auditory hair cells. In 4-week-old mice, three outer hair cells (OHC) and one inner hair cell (IHC) were clearly observed (Figure 5d). In addition, even after 3 months, no damage to hair cells was observed when there was no oxidative stress (Figure 5e). The results of the histological analysis showed that there was little damage to these cells under the influence of GI (Figure 5f), moderate damage under HFD (Figure 5g), and severe damage under hypoxic conditions (Figure 5h). In addition, the analysis revealed that an OHC was close to cell death in the dual- and triple-exposure conditions (Figure 5i–k). For quantitative evaluation, we assessed the survival rate of hair cells based on the histological images from each group (Figure 5l). The survival rate was over 80% in the single condition groups and 50% in the dual condition groups, but it reduced to less than 20% when the hypoxic condition was included. In other words, oxidative stress caused by hypoxia caused damage to hair cells and led to hearing loss.

We observed the appearance of hair cells to further examine the damage caused to them by oxidative stress. The function and survival of auditory hair cells were determined by observing the presence of stereocilia, based on previous literature [27]. Under hypoxic conditions, the cilia on the OHCs had partially disappeared (Figure 6). In addition, the damage to hair cells was severe when HFD and GI conditions were included, i.e., a triple-exposure condition. It was observed that the stereocilia disappeared almost entirely in this case, implying that auditory hair cells are damaged by oxidative stress under these conditions.

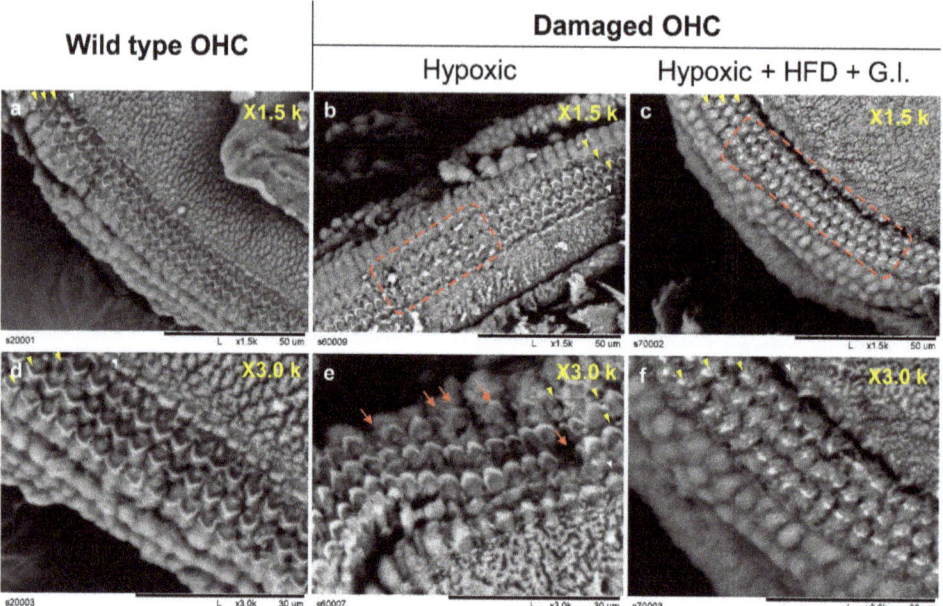

Figure 6. Images of OHCs and IHCs that survived in the explant model recorded by SEM. The yellow arrow indicates three OHC lines, and the white arrow indicates an IHC line. The red arrows indicate damaged hair cells. It was observed that the morphology of cilia disappeared on the line. The red dotted line indicates an extensive area of damaged hair cells. (**a–c**) microscope magnification ×1.5 k, scale bar = 50 µm; (**d–f**) microscope magnification ×3.0 k, scale bar = 30 µm. (**a,d**) show OHC images from a young mouse (4 weeks). (**b,e**) show OHCs damaged by oxidative stress due to hypoxia. (**c,f**) show OHCs damaged by oxidative stress due to hypoxia, HFD, and GI. Abbreviations: OHC, outer hair cells; IHC, inner hair cells; SEM, scanning electron microscopy; HFD, high-fat diet; GI, galactose injection.

2.5. Expression of Age-Related Factors in Cochlea

After confirming the occurrence of hearing loss due to the damage caused to hair cells by the three kinds of environmental stresses, we assessed whether factors of aging were expressed in the auditory organ. We also sought to demonstrate the age-related hearing loss caused by environmental stresses in our animal model by identifying factors that are typically expressed in ARHL. The genes *ApoE* [30–32] and *Edn1* [33,34] are expressed under persistent oxidative stress conditions and have been reported to be associated with vascular aging (Figure 7). In addition, *Ucp2* is the most important gene among those analyzed, and it has been reported to be expressed in mitochondrial dysfunction [18]. *Cdh23* is a gene typically expressed during ARHL [35,36]. Finally, *Kcnq4*, *Myo7a*, *Myo6*, and *Slc26a4* have been reported to be associated with the potassium channel and molecular physiological mechanisms of auditory organs [5,7,36]. All these genes are expressed during aging and are important markers that can be used to determine the cause of the expression of these genes [37].

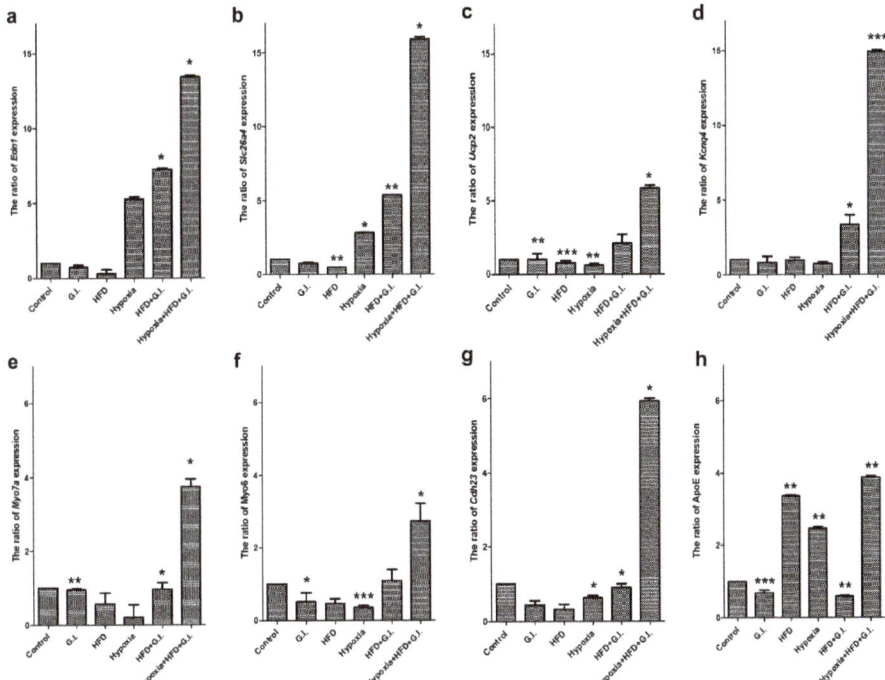

Figure 7. Expression of aging-related factors determined by real-time qPCR. (**a**) *Edn1*, (**b**) *Slc26a4*, (**c**) *Ucp2*, (**d**) *Kcnq4*, (**e**) *Myo7a*, (**f**) *Myo6*, (**g**) *Cdh23*, and (**h**) *ApoE*. Samples from each group show aspects of control, GI, HFD, and hypoxia (single condition), and HFD + GI, hypoxia + HFD + GI (complex conditions) from the left side. * $p < 0.05$, ** $p < 0.01$, *** $p < 0.0001$. Abbreviations: qPCR, quantitative polymerase chain reaction; HFD, high-fat diet; GI, galactose injection.

The expression of all the selected genes increased significantly under the triple-exposure condition (Figure 7). Ion channel-related proteins in the auditory organs, such as *Slc26a4* (Figure 7b) and *Kcnq4* (Figure 7d), were overexpressed. Importantly, the expression of *Ucp2*, which is expressed during mitochondrial dysfunction due to oxidative stress, was significantly increased compared to that of other genes (Figure 7c). The expression of *Myo7a* and *Myo6* increased significantly due to the damage to the auditory organs (Figure 7e,f). Furthermore, the expression of *Cdh23*, which is the most expressed gene during the aging of auditory organs, was found to be increased as well (Figure 7g). HFD is thought to induce the expression of *ApoE* and *Edn1*, which, although not very effective, are believed to contribute to hypoxic damage (Figure 7a). In the case of *ApoE*, the results of HFD and intermittent hypoxia alone showed similar expression levels of RNA as those of exposure to all three conditions (Figure 7h). It was expected that HFD would induce hyperlipidemia in the blood vessels of the auditory organs. An imbalance in nutritional supply due to reduced blood flow has also been reported as a cause of hearing loss. Therefore, when the GI, intermittent hypoxic condition, and HFD stimulations were not performed alone, the expression of aging factors was largely observed.

3. Discussion

ARHL is a critical health condition that affects the aging population, and its onset varies based on the individual's lifestyle, including eating and sleeping habits, noise exposure, and use of ototoxic drugs [4,11]. Previous studies have utilized specific genetically engineered mice or animal models of aging induced by drug injection, but these studies have been conducted without considering the changing conditions of the surrounding environment. This study describes the changes in hearing and histological phenotypes of hearing organs based on lifestyle. Herein, we show that the expression of genes associated with aging-related deafness is largely induced over a short period of time, and these genes can be explored further in preventive or therapeutic research. In other words, since it is necessary to devise an animal model suitable for such studies, we proposed an animal model that, when exposed to environmental stresses, results in hearing loss.

Hearing measurements can be obtained in an easier manner using the C57BL/6 mice model than the other models. A recent study showed that aging is caused by oxidative stress due to changes in lifestyle, and the same study also described strategies to prevent ARHL and develop regenerative therapeutic substances [38]. This study aimed to reveal the phenotypes associated with hearing loss in a mouse model without other diseases, such as diabetes or vascular diseases. In our study, we observed that mice exposed to environmental stress for more than 3 months showed symptoms of diabetes and vascular disease; however, we did not investigate these observations further since they were beyond the scope of our study. In addition, persistent environmental stress is associated with poor quality of life, difficulty in communication, impaired activity in daily life, dementia, and cognitive dysfunction [15].

In this study, we used three kinds of environmental stress stimuli. First, a hypoxia chamber was designed based on a study of hearing loss in sleep disorders such as OSAS [16]. When oxygen saturation decreases in the body during sleep, hearing ability decreases to 60 dB or less in patients over 60 years of age [15]. We demonstrated an aged mouse model with deafness caused by the variation in confirmation of stratum corneum and wrinkles in the mouse model of oxidative stress. Changes in lifestyle that increase SOD activity in the serum and a reduction in atmospheric oxygen significantly influence aging. *Cdh23* was also increasingly expressed in the triple-exposure group (Figure 6) [39]. However, although a change in the amount of RNA was observed in *Cdh23* in this study, studies are needed to identify more accurate gene mutations. Therefore, we have suggested that environmental oxidative stress can alter the phenotype of hearing and affect certain genes. The loss of auditory hair cells and reduction in hearing ability were not significantly influenced by a single stimulus. However, when two or more stimuli were added, hearing loss was observed to occur over a short period of time. HFD significantly increases the content of fat in the body, affects sugar metabolism, restricts blood vessels, and causes metabolic diseases [19]. These effects could be demonstrated by the expression of *Edn1* and *ApoE* in cells within the hearing organ. HFD caused metabolic abnormalities in mice exposed to hypoxic conditions. Finally, 500 mg/kg galactose was injected into some mice to induce aging through metabolic abnormalities in the body, and the effects of this administration were observed in those also exposed to HFD and hypoxic conditions. By determining the expression of *Ucp2* under all environmental stimuli, it was confirmed that mitochondrial dysfunction was caused by oxidative stress [12,14]. Mitochondrial dysfunction has been observed to induce apoptosis in many studies [9,19], and we obtained similar results through histological analysis in this study. Thus, we discussed that the reduction of frequencies was influenced when the blood vessels were damaged, and substance exchange in the bloodstream was poor because of the hypoxic condition and HFD. In summary, aging and physiological changes were induced by the three lifestyle conditions considered in this study (Figure 8).

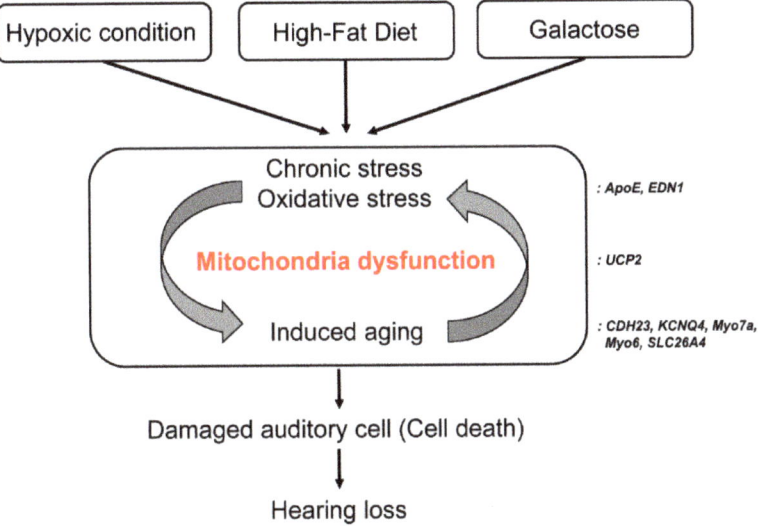

Figure 8. A schematic diagram of the aging mouse model exposed to three environmental stress factors. The three factors (hypoxia, HFD, and GI) cause mitochondrial dysfunction by inflicting oxidative stress on cells. Aged auditory hair cells accumulate due to irritation, followed by cell death and hearing loss. Abbreviations: HFD, high-fat diet; GI, galactose injection.

Hypoxia has the greatest effect on hearing loss induction. Meanwhile, HFD and GI induce cell nutrient supply abnormalities due to the metabolic changes they cause in the body, which promotes the aging of cells (Table 2). In this paper, it was suggested that the aging of animals due to environmental changes can be accelerated when oxidative stress is superimposed, and that hearing loss can rapidly increase after 2 months. We discussed that it is necessary to reduce oxidative stress or reduce environmental stress as candidates for therapeutic agents to slow the onset of aging hearing loss.

Table 2. Phenotypic changes caused by exposure to three environmental stresses (hypoxia, HFD, GI).

	Merged Condition			Effect of a Single Factor		
Phenotype	Triple	Dual	Single	Hypoxia	HFD	GI
Body weight	+++	++	+	++	+++	+
Skin thickness	+++	++	+	++	+++	+
Hair cell loss	+++	++	+	+++	++	+
Oxidative stress	+++	++	+	+++	++	+
Hearing loss	+++	++	+	+++	++	+
Age-related gene expression	+++	++	+	+++	++	+

Abbreviations: HFD, high-fat diet; GI, galactose injection.

4. Materials and Methods

4.1. Experimental Groups

A total of 72 male mice (*C57BL/6*) were divided into eight groups based on whether they were exposed to any of the three different sources of intermittent oxidative stress or not (nonexposed mice were used as controls; Figure S3). The different groups were as follows: Group 1 (G1), normoxic, normally fed (NF); Group 2 (G2), normoxic, NF, GI; Group 3 (G3), normoxic, HFD; Group 4 (G4), normoxic, HFD, GI; Group 5 (G5), hypoxic, NF; Group 6 (G6), hypoxic, NF, GI; Group 7 (G7), hypoxic, HFD; Group 8 (G8), hypoxic, HFD, GI. Additionally, young mice (male, 4 weeks, $n = 9$) were used as controls. The body weight of the mice was monitored throughout the experiment as an indicator of health.

4.2. Animal Procedures

C57BL/6 male mice (12 weeks old) were used in this study. The animal protocols used in this work were evaluated and approved by the by the institutional animal care and use committee in the animal laboratory of Yonsei University in Wonju College of Medicine (Protocol YWC-181001, Permit code: 181001-2, 2 September 2019). All animals were kept at room temperature with a 12-h light/dark cycle under different oxygen conditions, including normoxic and intermittent hypoxic conditions. They were classified according to exposure to three environmental conditions that were combinatory, leading to classification into eight groups. Groups G1 to −4 were kept under normoxic conditions with an oxygen concentration of 20%, while groups G5 to −8 were kept in a hypoxic chamber with an oxygen concentration of 5% for 12 h/day. In addition, the mice were divided into NF (NIH-41, autoclaved, Zeigler Bros Inc., Gardners, PA, USA) [40] and HFD groups [19]. The HFD groups was prepared as previously reported [18]. All materials and supporting data are listed in Table S1. Mice in groups G3, G4, G7, and G8 were fed an HFD with a fat content of 32% (Table S2), including vitamins (Table S3), to generate oxidative stress in the body, while mice of the G1, G2, G5, and G6 groups were NF (Table S4). The body metabolism changes during HFD, which promotes the aging of cells (Table S5).

In addition, mice in groups G2, G4, G6, and G8 were used to evaluate the effect of the promotion of aging through GI (500 mg/kg), which causes chronic oxidative stress and mitochondrial dysfunction. D-galactose (G0750, Sigma-Aldrich, St.Louis, MO, USA) was dissolved in a 0.9% saline solution and subcutaneously injected to induce aging in several groups (500 mg/kg) while other groups were injected with an equal volume of vehicle (0.9% saline). Body weight was measured weekly to monitor changes. Furthermore, the threshold of hearing was evaluated by measuring ABR every 2 weeks. To check the oxidative stress in the body, serum samples were collected every month.

4.3. Hypoxia Chamber Design

The hypoxia chamber was designed to inflict chronic oxidative stress in the mice (Figure S4). This chamber was made of acrylic sheets and consisted of a fan that automatically injected fresh air and nitrogen into the upper part of the chamber and dispersed the air (Figure S5). The chamber (340 × 240 × 60 mm, internal volume 4.9 L) was designed to control oxygen concentration via nitrogen injection with a LCI system (Live Cell Instrument Co., Seoul, Korea) in accordance with previous literature [16,41]. This chamber automatically maintained the oxygen concentration at either about 20% or 5% using nitrogen at a 12-h time split. Nitrogen was automatically injected every 2 min during the 12 h period to decrease the oxygen concentration to 5%. After 12 h, fresh air was injected to allow sufficient oxygen supply for 12 h. In total, a 24-h reaction was performed in each cycle, and the concentration of oxygen was recorded every second per day (Figure S4b,c). All the used gas was discharged out of the building via tubes, and an oxygen indicator was used to check the amount of oxygen in the hypoxia chamber. Inside the chamber, walls were created to divide the NF and HFD groups to distinguish the type of feeding (Figure S4d). The cages were cleaned once a week, and the food, water, and mice feces were removed.

4.4. Auditory Brainstem Response

All mice were anesthetized with 100 mg/kg ketamine (Yuhan-Kimberly, Seoul, Korea) and 10 mg/kg xylazine hydrochloride (Rompun, Bayer, Ansan, Korea) by intraperitoneal injection before ABR recording. Auditory brainstem responses (ABR) are auditory evoked potentials derived from the activity of the auditory nerve and the central auditory pathways in response to transient sound (auditory clicks or tone pips). The thresholds of the ABR wave V were determined by progressively attenuating the sound intensity in 5 dB steps from 80 dB SPL until wave V was no longer distinguishable from the noise floor in recorded traces.

Mice were tested in a sound-attenuating chamber with a built-in Faraday cage, and an isothermal pad was used to maintain the body temperature. The TDT RZ6/BioSigRZ system (Tucker Davis Technologies, Alachua, FL, USA) was used for stimulus generation, data management, and ABR collection [42]. Subdermal electrodes were placed in each mouse for data collection. The reference electrode, which was on the same side as the stimulus, was placed axial to the pinnae, while the ground electrode was placed in the ipsilateral ear. Meanwhile, the active electrodes were placed at the vertex. The ABR test was conducted every 2 weeks to assess the stability of the experimental group.

4.5. Superoxide Dismutase (SOD) Activity Test

SOD was rapidly measured using blood collected from the retro-orbital plexus of mice in each group. The collected blood was allowed to clot in an anticoagulant tube for 30 min at 25 °C (room temperature, RT). Purified serum was obtained after the blood was centrifuged at 2000× g for 15 min at 4 °C. All samples were stored at −80 °C for a month. Working samples were diluted in the ratio of 1:5 with sample buffer before assaying for SOD activity. The SOD Assay kit (No. 706002, Cayman Che., MI, USA) uses a tetrazolium salt for the detection of superoxide radicals generated by xanthine oxidase and hypoxanthine [43]. For each sample, SOD activity was calculated using the equation obtained from the linear regression of the standard curve, replacing the linearized rate. One unit was defined as the amount of enzyme required to represent 50% displacement of the superoxide radical. SOD activity was measured according to the manufacturer's method.

4.6. Histological Analysis

All mice were sacrificed by cervical dislocation, and both cochleae were dissected. The cochleae were perfused with a fixative containing 4% paraformaldehyde in phosphate-buffered saline (PBS; pH 7.4) at RT. The apical portion of the bony cochlea was gently opened to allow the fixative to perfuse through the tissues. The cochleae were decalcified by immersion in a Calci-Clear rapid decalcifier (National Diagnostics, Atlanta, GA, USA) for 24 h. Thereafter, the cochleae were embedded in a compound at optimal cutting temperature (Leica Microsystems, Bensheim, Germany), and cut into 2- to 5-μm-thick sections in a LEICA RM2145 (Leica Biosystems, Wetzlar, German). The cut sections were subjected to standard hematoxylin and eosin (H&E) staining (1–3 min of incubation in hematoxylin, and staining with eosin for 30–60 s).

4.7. Immunostaining

The cochlear sections were prepared on 5-μm-thick gelatine-coated slides by fixing them with 4% paraformaldehyde for 15 min and allowing them to dry at RT. The specimens were incubated in 5% normal goat serum for 1 h at RT to prevent nonspecific labeling. Then, the specimens were incubated with the primary antibody, MYO7A (1:200, ab3481, Abcam, UK), for 1 h at 4 °C [44–46]. Thereafter, the specimens were washed with PBS three times for five min each time, followed by incubation with a secondary antibody, goat anti-rabbit IgG H&L (Alexa Fluor® 488; 1:1000, ab150077, Abcam, UK), for 1 h at RT. After washing the samples three times for five min with PBS again, they were finally immobilized with a mounting solution containing DAPI (4′,6-diamidino-2-phenylindole). All the samples were observed by confocal microscopy (Carl Zeiss Microscopy GmbH, Jena, Germany), and images were analyzed using the software ZEN lite ver. 2.3 (ZEN lite, Jena, Germany).

4.8. Scanning Electron Microscope (SEM)

The cochlea was isolated to observe the morphology of the hair cells. The cochlea was extracted from the auditory organ and fixed in 2.5% glutaraldehyde for 2 h at 4 °C. The specimens were then fixed in 1% osmium tetroxide (OsO_4) after being washed twice with 0.1 M cacodylate buffer. The dehydration steps were performed using 50%, 70%, 80%, 90%, and 100% ethanol. Then, the samples were set to react with 3-methylbutyl acetate (Isoamyl acetate, Hanawa, Japan) for 15 min at RT. The samples were dried using hexamethyldisilazane (cat. 440191, Sigma-Aldrich, USA) for 15 min at RT. All samples were air-dried overnight on covered filter papers with a lid. The samples were gold-coated to observe the morphology of the cochlea using a tabletop microscope (TM-1000, Hitachi Ltd., Tokyo, Japan) [46].

4.9. Real-Time PCR

Real-time PCR was performed to determine the induction of aging and hearing loss by analyzing the expression of various genes in the liver, kidney, and cochlea. Total RNA was extracted using TRIzol (Thermo Fisher Scientific, San Diego, CA, USA). To prepare the mRNA samples, 2 µL of mRNA and 8 µL of reverse transcriptase reagents, which comprised 1 µL of 10× enzyme mix, 2 µL of 5× enzyme reaction buffer, and 5 µL of nuclease-free water, were used to prepare a 10-µL mixture according to the manufacturer's protocol. cDNA was diluted in a ratio of 1:10 with 90 µL nuclease-free water for microRNA real-time PCR. RT-PCR was performed using the Applied Biosystems 7900 HT sequence detection system (Thermo Fisher Sci. San Diego, CA, USA). Samples were subjected to reverse transcription using the SYBR Select master mix (Applied Biosystems, Calrsbad, CA, USA), following the manufacturer's protocol. The sequences of the primers used were as follows (Table S6): apo-lipoprotein E (*ApoE*), forward: 5′-GGT TCG AGC CAA TAG TGG AA–3′, and reverse: 5′-ATG GAT GTT GCA GGA CA-3′; Cadherin-23 (*Cdh23*), forward: 5′-ATG GAG AGC CCT CTG GAA AT-3′, and reverse: 5′-ACC CAC AAA GGC TGT ACT GG-3′; eosinophil-derived neurotoxin 1 (*Edn1*), forward: 5′-ACA CCG TCC TCT TCG TTT TG-3′, and reverse: 5′-GAG TC CTT GGA AAG TCA CG-3′; potassium voltage-gated channel subfamily Q member 4 (*Kcnq4*), forward: 5′-TGT TGG GAT CCG TGG TCT AT -3′, and reverse: 5′- GAGTTG GCA TCC TTC TCA GC-3′; myosin VIIA (*Myo7a*), forward: 5′-GAC AAC TCT AGC CGC TTT GG-3′, and reverse: 5′-GAC ACG TGA CTT CTC CAG CA-3′; myosin VI (*Myo6*), forward: 5′-AGA CCA CTT CCG GCT CAC TA-3′, and reverse: 5′- TGG GTT GTC TCG TAG CAC AC-3′; uncoupling protein 2 (*Ucp2*), forward: 5′-CTC AAA GCA GCC TCC AGA AC-3′, and reverse: 5′-ACA TCT GTG GCC TTG AAA CC-3′; solute carrier family 26 member 4 (*Slc26a4*), forward: 5′-TCA TTG CCT TGG GAA TAA GC-3′, and reverse: 5′-GGC AAC CAT CAC AAT CAC AG-3′; *18S* rRNA, forward: 5′-CAT TCG AAC GTC TGC CCT AT-3′, and reverse: 5′-GTT TCT CAG GCT CCC TCT CC-3′. The total 10 µL sample for real-time PCR contained 1 µL cDNA, 5 µL of premix, 1 µL each of 10 pmol forward and reverse primers, and 3 µL of nuclease-free water. The PCR conditions comprised preamplification at 95 °C for three min, 40 cycles of 95 °C for 10 s, and then 60 °C for 60 s, and melting curve analysis. All processes were performed in duplicate. The normalization of mRNA expression level was calculated using *18S* rRNA.

4.10. Statistical Analysis

Statistical analysis was performed using SPSS statistical package version 21.0 (SPSS Inc. Chicago, IL, USA). Descriptive results of continuous variables were expressed as the mean ± standard deviation for normally distributed variables. Mean hearing thresholds were compared by two-way ANOVA. In addition, the sensitivity and specificity of the statistically significant mRNAs were analyzed by the Mann–Whitney U-test with GraphPad PRISM version 5.0 (GraphPad Inc., La Jolla, CA, USA). *p*-values less than 0.05 were considered to be statistically significant.

5. Conclusions

Interestingly, exposure to HFD or GI as a single condition showed no significant hearing loss. However, when hypoxic stimulation was added, the dual condition showed intermediate effects, and the triple-exposure condition showed the maximum effects. In addition, OHC loss for high sound frequencies occurs when the blood vessels are damaged and the exchange of substances in the bloodstream is poor. This can cause ion channel abnormalities and genetic defects in the auditory organs. With the new model developed in this study, which causes natural short-term induction of

ARHL due to oxidative stress through changes in the lifestyle, we could observe the age-related markers and phenotypes associated with ARHL. The animal model used and results reported in this study can aid in the development of strategies for the prevention and treatment of ARHL. With the increase in the aged population, advances in medical technologies and research on hearing loss are warranted.

Supplementary Materials: The following are available online at http://www.mdpi.com/1422-0067/21/19/7068/s1, Figure S1: Phenotype of mice groups, Figure S2: Two-way ANOVA of hearing threshold at three frequencies (8, 16, and 24 kHz) depending on the duration, respectively. Figure S3: Overall design, including the mouse housing conditions and ABR test. Figure S4: Hypoxia chamber design for oxidative stress., Figure S5: Overall appearance of the hypoxic chamber. Table S1: Thickness of the dermis and fat layers between different groups. Table S2: Ingredient Composition of High-Fat Diet 32 (HFD32). Table S3: Ingredient composition of AIN93-VX vitamin mix and AIN93G mineral mix. Table S4: Ingredients and nutrient composition in experimental chows (NIH-41). Table S5: Compared guaranteed analysis between NIH41 and HFD32 (%). Table S6: Primers of target genes for aging.

Author Contributions: Conceptualization, D.J.P.; methodology, D.J.P., S.H., J.S.C., S.H.L., and J.-E.P.; software, D.J.P. and S.H.; ata curation, S.H.; Fofrmal analysis, J.S.C.; resources, Y.J.S.; writing—original draft, D.J.P.; writing—review and editing, S.H., J.S.C., S.H.L., J.-E.P. and Y.J.S.; visualization, D.J.P.; project administration, Y.J.S.; funding acquisition, D.J.P. and Y.J.S. All authors have read and agreed to the published version of the manuscript.

Funding: This research received no external funding.

Conflicts of Interest: The authors declare no potential conflicts of interest with respect to the authorship and/or the publication of this article.

Abbreviations

ABR	Auditory brainstem response
ARHL	Age-related hearing loss
GI	Galactose injection
H&E	Haematoxylin and eosin
HFD	High-fat diet
IHC	Inner hair cell
KHIDI	Korea Health Industry Development Institute
NF	Normally fed
OC	Organ of Corti
OHC	Outer hair cell
OSAS	Obstructive sleep apnoea syndrome
ROS	Reactive oxidative stress
RT	Room temperature

References

1. Bowl, M.R.; Dawson, S.J. The mouse as a model for age-related hearing loss-a mini-review. *Gerontology* **2015**, *61*, 149–157. [CrossRef] [PubMed]
2. Yamasoba, T.; Lin, F.R.; Someya, S.; Kashio, A.; Sakamoto, T.; Kondo, K. Current concepts in age-related hearing loss: Epidemiology and mechanistic pathways. *Hear. Res.* **2013**, *303*, 30–38. [CrossRef] [PubMed]
3. Zelaya, C.E.; Lucas, J.W.; Hoffman, H.J. *Self-Reported Hearing Trouble in Adults Aged 18 and Over: United States, 2014*; Nchs Data Brief, No 214; National Center for Health Statistics: Hyattsville, MD, USA, 2015.
4. Someya, S.; Xu, J.Z.; Kondo, K.; Ding, D.L.; Salvi, R.J.; Yamasoba, T.; Rabinovitch, P.S.; Weindruch, R.; Leeuwenburgh, C.; Tanokura, M.; et al. Age-related hearing loss in c57bl/6j mice is mediated by bak-dependent mitochondrial apoptosis. *Proc. Natl. Acad. Sci. USA* **2009**, *106*, 19432–19437. [CrossRef] [PubMed]
5. Alimardani, M.; Hosseini, S.M.; Khaniani, M.S.; Haghi, M.R.; Eslahi, A.; Farjami, M.; Chezgi, J.; Derakhshan, S.M.; Mojarrad, M. Targeted mutation analysis of the slc26a4, myo6, pjvk and cdh23 genes in iranian patients with ar nonsyndromic hearing loss. *Fetal Pediatr. Pathol.* **2019**, *38*, 93–102. [CrossRef]
6. Seidman, M.D.; Ahmad, N.; Joshi, D.; Seidman, J.; Thawani, S.; Quirk, W.S. Age-related hearing loss and its association with reactive oxygen species and mitochondrial DNA damage. *Acta Otolaryngol. Suppl.* **2004**, *552*, 16–24. [CrossRef]

7. Holme, R.H.; Steel, K.P. Stereocilia defects in waltzer (cdh23), shaker1 (myo7a) and double waltzer/shaker1 mutant mice. *Hear. Res.* **2002**, *169*, 13–23. [CrossRef]
8. Chen, H.; Tang, J. The role of mitochondria in age-related hearing loss. *Biogerontology* **2014**, *15*, 13–19. [CrossRef]
9. Johnson, K.R.; Tian, C.; Gagnon, L.H.; Jiang, H.; Ding, D.; Salvi, R. Effects of cdh23 single nucleotide substitutions on age-related hearing loss in c57bl/6 and 129s1/sv mice and comparisons with congenic strains. *Sci. Rep.* **2017**, *7*, 44450. [CrossRef]
10. White, K.; Kim, M.J.; Han, C.; Park, H.J.; Ding, D.; Boyd, K.; Walker, L.; Linser, P.; Meneses, Z.; Slade, C.; et al. Loss of idh2 accelerates age-related hearing loss in male mice. *Sci. Rep.* **2018**, *8*, 5039. [CrossRef]
11. Ren, H.M.; Ren, J.; Liu, W. Recognition and control of the progression of age-related hearing loss. *Rejuvenation Res.* **2013**, *16*, 475–486. [CrossRef]
12. Liu, X.Z.; Yan, D. Ageing and hearing loss. *J. Pathol.* **2007**, *211*, 188–197. [CrossRef] [PubMed]
13. Kim, S.H.; Yeo, S.G. Presbycusis. *Hanyang Med. Rev.* **2015**, *35*, 78–83. [CrossRef]
14. Hildesheimer, M.; Rubinstein, M.; Nuttal, A.L.; Lawrence, M. Influence of blood viscosity on cochlear action potentials and oxygenation. *Hear. Res.* **1982**, *8*, 187–198. [CrossRef]
15. Nash, S.D.; Cruickshanks, K.J.; Klein, R.; Klein, B.E.; Nieto, F.J.; Huang, G.H.; Pankow, J.S.; Tweed, T.S. The prevalence of hearing impairment and associated risk factors: The Beaver Dam Offspring Study. *Arch. Otolaryngol. Head Neck Surg.* **2011**, *137*, 432–439. [CrossRef] [PubMed]
16. Seo, Y.J.; Park, S.Y.; Chung, H.J.; Kim, C.H.; Lee, J.G.; Kim, S.H.; Cho, H.J. Lowest oxyhemoglobin saturation may be an independent factor influencing auditory function in severe obstructive sleep apnea. *J. Clin. Sleep Med.* **2016**, *12*, 653–658. [CrossRef]
17. Hao, S.; Wang, L.; Zhao, K.; Zhu, X.; Ye, F. rs1894720 polymorphism in miat increased susceptibility to age-related hearing loss by modulating the activation of mir-29b/sirt1/pgc-1alpha signaling. *J. Cell. Biochem.* **2019**, *120*, 4975–4986. [CrossRef]
18. Fujimoto, C.; Yamasoba, T. Oxidative stresses and mitochondrial dysfunction in age-related hearing loss. *Oxid. Med. Cell. Longev.* **2014**, *2014*, 582849. [CrossRef]
19. Fujita, T.; Yamashita, D.; Uehara, N.; Inokuchi, G.; Hasegawa, S.; Otsuki, N.; Nibu, K. A high-fat diet delays age-related hearing loss progression in c57bl/6j mice. *PLoS ONE* **2015**, *10*, e0117547. [CrossRef]
20. Kume, S.; Uzu, T.; Horiike, K.; Chin-Kanasaki, M.; Isshiki, K.; Araki, S.; Sugimoto, T.; Haneda, M.; Kashiwagi, A.; Koya, D. Calorie restriction enhances cell adaptation to hypoxia through sirt1-dependent mitochondrial autophagy in mouse aged kidney. *J. Clin. Investig.* **2010**, *120*, 1043–1055. [CrossRef]
21. Mitchell, P.; Gopinath, B.; McMahon, C.M.; Rochtchina, E.; Wang, J.J.; Boyages, S.C.; Leeder, S.R. Relationship of type 2 diabetes to the prevalence, incidence and progression of age-related hearing loss. *Diabet. Med.* **2009**, *26*, 483–488. [CrossRef]
22. Guo, B.; Guo, Q.; Wang, Z.; Shao, J.B.; Liu, K.; Du, Z.D.; Gong, S.S. D-galactose-induced oxidative stress and mitochondrial dysfunction in the cochlear basilar membrane: An in vitro aging model. *Biogerontology* **2020**, *21*, 311–323. [CrossRef] [PubMed]
23. Ho, S.C.; Liu, J.H.; Wu, R.Y. Establishment of the mimetic aging effect in mice caused by d-galactose. *Biogerontology* **2003**, *4*, 15–18. [CrossRef] [PubMed]
24. Liao, C.H.; Chen, B.H.; Chiang, H.S.; Chen, C.W.; Chen, M.F.; Ke, C.C.; Wang, Y.Y.; Lin, W.N.; Wang, C.C.; Lin, Y.H. Optimizing a male reproductive aging mouse model by d-galactose injection. *Int. J. Mol. Sci.* **2016**, *17*, 98. [CrossRef] [PubMed]
25. Parameshwaran, K.; Irwin, M.H.; Steliou, K.; Pinkert, C.A. D-galactose effectiveness in modeling aging and therapeutic antioxidant treatment in mice. *Rejuvenation Res.* **2010**, *13*, 729–735. [CrossRef]
26. Alameda, J.P.; Ramirez, A.; Garcia-Fernandez, R.A.; Navarro, M.; Page, A.; Segovia, J.C.; Sanchez, R.; Suarez-Cabrera, C.; Paramio, J.M.; Bravo, A.; et al. Premature aging and cancer development in transgenic mice lacking functional cyld. *Aging* **2019**, *11*, 127–159. [CrossRef]
27. Bourguignon, L.Y.; Wong, G.; Xia, W.; Man, M.Q.; Holleran, W.M.; Elias, P.M. Selective matrix (hyaluronan) interaction with cd44 and rhogtpase signaling promotes keratinocyte functions and overcomes age-related epidermal dysfunction. *J. Dermatol. Sci.* **2013**, *72*, 32–44. [CrossRef]
28. Orioli, D.; Dellambra, E. Epigenetic regulation of skin cells in natural aging and premature aging diseases. *Cells* **2018**, *7*, 268. [CrossRef]

29. Raynor, L.A.; Pankow, J.S.; Miller, M.B.; Huang, G.H.; Dalton, D.; Klein, R.; Klein, B.E.; Cruickshanks, K.J. Familial aggregation of age-related hearing loss in an epidemiological study of older adults. *Am. J. Audiol.* **2009**, *18*, 114–118. [CrossRef]
30. Guo, Y.; Zhang, C.; Du, X.; Nair, U.; Yoo, T.J. Morphological and functional alterations of the cochlea in apolipoprotein e gene deficient mice. *Hear. Res.* **2005**, *208*, 54–67. [CrossRef]
31. Kim, Y.Y.; Chao, J.R.; Kim, C.; Kim, B.; Nguyen, P.T.T.; Jung, H.; Chang, J.; Lee, J.H.; Suh, J.G. Hearing loss through apoptosis of the spiral ganglion neurons in apolipoprotein e knockout mice fed with a western diet. *Biochem. Biophys. Res. Commun.* **2020**, *523*, 692–698. [CrossRef]
32. Kurniawan, C.; Westendorp, R.G.; de Craen, A.J.; Gussekloo, J.; de Laat, J.; van Exel, E. Gene dose of apolipoprotein e and age-related hearing loss. *Neurobiol. Aging* **2012**, *33*, 2230.e7–2230.e12. [CrossRef] [PubMed]
33. Bondurand, N.; Dufour, S.; Pingault, V. News from the endothelin-3/ednrb signaling pathway: Role during enteric nervous system development and involvement in neural crest-associated disorders. *Dev. Biol.* **2018**, *444* (Suppl. S1), S156–S169. [CrossRef] [PubMed]
34. Uchida, Y.; Sugiura, S.; Nakashima, T.; Ando, F.; Shimokata, H. Endothelin-1 gene polymorphism and hearing impairment in elderly japanese. *Laryngoscope* **2009**, *119*, 938–943. [CrossRef]
35. Usami, S.I.; Nishio, S.Y.; Moteki, H.; Miyagawa, M.; Yoshimura, H. Cochlear implantation from the perspective of genetic background. *Anat. Rec.* **2020**, *303*, 563–593. [CrossRef] [PubMed]
36. Park, H.J.; Shaukat, S.; Liu, X.Z.; Hahn, S.H.; Naz, S.; Ghosh, M.; Kim, H.N.; Moon, S.K.; Abe, S.; Tukamoto, K.; et al. Origins and frequencies of slc26a4 (pds) mutations in east and south asians: Global implications for the epidemiology of deafness. *J. Med. Genet.* **2003**, *40*, 242–248. [CrossRef] [PubMed]
37. Muller, U.; Barr-Gillespie, P.G. New treatment options for hearing loss. *Nat. Rev. Drug Discov.* **2015**, *14*, 346–365. [CrossRef]
38. Wang, J.; Puel, J.L. Presbycusis: An update on cochlear mechanisms and therapies. *J. Clin. Med.* **2020**, *9*, 218. [CrossRef]
39. Bouzid, A.; Smeti, I.; Chakroun, A.; Loukil, S.; Gibriel, A.A.; Grati, M.; Ghorbel, A.; Masmoudi, S. Cdh23 methylation status and presbycusis risk in elderly women. *Front. Aging Neurosci.* **2018**, *10*, 241. [CrossRef]
40. Reeves, P.G.; Nielsen, F.H.; Fahey, G.C., Jr. Ain-93 purified diets for laboratory rodents: Final report of the american institute of nutrition ad hoc writing committee on the reformulation of the ain-76a rodent diet. *J. Nutr.* **1993**, *123*, 1939–1951. [CrossRef]
41. Seo, Y.J.; Ju, H.M.; Lee, S.H.; Kwak, S.H.; Kang, M.J.; Yoon, J.H.; Kim, C.H.; Cho, H.J. Damage of inner ear sensory hair cells via mitochondrial loss in a murine model of sleep apnea with chronic intermittent hypoxia. *Sleep* **2017**, *40*, zsx106. [CrossRef]
42. Ju, H.M.; Lee, S.H.; Choi, J.S.; Seo, Y.J. A simple model for inducing optimal increase of sdf-1 with aminoglycoside ototoxicity. *Biomed. Res. Int.* **2017**, *2017*, 4630241. [CrossRef] [PubMed]
43. Chatuphonprasert, W.; Lao-Ong, T.; Jarukamjorn, K. Improvement of superoxide dismutase and catalase in streptozotocin-nicotinamide-induced type 2-diabetes in mice by berberine and glibenclamide. *Pharm. Biol.* **2013**, *52*, 419–427. [CrossRef] [PubMed]
44. Kim, Y.Y.; Nam, H.; Jung, H.; Kim, B.; Suh, J.G. Over-expression of myosin7a in cochlear hair cells of circling mice. *Lab. Anim. Res.* **2017**, *33*, 1–7. [CrossRef] [PubMed]
45. Riva, C.; Donadieu, E.; Magnan, J.; Lavieille, J.P. Age-related hearing loss in cd/1 mice is associated to ros formation and hif target proteins up-regulation in the cochlea. *Exp. Gerontol.* **2007**, *42*, 327–336. [CrossRef] [PubMed]
46. Potter, P.K.; Bowl, M.R.; Jeyarajan, P.; Wisby, L.; Blease, A.; Goldsworthy, M.E.; Simon, M.M.; Greenaway, S.; Michel, V.; Barnard, A.; et al. Novel gene function revealed by mouse mutagenesis screens for models of age-related disease. *Nat. Commun.* **2016**, *7*, 12444. [CrossRef] [PubMed]

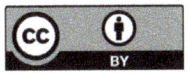 © 2020 by the authors. Licensee MDPI, Basel, Switzerland. This article is an open access article distributed under the terms and conditions of the Creative Commons Attribution (CC BY) license (http://creativecommons.org/licenses/by/4.0/).

Chronic Oral Selegiline Treatment Mitigates Age-Related Hearing Loss in BALB/c Mice

Judit Szepesy [1,2], Viktória Humli [1], János Farkas [1], Ildikó Miklya [1], Júlia Tímár [1], Tamás Tábi [3], Anita Gáborján [2], Gábor Polony [2], Ágnes Szirmai [2], László Tamás [2], László Köles [1,4], Elek Sylvester Vizi [1,5] and Tibor Zelles [1,5,*]

1. Department of Pharmacology and Pharmacotherapy, Semmelweis University, H-1089 Budapest, Hungary; szepesy.judit@med.semmelweis-univ.hu (J.S.); humli.viktoria@med.semmelweis-univ.hu (V.H.); farkas.janos2@med.semmelweis-univ.hu (J.F.); miklya.ildiko@med.semmelweis-univ.hu (I.M.); timar.julia@med.semmelweis-univ.hu (J.T.); koles.laszlo@med.semmelweis-univ.hu (L.K.); esvizi@koki.mta.hu (E.S.V.)
2. Department of Otorhinolaryngology, Head and Neck Surgery, Semmelweis University, H-1083 Budapest, Hungary; gaborjan.anita@gmail.com (A.G.); polony.gabor@med.semmelweis-univ.hu (G.P.); szirmai.agnes@med.semmelweis-univ.hu (Á.S.); tamas.laszlo@med.semmelweis-univ.hu (L.T.)
3. Department of Pharmacodynamics, Semmelweis University, H-1089 Budapest, Hungary; tabi.tamas@pharma.semmelweis-univ.hu
4. Department of Oral Biology, Semmelweis University, H-1089 Budapest, Hungary
5. Laboratory of Molecular Pharmacology, Institute of Experimental Medicine, H-1083 Budapest, Hungary
* Correspondence: zelles.tibor@med.semmelweis-univ.hu; Tel.: +36-1-210-4412

Abstract: Age-related hearing loss (ARHL), a sensorineural hearing loss of multifactorial origin, increases its prevalence in aging societies. Besides hearing aids and cochlear implants, there is no FDA approved efficient pharmacotherapy to either cure or prevent ARHL. We hypothesized that selegiline, an antiparkinsonian drug, could be a promising candidate for the treatment due to its complex neuroprotective, antioxidant, antiapoptotic, and dopaminergic neurotransmission enhancing effects. We monitored by repeated Auditory Brainstem Response (ABR) measurements the effect of chronic per os selegiline administration on the hearing function in BALB/c and DBA/2J mice, which strains exhibit moderate and rapid progressive high frequency hearing loss, respectively. The treatments were started at 1 month of age and lasted until almost a year and 5 months of age, respectively. In BALB/c mice, 4 mg/kg selegiline significantly mitigated the progression of ARHL at higher frequencies. Used in a wide dose range (0.15–45 mg/kg), selegiline had no effect in DBA/2J mice. Our results suggest that selegiline can partially preserve the hearing in certain forms of ARHL by alleviating its development. It might also be otoprotective in other mammals or humans.

Keywords: age-related hearing loss; selegiline; chronic oral treatment; hearing protection; mouse model

1. Introduction

In line with the globally increasing life expectancy, prevalence of aging-associated diseases and their health care costs are also increasing. The main age-related disorders are Alzheimer's-disease, stroke, cancer, and atherosclerosis; however, the risk of age-related hearing loss (ARHL) rises as well.

ARHL, also known as presbycusis, is the most common form of sensorineural hearing losses (SNHLs), the prevalence of which is increasing [1]. According to the World Health Organization (WHO), approximately one in three people over the age of 65 years suffer from a certain degree of hearing loss [2]. Due to a decline in hearing ability and speech understanding in noisy environments [3], ARHL threatens personal autonomy, resulting in major difficulties in daily life and, ultimately, social isolation and depression [4].

Underlying factors of cochlear aging include genetic susceptibility, otological disorders, and environmental factors, for example, increased noise exposure [5,6]. The main pathological processes presumed to play a crucial role in the development of ARHL are ischemia, excitotoxicity [6], increased level of reactive oxygen species (ROS) [7], apoptosis [8], and low-grade inflammation [9,10]. As a result, age-related degeneration of stria vascularis, auditory hair cells (HCs), and spiral ganglion neurons (SGNs) could be primarily observed [6,11,12].

The pathophysiology and the genetic architecture of ARHL are generally investigated in different inbred mouse strains due to the fact that mice possess cochlear anatomy [13], physiology, pathophysiology [13,14], and a pattern of ARHL [5,15] similar to humans. In addition, there are many strains of mice with different vulnerabilities to ARHL due to divergent genetic backgrounds [5,8].

Different lines of BALB/c and DBA/2J mice are widely used as murine models in ARHL research [16]. Both strains exhibit the characteristic patterns of human presbycusis [16,17] such as age-related elevation of hearing thresholds beginning at higher frequencies, degeneration of outer hair cells (OHCs) and SGNs beginning at basal cochlear regions, and furthermore, less severe loss of inner hair cells (IHCs) [16]. However, strain-specific variation can be observed in the development of ARHL. In DBA/2J mice, hearing loss progresses more rapidly due to the presence of multiple ARHL-related genes [16].

Although various hearing aids and cochlear implants have been proven to be effective therapies in certain clinical cases, due to its high prevalence and lack of specific pharmacological treatment, ARHL represents an unmet clinical need. Current pharmacotherapeutic approaches in ARHL research focus on testing potential otoprotective drug agents primarily with antioxidant, antiapoptotic or neuroprotective effects, reviewed by Jing Wang and Jean-Luc Puel [8]. Since current drug development programs have not reached phase 3 clinical trials according to (ClinicalTrials.gov; accessed on 24 January 2021) and EudraCT databases, there is still room for exploring novel therapeutical avenues.

Selegiline [(−)deprenyl], a selective and irreversible inhibitor of monoamine oxidase B (MAO-B) [18], was approved for the treatment of Parkinson disease and major depressive disorder [19] by the Food and Drug Administration (FDA) decades ago. Selegiline increases the level of catecholamines; furthermore, neuroprotective, antioxidant, and antiapoptotic effects of this compound has been evidenced as well [20,21]. These properties make selegiline a promising candidate for the treatment of different forms of SNHLs including ARHL. Although the idea of otoprotection in mammals by selegiline was raised and patented (US5561163, EP 0 831 798 B1), it is based on the generalization of the result of a moderately controlled, not-thorough study on outpatient elderly dogs. The study lacked a control group, their hearing was assessed by inadequate behavioral response to sounds such as command and owners' acknowledgments, and it lasted 1 to 3 months for different dogs [22]. An accurate examination of the potential otoprotective effect of selegiline in ARHL is still missing.

The aim of the present study was to perform a comprehensive investigation of the efficacy of selegiline in preventing or mitigating the deterioration of hearing by age. Here we show that chronic administration of selegiline until the age of week 49 (~1 year) in the dose of 4 mg/kg reduced the progression of ARHL in BALB/c, but not in DBA/2J mice.

2. Results

2.1. Effect of Chronic Oral Administration of Selegiline on Hearing Function in BALB/c and DBA/2J Mice

Hearing thresholds of mice were measured at different frequencies and time points to investigate the effect of different doses of selegiline on ARHL in BALB/c and DBA/2J mice. The experimental protocol is presented in Figure 1. See Section 4.3 for the details of the experimental design of auditory measurements and drug administration.

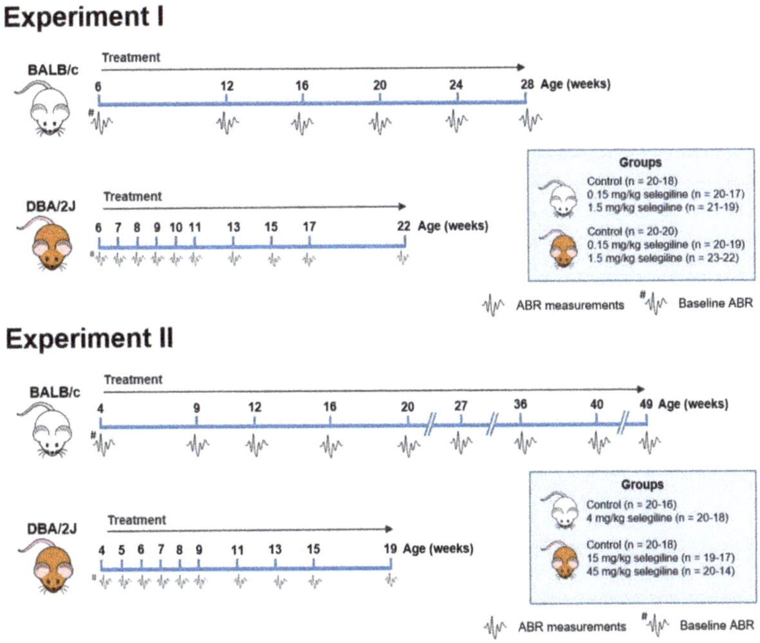

Figure 1. Flow chart showing the treatment protocol and time points of Auditory Brainstem Response (ABR) measurements in BALB/c and DBA/2J mice. Selegiline was dissolved in tap water and freely available for the mice throughout the entire experiment. The daily dose of selegiline was set to a given value (0.15, 1.5, 4, 15, and 45 mg/kg). ABR measurements are indicated by the tiny waveforms. The first ABR measurement (baseline hearing threshold) was performed one day before the onset of selegiline administration. The whole study was carried out in two subsets. The insets show the treatment groups. The number of mice at the start and at the end of the experiments is indicated in parentheses. Experiment I. 0.15 and 1.5 mg/kg selegiline were administered to both BALB/c and DBA/2J mice. The control group received tap water, the solvent of selegiline. In the case of DBA/2J mice, ABR measurements were performed more frequently at the beginning of the experimental period. Experiment II. 4 mg/kg of selegiline was administered to BALB/c mice, and 15 and 45 mg/kg doses to DBA/2J. The dose reduction in BALB/c mice and omission of the 4th treatment group were necessary because this strain lessened its water intake at higher concentrations of selegiline in tap water.

In Experiment II, selegiline, in concentration calculated for ingesting the maximum target dose of 45 mg/kg, caused a substantial reduction in drinking volume to 0.58 mL/mouse/day in BALB/c mice. Testing different concentrations of selegiline in the tap water in parallel with the measurement of water consumption, we chose the 0.05 mg/mL concentration providing an average daily fluid intake of approximately 2 mL/mouse with a 4 mg/kg dose of selegiline.

2.1.1. Experiment I (0.15 and 1.5 mg/kg Selegiline)

In control BALB/c mice, hearing thresholds progressed gradually with age at all measured frequencies. Auditory threshold shift at 28 weeks of age was 15.29 ± 3.11 dB, 15.88 ± 2.11 dB, and 33.53 ± 2.96 dB at 4.1, 8.2 kHz and 16.4 kHz, respectively, whereas no change was detected using click stimulus (Figure 2A). 0.15 mg/kg selegiline did not influence the thresholds, except enhancements at 16 weeks of age with the click stimulus and at 24 weeks of age at 16 kHz, which seemed rather incidental. A small, but tendentious decrease of the threshold shifts was detected at the dose of 1.5 mg/kg at 8.2 kHz with statistically significant values at ages of 12, 16, and 28 weeks. A similar decrease was measured at the last measuring age, week 28, at 16 kHz (Figure 2A).

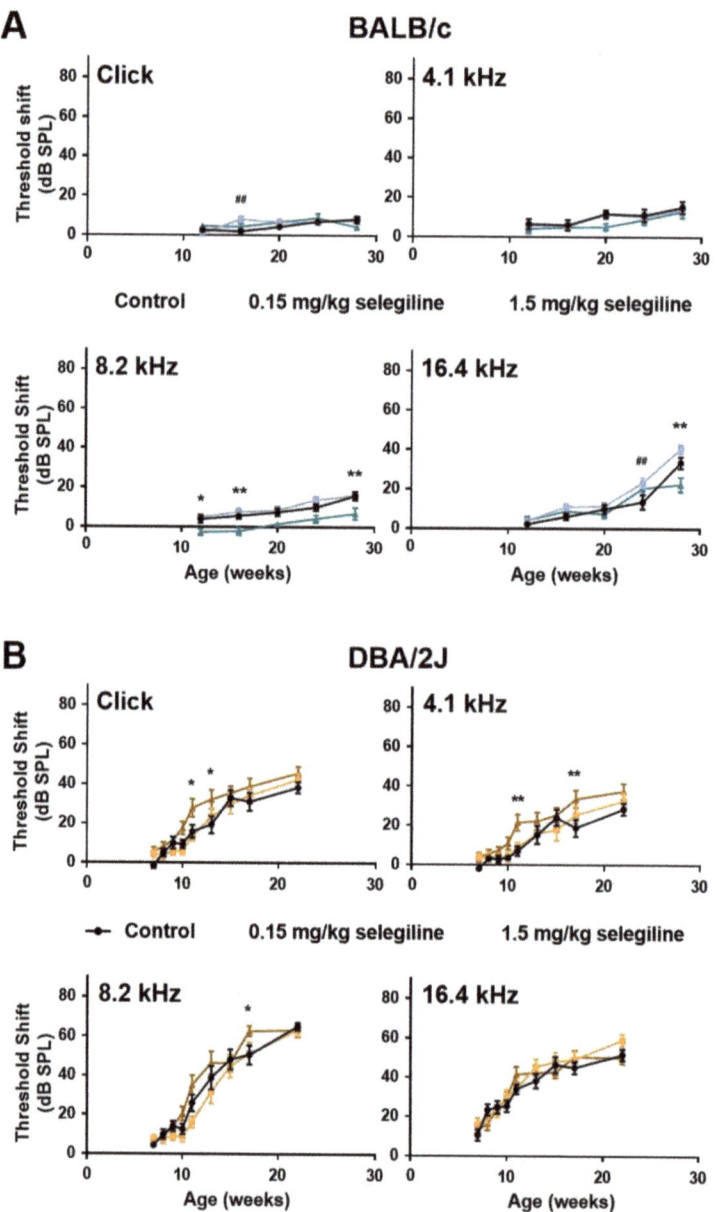

Figure 2. Effect of chronic oral selegiline administration on age-related hearing loss in BALB/c and DBA/2J mice. The drug was added to drinking water. The hearing function was followed by repeated ABR measurements in both the click and tone burst (Figure 1). Treatment of BALB/c (**A**) and DBA/2J (**B**) mice with 0.15 and 1.5 mg/kg selegiline. Data represents mean ± SEM. Two-way ANOVA followed by Bonferroni post-hoc test. 0.15 mg/kg (## $p < 0.01$) and 1.5 mg/kg (* $p < 0.05$, ** $p < 0.01$) selegiline vs. control (see Section 4).

In DBA/2J mice, early-onset hearing loss could be observed both with click stimulus and pure tones of different frequencies (Figure 2B). Average threshold shift values were similar in control and 0.15 mg/kg selegiline-treated animals at all time points and measured frequencies, and the same observation applies to click stimulus. Surprisingly, 1.5 mg/kg selegiline enhanced the threshold shifts at 4.1 and 8.2 kHz as well as at click stimulus significantly at some ages (Figure 2B).

These data show that 1.5 mg/kg selegiline has a small but significant protective effect at 8.2 kHz on ARHL in BALB/c mice. In contrast, this dose has rather potentiated the age-dependent threshold shift elevation in DBA/2J mice.

2.1.2. Experiment II (4 and 15, 45 mg/kg Selegiline)

In control BALB/c mice, ABR thresholds gradually increased with age at both click stimulus and the three test frequencies (Figure 3A). The highest threshold shift was detected at 16.4 kHz. In the 4 mg/kg selegiline-treated group, threshold shifts at click and at 4.1 kHz were nearly identical to control values during the whole experiment (almost 12 months). At 8.2 and 16.4 kHz, a significant decrease in the threshold shifts was seen after selegiline administration from the 27th weeks of age, compared to the control (Figure 3A).

ABR testing of DBA/2J mice was more frequent at the beginning and covered a shorter time window because of the highly accelerated ARHL in this strain. In these mice, the degree of hearing loss was nearly identical in control and selegiline-treated animals (Figure 3B). Small, but significant elevations appeared at three time points for 45 mg/kg selegiline (at 13 and 19 weeks of age at 4.1 kHz, and at 5 weeks of age at 16 kHz).

These data show that chronic oral administration of 4 mg/kg selegiline significantly alleviated the progressive elevation of hearing thresholds from the age of 27 weeks in BALB/c mice at higher frequencies, while even significantly higher doses failed to influence the progression relevantly in DBA/2J mice.

2.2. Effect of Chronic Oral Selegiline Administration on Water Intake, Body Weight and Survival Rate of BALB/c and DBA/2J Mice

2.2.1. Changes in Water Intake

Lower doses of selegiline caused a slight decrease in water intake of BALB/c mice in about the last third of the 22-week treatment period. At 28 weeks of age, average fluid consumption of the 0.15 and 1.5 mg/kg selegiline-treated mice was 4.44 and 3.72 mL/day, compared to 5.40 mL/day water intake of control animals. In DBA/2J mice the fluid consumption was similar in all experimental groups (Figure 4A, Experiment I). Statistical analysis of data was not feasible because of the group-housing of mice (10 mice per cage, see Section 4.3).

In Experiment II, water intake of control BALB/c mice was gradually increased during the 4–49 weeks of age experimental period from a daily intake of 2.74–3.31 mL to 8.12–8.85 mL. In contrast, the average daily intake of the 4 mg/kg selegiline-treated group was 1.61–2.14 mL during the entire treatment period. Despite this difference in fluid intake, both experimental groups were in a good general condition. In DBA/2J mice, average fluid consumption was similar in all experimental groups until about the 9th week of treatment, when mice treated with 45 mg/kg selegiline tended to consume more fluid than control animals (Figure 4B, Experiment II).

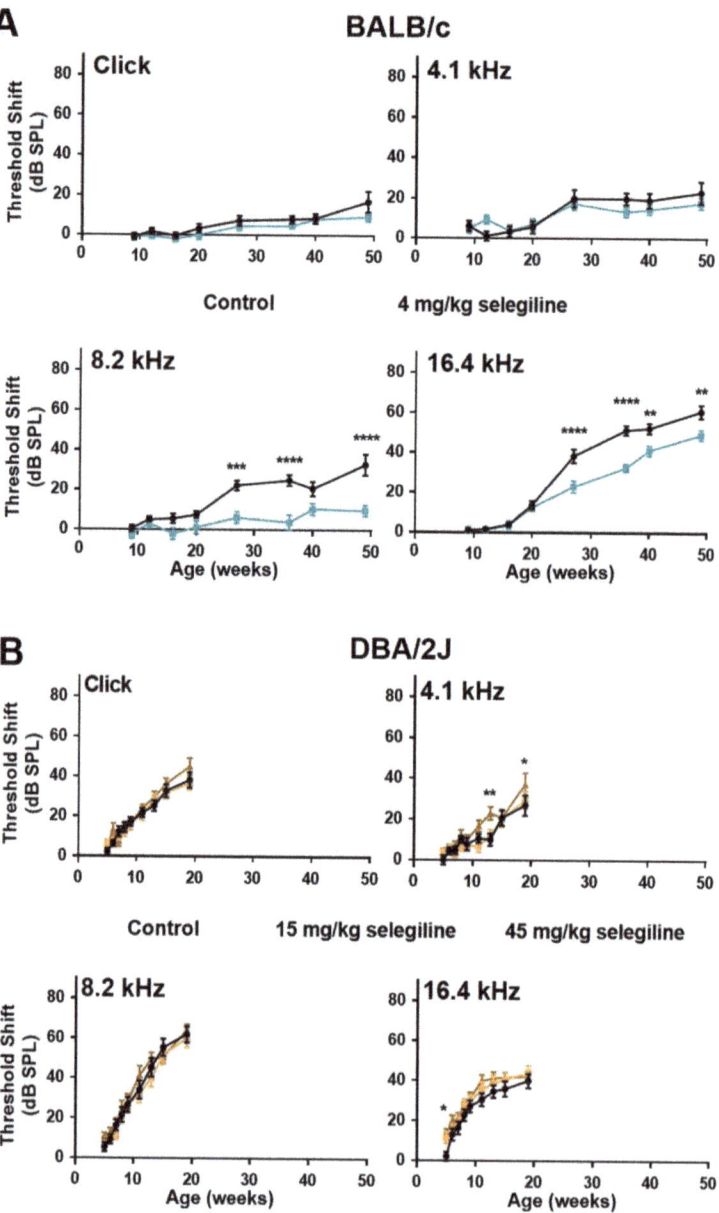

Figure 3. Higher doses of chronic oral selegiline administration alleviated the age-related hearing loss in BALB/c, but not in DBA/2J mice. The drug was added to drinking water. The hearing function was followed by repeated ABR measurements during the age of 4–49 weeks in BALB/c and 4-19 weeks in DBA/2J mice (see protocol in Figure 1). (**A**) Administration of 4 mg/kg selegiline to BALB/c mice. (**B**) Treatment of DBA/2J mice with 15 and 45 mg/kg selegiline. Data represents mean ± SEM. Two-way ANOVA followed by Bonferroni post-hoc test. 4 or 45 mg/kg selegiline vs. control in BALB/c and DBA/2J mice, respectively (* $p < 0.05$, ** $p < 0.01$, *** $p < 0.001$, **** $p < 0.0001$; see Section 4).

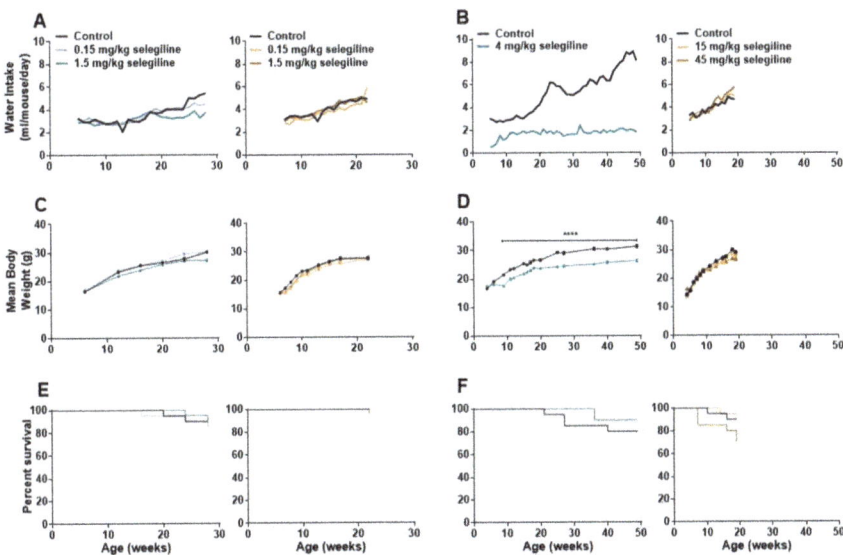

Figure 4. Changes in water consumption, body weight, and analysis of survival during the long term oral treatment by different concentrations of selegiline in BALB/c and DBA/2J mice. Selegiline was administered in tap water. The water intake/day was measured for a whole cage of 10 mice, and the ml/mouse/day values were calculated from that. (**A**) Effect of 0.15 and 1.5 mg/kg (Experiment I) and (**B**) 4 mg/kg and 15 and 45 mg/kg selegiline (Experiment II) on the water intake in BALB/c and DBA/2J mice. (**C**) Effect of the lower (0.15 and 1.5 mg/kg; Experiment I) and (**D**) higher (4 mg/kg and 15 and 45 mg/kg; Experiment II) doses of selegiline on weight gain in BALB/c and DBA/2J mice (**** $p < 0.0001$). (**E,F**) The Kaplan-Meier plots show the effect of different doses of per os selegiline on survival rate in BALB/c and DBA/2J mice (compared to control by Mantel-Cox and Gehan-Breslow-Wilcoxon tests; see details in Methods).

2.2.2. Changes in Body Weight

Body weights of mice were measured regularly during both Experiment I and II. The control group of BALB/c mice in Experiment I showed a weight gain from 16.40 ± 0.18 g (6 weeks of age) to 30.11 ± 0.34 g (28 weeks of age). Treatment of 1.5 mg/kg selegiline caused a slight, but significant reduction in weight gain ($p < 0.01$ at ages of 12 and 16 weeks and $p < 0.0001$ at age 28 week). 0.15 mg/kg selegiline had no effect. The average weight of control DBA/2J mice increased from 15.7 ± 0.26 g to 27.70 ± 0.51 g (from age of 6 to 22 weeks). Drinking of 0.15 mg/kg selegiline resulted in a slight, but significant reduction in weight gain ($p < 0.05$–$p < 0.0001$ between ages of 7 to 17 weeks). Despite the statistical significance, this weight gain fits well into the range of normal weight gain in this substrain [23] (Figure 4C, Experiment I).

Weight of control BALB/c mice in Experiment II increased from 16.70 ± 0.30 g (4 weeks of age) to 31.37 ± 0.51 g (49 weeks of age). Four mg/kg selegiline treatment significantly reduced the gain of body weight compared to the control during the entire experiment (17.53 ± 0.32 g at 4 and 26.35 ± 0.49 g at 49 weeks of age). The difference was in the 10–18% range, which is in accordance with the ethical guidelines on animal experimentation [24–26]. This gain of weight in the selegiline-treated group fits into the range of normal weight gain represented on the growth chart of 3 to 15 week-old BALB/cAnNCrl mice of Charles River Laboratories [23] from where these animals were purchased. Moreover, selegiline-treated mice did not exhibit any signs of pain or distress. The appearance and the natural behavior of the animals were normal during the entire period of the experiment. This reduction could be explained by the avoidance of drinking due to taste preferences in BALB/c mice [27]. In Experiment II, the body weight of control mice increased from 14.40 ± 0.54 g (4 weeks of age) to 29.11 ± 0.43 g (19 weeks of age) in the DBA/2J strain. The rate of weight gain of the 15 mg/kg selegiline treated group, 14.00 ± 0.63 g to 28.12 ± 0.55 g, did not differ from that of the control. Daily oral administration of 45 mg/kg selegiline resulted in a significant decrease of weight gain in time points between the 13th to the 19th week of age ($p < 0.05$–$p < 0.001$). Overall, body weight of this treatment group increased from 16.50 ± 0.52 g to 26.86 ± 0.65 g (Figure 4D, Experiment II).

2.2.3. Survival Rate

As shown in Figure 4E, the survival rates in BALB/c mice were similar in all experimental groups. There was no significant difference between control (90%) and the 0.15 or the 1.5 mg/kg selegiline-treated mice (85% and 90.5%, respectively) at 28 weeks of age (Kaplan-Meier test with log rank (Mantel-Cox) and the Gehan-Breslow-Wilcoxon tests). DBA/2J mice treated with 0.15 mg/kg and 1.5 mg/kg selegiline showed a survival rate of 95% and 95.7% at 22 weeks of age, respectively, while all animals survived in the control group. These results showed no beneficial effect of chronic oral treatment of 0.15 or 1.5 mg/kg selegiline on survival in either mouse strains.

In Experiment II, the survival rate of 4 mg/kg selegiline-treated BALB/c mice was 90% following 45 weeks of treatment and showed no significant difference compared to control mice with a survival rate of 80% (Figure 4F). In DBA/2J mice, the portion of survival was 90%, and 15 mg/kg selegiline treatment did not affect that (89.5%). Mice treated with 45 mg/kg selegiline exhibited only 70% survival at the end of the experiment with no significant difference compared to the other two groups. Although, selegiline administration did not prolong the survival of BALB/c and DBA/2J mouse strains significantly, a slight increase in the survival rate in BALB/c mice and a moderate decrease in the survival in DBA/2J mice with the highest used doses might be observed.

2.3. *Effect of 4 mg/kg Selegiline on Locomotor Activity*

We tested the otoprotective dose of selegiline (4 mg/kg) on the behavior of BALB/c mice (Figure 5). The horizontal activity (ambulation) decreased (A–B), while the vertical activity was enhanced (D–E). In general, there was no change in the total activity indicated by the lack of difference in the immobility time and local movement time (C–F).

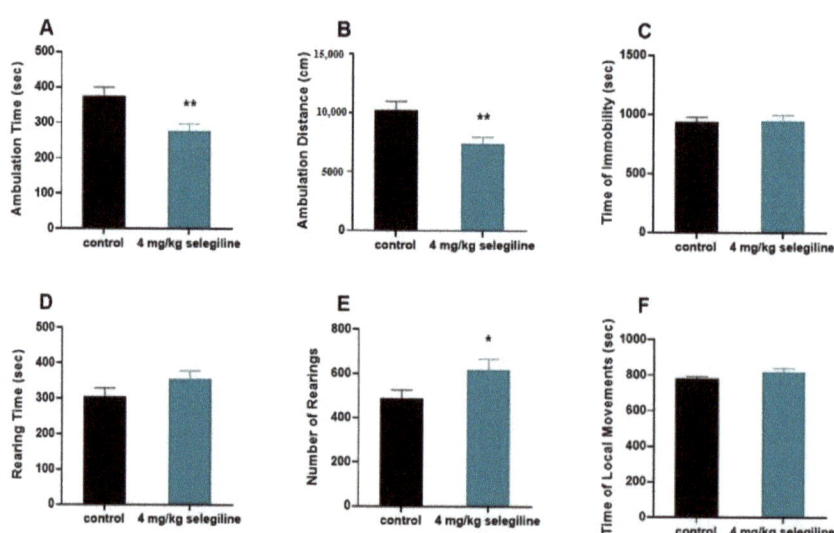

Figure 5. Effect of selegiline (4 mg/kg) on various patterns of locomotor activity of BALB/c mice. The horizontal activity (ambulation; (**A**,**B**)), the vertical activity (**D**,**E**), and the immobility time and local movement time (**C**,**F**) were tested. The observation period lasted 40 min. The control group received tap water ($n = 9$). The treatment group received 4 mg/kg selegiline dissolved in their drinking water ($n = 9$). All data are presented as mean ± S.E.M. Unpaired *t*-test, * $p < 0.05$, ** $p < 0.01$.

3. Discussion

Specific pharmacotherapy for ARHL is still missing. A number of animal studies have found that targeting the factors involved in the pathomechanism [6,28,29] can be a promising therapeutic direction. Antioxidant therapy, such as administration of N-acetylcysteine [30,31], application of apoptosis inhibitors like X-Linked Inhibitor of Apoptotic Protein [32], or neuroprotective compounds [8], have a protective effect on ARHL, but none of these drugs were involved in phase 3 clinical trials according to (ClinicalTrials.gov; accessed on 24 January 2021) and EudraCT databases. The FDA-approved antiparkinsonian drug selegiline is known as an anti-aging drug [33], has complex neuroprotective, antioxidant, and antiapoptotic effects [34–36]. Therefore, we considered it relevant to examine whether selegiline shows a positive impact on presbycusis and lessen the progression of the disorder.

The potential otoprotective effect of different doses of selegiline on ARHL was tested in two mouse strains. BALB/c mice show a massive age-related decline in auditory functions by the age of 10 months [16,17], but age-related changes in the auditory function of this strain gradually increase from 4 weeks of age, primarily at higher frequencies, and lead to clearly noticeable elevation of hearing threshold values from the age of 24–28 weeks. In DBA/2J mice, age-related hearing impairment already begins after weaning, and this strain exhibits severe loss of auditory functions by 12 weeks of age [16,17,37].

Since individual differences in the time course of ARHL also occur in humans, investigation of potential otoprotective drug candidates against ARHL in mouse strains with different progression of hearing loss increases the translational value of findings. In addition, involvement of two different mouse strains improves the generalizability of study results [38].

Based on the progression rate of hearing loss, we considered that chronic administration of selegiline from a young age might be more beneficial. Administration of selegiline at the dose of 4 mg/kg alleviated the progression of ARHL in BALB/c mice. This protection was pronounced at higher frequencies from the age of 27 weeks, including the most sensitive frequency range of mice [39], and preserved throughout the experiment. In contrast, the protective effect of selegiline cannot be observed in DBA/2J mice. BALB/c strain is homozygous for the Ahl1 allele, while the larger susceptibility of DBA/2J strain for ARHL is due to the presence of Ahl1, Ahl8, and Ahl9 genes [40–42]. Differences in the efficacy of selegiline would presumably be due to the presence of more ARHL predisposing genes in DBA/2J strain, which might cause the higher progression rate, severity, and probably a more complex pathology leading to ARHL.

The question arises which beneficial properties of selegiline might be behind the otoprotective effect. It is known that degeneration of outer hair cells (OHCs) and spiral ganglion neurons (SGNs) is one of the main characteristic patterns of ARHL [16]. In DBA/2J mice, age-dependent loss of OHCs and SGNs are extremely severe and occur already in young mice [16]. Early loss of auditory function in this strain is most likely associated with early degeneration of OHCs [16]. On the contrary, in the BALB/c strain, loss of SGNs begins after 4 months and progresses gradually [16,43,44]. After several weeks, this neural loss may manifest in the elevation of hearing thresholds. Willott et al. found that loss of OHCs starts between 50 days and 4 months of age at the cochlear base. The middle regions are affected less, and only by 10 months [16]. In our experiments, a significant decrease in the progression of the elevation of hearing thresholds in the 4 mg/kg selegiline-treated group was seen at 8.2 and 16.4 kHz from 27 weeks of age. The time of appearance of this protective effect correlates with the time course of SGN loss in BALB/c mice. Therefore, selegiline-induced neuroprotection might be one of the main contributors to its otoprotective effect observed in ARHL.

A further mechanism involved in the otoprotective effect of selegiline might be its dopamine (DA) release enhancing action. The excessive release of glutamate (Glu) from inner hair cells (IHCs) in different forms of SNHLs, including the ARHL, initiates to the excitotoxic damage of the primary auditory neurons and their synapse with the IHCs [45–47].

This excitotoxic overactivation is inhibited by DA released from the lateral olivocochlear (LOC) efferents forming axodendritic synapses on the auditory neurons, thereby protecting the IHC-afferent nerve synapse [47–51]. Changes in the cochlear dopaminergic system in aging animals have been previously described. Vicente-Torres et al. reported that the concentration of DA and its metabolites were enhanced in the cochlea in older rats, and this increase could constitute a compensatory mechanism against the age-related loss of afferent type I neurons [52]. Theoretically, any drug that boosts the function of the LOC-DA system could provide preventive or curative effects on ARHL [51,53,54]. Selegiline, through the inhibition of MAO enzyme, affects dopaminergic neuronal transmission and enhances the release of DA in the nervous system [34,55]. Polony et al. showed that rasagiline, a congener of selegiline [35], by blocking the metabolism and uptake of DA, enhanced the release of DA from LOC terminals in mouse cochlear preparation and ameliorated the hearing impairment induced by an aminoglycoside antibiotic [51]. Furthermore, this otoprotective effect might persist during long-term selegiline treatment because of the lack of alteration in the sensitivity of DA receptors [56].

The ineffectiveness of selegiline in DBA/2J strain does not diminish the significance of its otoprotective effect in BALB/c mice. As different subtypes of ARHL are present in different mouse strains of ARHL models, individual genetic predispositions related to age-related auditory degeneration can be observed in humans [57–60]. This results in subpopulations of treatment-resistant and treatment-responsive patients [8]. Selegiline might show an otoprotective effect in some, but not all of these clusters, depending on the individual genetic background (personalized medicine).

Besides otoprotection, administration of selegiline showed the unexpected effect of reduced water intake and a decreased weight gain of mice with a pronounced presence in the BALB/c substrain.

Selegiline was dissolved in drinking water and administered chronically. This way of drug application eliminates the trauma and also the risk of infections associated with daily parenteral injections or oral gavage. Furthermore, it is the preferred drug delivery route in human patients [61,62]. In several previous studies, selegiline was administered via this route to rodents, and it had no effect on fluid consumption [63–65]. In our experiments, contrary to the literature, the administration of selegiline in drinking water led to a reduction in drinking in BALB/c mice in a concentration-dependent manner. The planned doses of 15 or 45 mg/kg could not be reached in the BALB/c mice. On the contrary, decreased fluid consumption could not be observed in the DBA/2J strain. It has been described that the BALB/c6NCrlBL substrain exhibits lower preferences to higher molar concentrations of NaCl, citric acid, and quinine HCl as well [27]. Moreover, BALB/c mice show significant sensitivity to bitter taste [66]. According to a report by the National Toxicology Program, decreased water intake of BALB/c mice relates to the taste of the drinking solution [67]. Based on these findings, we hypothesize that the reduced fluid consumption was related to the special strain specific taste preference of BALB/c mice, i.e., this strain does not like the taste of selegiline-HCl.

There was also a decrease in weight gain in selegiline-treated BALB/c groups. It did not mean a real decrease in body weight, but a restraint on the weight gain that showed a correlation with the concentration of selegiline in the drinking water. Decreased fluid consumption of 4 mg/kg selegiline-treated BALB/c groups occurred even before initiation of the reduction in body weight gain. This may support the hypothesis that decreased weight gain might be the result of the decreased food consumption caused by the compensatory reduction of water intake. Reduced food intake is a protective response of the body to defend the fluid balance [68].

It has been reported that caloric restriction without malnutrition could reduce the severity of ARHL [69,70]. However, results on this topic are contradictory. Sweet et al. reported that caloric restriction could mitigate the progression of ARHL in CBA/J mice if the restriction occurs at the initial phase of degeneration of the auditory system [71]. Effects of dietary restriction on ARHL in different inbred mouse strains were also investigated by

Kenneth R. Henry [72]. In AKR mice, which strain shows early-onset hearing impairment, dietary restriction affected neither the life span nor the progression of ARHL. By contrast, AU/Ss mice on a restricted diet lived longer and had less severe ARHL compared to their littermate controls. Henry has emphasized that the relation between cochlear function and dietary restriction is genotype-dependent. Willot at al. found that strain specific ameliorative effects of caloric restriction on age-related cochlear degeneration, if it could be observed at all, are limited [73]. Although we cannot rule out the possibility of caloric restriction based otoprotection in BALB/c mice, contradictory results in the literature and the differences between the time course of the appearance of hearing protection and decreased body weight in our study argue against its potential otoprotective effect. Moreover, a number of studies found that decreased body weight of selegiline treated animals do not contribute to the life prolonging effect of selegiline [63,74–76].

Our results of survival analysis were less unexpected. Significant differences in longevity between control and selegiline-treated groups could be observed neither in DBA/2J nor in BALB/c mice. Although life prolonging effects of chronic selegiline treatment have been reported in rats, hamsters, and dogs, a number of studies failed to obtain positive longevity effects in mice [63,77].

The 4 mg/kg protective dose of selegiline in the BALB/c mice, by using the FDA guidance (https://www.fda.gov/media/72309/download; accessed on 24 August 2018) for mouse to human dose conversion, gives an approximate of 20 mg/day human equivalent dose. The use of a higher than human antiparkinsonian dose (5–10 mg/day) of selegiline raises the possibility of enhanced activity, a possible side effect of the drug in higher dose. Our behavioral study on 4 month-old BALB/c mice showing otoprotection for 4 mg/kg selegiline did not substantiate this notion. Though selegiline treatment affected the features of locomotor activity, namely enhanced the initial exploratory behavior (rearing) and in line with this reduced the ambulation, the lack of change in immobility and local movements, however, strongly speaks against a possible activity enhancing action of it. This supports its repositioning in higher dose to delay ARHL progression.

In the present study, we demonstrated that chronic oral administration of selegiline mitigated the development of age-related hearing loss in BALB/c, but not in the DBA/2J mice. Preserved hearing function of BALB/c mice could be explained by the neuroprotective, antiapoptotic, antioxidant, and DA neurotransmission enhancing (LOC) effects of selegiline. However, we cannot exclude the possible otoprotective effect of caloric restriction observed in our experiments. Strain differences indicate that the protective effect of selegiline depends on the host's genetic background. Direct translation of our results to clinical application would suggest that chronic selegiline treatment seems to be a reasonable therapy in certain types of human ARHL, taking into account individual genetic predisposition (personalized medicine).

4. Materials and Methods

4.1. Ethics Statement

Animal care and experimental procedures were approved by the National Scientific Ethical Committee on Animal Experimentation and the Semmelweis University's Institutional Animal Care and Use Committee (H-1089 Budapest, Hungary) and permitted by the Government Office of Pest County Division of Food Chain Safety and Animal Health Directorate (project identification code: PE/EA/1912-7/2017). Mice were handled with the principles of NIH guidelines (National Research Council (2011), Guide for the Care and Use of Laboratory Animals: Eighth Edition).

4.2. Experimental Animals and Housing Conditions

Experiments were performed on male BALB/cAnNCrl (#028) and male DBA/2J (#625) mice, hereafter referred to as BALB/c and DBA/2J. Animals were purchased from Charles River's facilities located in Germany and France, respectively (Charles River Laboratories, Wilmington, Massachusetts, 4 weeks of age at arrival). Animals were housed and maintained under a 12:12 h light–dark cycle and controlled environmental conditions (20–24 °C and 35–75% relative humidity) with ad libitum access to food and water throughout the entire duration of the experiment.

4.3. Experimental Design of Hearing Function Measurements and Selegiline Administration

In order to test the effect of a broader selegiline dose range and because of the high number of animals per group and the limits of ABR recordings per day, these measurements were divided into two separate experiments. Chronic administration of selegiline was achieved by adding Selegiline HCl (Chinoin Private Co. Ltd., Budapest, Hungary) to drinking water.

Experiment I. Six-week-old male BALB/c and DBA/2J mice were divided into 3 treatment groups each per strain: BALB/c: Control (n = 20–18), selegiline-treated 0.15 mg/kg (n = 20–17), and selegiline-treated 1.5 mg/kg (n = 21–19). DBA/2J: Control (n = 20–20), selegiline-treated 0.15 mg/kg (n = 20–19), and selegiline-treated 1.5 mg/kg (n = 23–22). The number of mice at the start and at the end of the experiment is indicated in parentheses. BALB/c mice were treated until the age of week 28, and their hearing function was monitored (ABR) regularly. DBA/2J mice were treated and monitored for a shorter time (weeks of age 6–22), because the progression of ARHL is more rapid in this strain, and their mean hearing thresholds at frequencies above 8 kHz are 80–90 dB by that age [16,78].

Selegiline administration was started right after the first measurement of auditory functions and continued until the last measurement of hearing thresholds. Selegiline was dissolved in drinking water (tap water). Body weight of each mouse and water intake of each cage were monitored every 3 days by weighing the mice and water bottles. Ten mice were housed per cage; therefore, individual water intake and oral ingestion of selegiline could not be determined, but per mouse ingestion of selegiline was calculated. The concentration of selegiline in the bottles was adjusted to set and keep the required dose in the actual treatment group. Based on these estimates, the following doses were administered: BALB/c mice (mean ± SD): 0.14 ± 0.05 mg/kg and 1.32 ± 0.41 mg/kg; DBA/2J mice (mean ± SD): 0.19 ± 0.08 mg/kg and 1.91 ± 0.75 mg/kg, referred to henceforth as the 0.15 mg/kg and 1.5 mg/kg doses, respectively. This inevitable variability in dose levels is inherent to the oral administration method, which avoids daily parenteral injections with stress and risk of infections, on the other side. Control animals received regular tap water.

Experiment II. In a second set of experiments, the effect of higher doses of selegiline was investigated. In BALB/c mice the tested period was also extended significantly (weeks of age 4–49).

Four-week-old male BALB/c and DBA/2J mice were divided into the following treatment groups. BALB/c: Control (n = 20–16), selegiline-treated 4 mg/kg (n = 20–18). DBA/2J: Control (n = 20–18), selegiline-treated 15 mg/kg (n = 19–17), and selegiline-treated 45 mg/kg (n = 20–14). The number of mice at the start and at the end of the experiment is indicated in parentheses. Hearing function was monitored (ABR) regularly. DBA/2J mice were treated and monitored for a shorter time (weeks of age 4–19), because of their more rapid progression of ARHL (Figure 3B).

The housing of mice, the way of selegiline administration, measurement of water consumption and body weight and the calculation and adjustment of selegiline concentration to achieve the required ingestion of the drug were identical to Experiment I. BALB/c mice, but not the DBA/2J strain, reduced their intake from water containing high concentrations of selegiline, and the highest ingested dose we could reach was 4 mg/kg. Therefore, we did not run a 4th treatment group in BALB/c mice. Based on the estimates, the following doses were administered: BALB/c mice (mean ± SD): 3.84 ± 0.55 mg/kg; DBA/2J mice (mean ± SD): 14.93 ± 2.81 mg/kg and 46.82 ± 11.35 mg/kg, referred to henceforth as the 4 mg/kg and 15 and 45 mg/kg doses, respectively. Control animals received regular tap water.

4.4. Auditory Brainstem Response (ABR) Recordings

ABR tests were performed to follow up changes in auditory function by measuring hearing thresholds as previously described [9,51]. In brief, mice were anesthetized with a mixture of ketamine-xylazine injection (100 mg/kg and 10 mg/kg, intraperitoneally, respectively). The core temperature of mice was maintained between 36 and 38 °C using a temperature-controlled heating pad (Supertech Instruments, H-7624 Pécs, Hungary). For recording evoked potentials, needle electrodes were placed subcutaneously at the vertex (active electrode), behind the right pinna (reference electrode), and at the rear leg (ground). Hearing tests were performed in an electrically shielded sound-proof chamber using an auditory research system developed by Tucker Davis Technologies (TDT system 3 with RX6 signal processor and RA16 Medusa Base Station; Tucker–Davis Technologies (TDT), Alachua, FL, USA). Auditory stimuli consisting of click (0.4 ms duration, with bandwidths of 0–50 kHz) and 4-, 8-, and 16 kHz tone bursts (3 ms duration, 0.2 ms rise/decay) were digitally generated in the SigGenRP software package (TDT, Alachua, FL, USA) and delivered into the right ear through an EC-1 electrostatic speaker in a closed acoustic system, controlled by the BioSigRP software (TDT, Alachua, FL, USA). All biological signals were amplified through RA4PA Medusa PreAmplifier (TDT, Alachua, FL, USA) connected to RA4LI Low Impedance Headstage (TDT, Alachua, FL, USA). Sound pressure levels (SPL) of the click stimulus were increased in 10-dB steps from 0 to 80 dB. In tone burst stimulation mode, the intensity was attenuated in 10 dB steps from 90 to 10 dB at each frequency. Attenuation was controlled by a PA5 Programmable Attenuator (TDT, Alachua, FL, USA). For calibrating the sound delivery system, a half-inch free field preamplifier integrated microphone was used (ACO Pacific Inc., Belmont, CA 94002, USA; Model 7017) with the application of the SigCalRP (TDT, Alachua, FL, USA) calibration software. Responses were amplified, filtered, and averaged 800 times in real-time. The hearing threshold was defined as the minimal intensity level at which an ABR waveform with an identifiable peak could be detected visually. Shifts in auditory thresholds were calculated for click and tone bursts by subtracting the auditory thresholds registered at the start of the experiment (baseline auditory threshold levels) from the hearing thresholds registered at different ages.

The tested frequency range of 4–16 kHz in mice corresponds approximately to the 1–4 kHz range in human beings [39]. This range is essential for normal speech perception and regularly tested during basic audiologic assessments [79–83], and also used in guidelines recommending the sound pressure level of hearing impairment that is required for prescribing hearing aids [84]. This matching in the practically relevant mouse-human frequency range provides a reliable translational value to our study.

4.5. Survival Analysis

Mice in each cage were controlled daily. The effect of different doses of selegiline on the survival of BALB/c and DBA/2J mice was analyzed by the Kaplan-Meier method, and the curves were compared by the log rank (Mantel-Cox) and Gehan-Breslow-Wilcoxon tests. Survival rate was plotted as the percent of survival.

4.6. Test of Locomotor Activity

Locomotor activity of some control ($n = 9$) and selegiline treated (1 mg/kg; $n = 9$) BALB/c mice at their 4 months of age in Experiment II were measured by "CONDUCTA System for behavioral and activity studies" (Experimetria Ltd., H-1062 Budapest, Hungary). The apparatus consists of three black-painted testing boxes (40 × 50 × 50 cm each) set in an isolated room. Three animals could be tested in parallel without any connection between them. One animal was placed in one box. Ambulation (walking, running) time and distance, rearing, local movement, and immobility time were recorded individually for each box. The movements of mice were detected by high-density arrays of infrared diodes. The observation started immediately without any habituation and lasted 40 min.

Mice were absolutely naïve to the apparatus, and they were placed into the experimental box only once.

4.7. Data Analysis

Change of the auditory thresholds was expressed as a threshold shift. Two-way ANOVA followed by the Bonferroni post-hoc test was performed to determine the statistical significance in the 6.01 version of GraphPad Prism. Calculations were computed separately at every frequency and click stimulation. One-way ANOVA followed by Bonferroni post-hoc test was used to compare body weights between control and selegiline-treated animals. Survival rate differences were analyzed by Kaplan-Meier method with log rank (Mantel-Cox) and Gehan-Breslow-Wilcoxon tests using GraphPad Prism (v.6.01). Analyses of locomotor activity were performed using GraphPad Prism v.8.0.1. Statistical significance of difference between mean values was evaluated by Unpaired Student's *t*-test. Data are expressed as mean ± standard error of the mean (SEM). For all comparisons, levels of significance are as follows: * $p < 0.05$, ** $p < 0.01$, *** $p < 0.001$, **** $p < 0.0001$.

Author Contributions: Conceptualization, J.S., V.H., E.S.V. and T.Z.; methodology, J.S., V.H. and T.Z.; validation, J.S., V.H. and T.Z.; formal analysis, J.S., I.M., J.T. and T.T.; investigation, J.S., V.H., I.M., J.T. and T.T.; resources, A.G., G.P., Á.S., L.T., L.K., E.S.V. and T.Z.; data curation, J.S., J.F. and T.Z.; writing—original draft preparation, J.S. and T.Z.; writing—review and editing, J.S., J.T., A.G., G.P., Á.S., L.T., L.K., E.S.V. and T.Z.; visualization, J.S. and J.F.; supervision, T.Z.; project administration, J.S., V.H. and T.Z.; funding acquisition, L.K. and T.Z. All authors have read and agreed to the published version of the manuscript.

Funding: This work was supported by the Hungarian Scientific Research Fund (NKFIH, K128875) and the Higher Education Institutional Excellence Program of the Ministry of Human Capacities in Hungary, within the framework of the Neurology thematic program of Semmelweis University (FIKP 2020).

Acknowledgments: Selegiline was a generous gift of Sanofi/Chinoin, Budapest, Hungary.

Conflicts of Interest: The authors declare no conflict of interest.

References

1. Gopinath, B.; Rochtchina, E.; Wang, J.J.; Schneider, J.; Leeder, S.R.; Mitchell, P. Prevalence of age-related hearing loss in older adults: Blue mountains study. *Arch. Intern. Med.* **2009**, *169*, 415–416. [CrossRef]
2. World Health Organization. Deafness and Hearing Loss. Available online: https://www.who.int/news-room/fact-sheets/detail/deafness-and-hearing-loss (accessed on 2 March 2021).
3. Peelle, J.E.; Wingfield, A. The Neural Consequences of Age-Related Hearing Loss. *Trends Neurosci.* **2016**, *39*, 486–497. [CrossRef] [PubMed]
4. Dalton, D.S.; Cruickshanks, K.J.; Klein, B.E.K.; Klein, R.; Wiley, T.L.; Nondahl, D.M. The Impact of Hearing Loss on Quality of Life in Older Adults. *Gerontologist* **2003**, *43*, 661–668. [CrossRef]
5. Van Eyken, E.; Van Camp, G.; Van Laer, L. The complexity of age-related hearing impairment: Contributing environmental and genetic factors. *Audiol. Neurotol.* **2007**, *12*, 345–358. [CrossRef]
6. Gates, G.A.; Mills, J.H. Presbycusis. *Lancet* **2005**, *366*, 1111–1120. [CrossRef]
7. Someya, S.; Tanokura, M.; Weindruch, R.; Prolla, T.; Yamasoba, T. Effects of Caloric Restriction on Age-Related Hearing Loss in Rodents and Rhesus Monkeys. *Curr. Aging Sci.* **2010**, *3*, 20–25. [CrossRef] [PubMed]
8. Wang, J.; Puel, J.L. Toward cochlear therapies. *Physiol. Rev.* **2018**, *98*, 2477–2522. [CrossRef]
9. Szepesy, J.; Miklós, G.; Farkas, J.; Kucsera, D.; Giricz, Z.; Gáborján, A.; Polony, G.; Szirmai, Á.; Tamás, L.; Köles, L.; et al. Anti-PD-1 Therapy Does Not Influence Hearing Ability in the Most Sensitive Frequency Range, but Mitigates Outer Hair Cell Loss in the Basal Cochlear Region. *Int. J. Mol. Sci.* **2020**, *21*, 6701. [CrossRef]
10. Watson, N.; Ding, B.; Zhu, X.; Frisina, R.D. Chronic inflammation—Inflammaging—In the ageing cochlea: A novel target for future presbycusis therapy. *Ageing Res. Rev.* **2017**, *40*, 142–148. [CrossRef]
11. Schuknecht, H.F.; Gacek, M.R. Cochlear pathology in presbycusis. *Ann. Otol. Rhinol. Laryngol.* **1993**, *102*, 1–16. [CrossRef]
12. Otte, J.; Schuknecht, H.F.; Kerr, A.G. Ganglion cell populations in normal and pathological human cochleae. Implications for cochlear implantation. *Laryngoscope* **1978**, *88*, 1231–1246. [CrossRef]
13. Steel, K.P. Similarities between mice and humans with hereditary deafness. *Ann. N. Y. Acad. Sci.* **1991**, *630*, 68–79. [CrossRef]
14. Steel, K.P.; Bock, G.R. Hereditary inner-ear abnormalities in animals. Relationships with human abnormalities. *Arch. Otolaryngol.* **1983**, *109*, 22–29. [CrossRef]

15. Keithley, E.M.; Canto, C.; Zheng, Q.Y.; Fischel-Ghodsian, N.; Johnson, K.R. Age-related hearing loss and the ahl locus in mice. *Hear. Res.* **2004**, *188*, 21–28. [CrossRef]
16. Willott, J.F.; Turner, J.G.; Carlson, S.; Ding, D.; Seegers Bross, L.; Falls, W.A. The BALB/C mouse as an animal model for progressive sensorineural hearing loss. *Hear. Res.* **1998**, *115*, 162–174. [CrossRef]
17. Ralls, K. Auditory sensitivity in mice: Peromyscus and Mus musculus. *Anim. Behav.* **1967**, *15*, 123–128. [CrossRef]
18. Knoll, J.; Magyar, K. Some puzzling pharmacological effects of monoamine oxidase inhibitors. *Adv. Biochem. Psychopharmacol.* **1972**, *5*, 393–408.
19. Alexander Bodkin, J.; Amsterdam, J.D. Transdermal Selegiline in Major Depression: A Double-Blind., Placebo-Controlled, Parallel-Group Study in Outpatients. *Am. J. Psychiatry* **2020**, *159*, 1869–1875. [CrossRef]
20. Miklya, I. The significance of selegiline/(-)-deprenyl after 50 years in research and therapy (1965–2015). *Mol. Psychiatry* **2016**, *21*, 1499–1503. [CrossRef]
21. Knoll, J. (-)Deprenyl-medication: A strategy to modulate the age-related decline of the striatal dopaminergic system. *J. Am. Geriatr. Soc.* **1992**, *40*, 839–847. [CrossRef]
22. Ruehl, W.W.; Entriken, T.L.; Muggenburg, B.A.; Bruyette, D.S.; Griffith, W.C.; Hahn, F.F. Treatment with L-deprenyl prolongs life in elderly dogs. *Life Sci.* **1997**, *61*, 1037–1044. [CrossRef]
23. Charles River Laboratories. Available online: https://www.criver.com/products-services/find-model/balbc-mouse?region=3631 (accessed on 2 March 2021).
24. Talbot, S.R.; Biernot, S.; Bleich, A.; van Dijk, R.M.; Ernst, L.; Häger, C.; Helgers, S.O.A.; Koegel, B.; Koska, I.; Kuhla, A.; et al. Defining body-weight reduction as a humane endpoint: A critical appraisal. *Lab. Anim.* **2020**, *54*, 99–110. [CrossRef]
25. Morton, D.B. A systematic approach for establishing humane endpoints. *ILAR J.* **2000**, *41*, 80–86. [CrossRef]
26. Morton, D.B.; Griffiths, P.H. Guidelines on the recognition of pain, distress and discomfort in experimental animals and a hypothesis for assessment. *Vet. Rec.* **1985**, *116*, 431–436. [CrossRef]
27. Kachele, D.L.; Lasiter, P.S. Murine strain differences in taste responsivity and organization of the rostral nucleus of the solitary tract. *Brain Res. Bull.* **1990**, *24*, 239–247. [CrossRef]
28. Someya, S.; Prolla, T.A. Mitochondrial oxidative damage and apoptosis in age-related hearing loss. *Mech. Ageing Dev.* **2010**, *131*, 480–486. [CrossRef]
29. Wang, J.; Puel, J.-L. Presbycusis: An Update on Cochlear Mechanisms and Therapies. *J. Clin. Med.* **2020**, *9*, 2018. [CrossRef]
30. Marie, A.; Meunier, J.; Brun, E.; Malmstrom, S.; Baudoux, V.; Flaszka, E.; Naert, G.; Roman, F.; Cosnier-Pucheu, S.; Gonzalez-Gonzalez, S. N-acetylcysteine Treatment Reduces Age-related Hearing Loss and Memory Impairment in the Senescence-Accelerated Prone 8 (SAMP8) Mouse Model. *Aging Dis.* **2018**, *9*, 664–673. [CrossRef] [PubMed]
31. Ding, D.; Jiang, H.; Chen, G.-D.; Longo-Guess, C.; Muthaiah, V.P.K.; Tian, C.; Sheppard, A.; Salvi, R.; Johnson, K.R. N-acetylcysteine prevents age-related hearing loss and the progressive loss of inner hair cells in γ-glutamyl transferase 1 deficient mice. *Aging* **2016**, *8*, 730–750. [CrossRef]
32. Ruan, Q.; Zeng, S.; Liu, A.; Chen, Z.; Yu, Z.; Zhang, R.; He, J.; Bance, M.; Robertson, G.; Yin, S.; et al. Overexpression of X-Linked Inhibitor of Apoptotic Protein (XIAP) reduces age-related neuronal degeneration in the mouse cochlea. *Gene Ther.* **2014**, *21*, 967–974. [CrossRef]
33. Kitani, K.; Minami, C.; Yamamoto, T.; Kanai, S.; Ivy, G.O.; Carrillo, M.-C. Pharmacological interventions in aging and age-associated disorders: Potentials of propargylamines for human use. *Ann. N. Y. Acad. Sci.* **2002**, *959*, 295–307. [CrossRef]
34. Ebadi, M.; Sharma, S.; Shavali, S.; El Refaey, H. Neuroprotective actions of selegiline. *J. Neurosci. Res.* **2002**, *67*, 285–289. [CrossRef]
35. Szökő, É.; Tábi, T.; Riederer, P.; Vécsei, L.; Magyar, K. Pharmacological aspects of the neuroprotective effects of irreversible MAO-B inhibitors, selegiline and rasagiline, in Parkinson's disease. *J. Neural Transm.* **2018**, *125*, 1735–1749. [CrossRef]
36. Tábi, T.; Vécsei, L.; Youdim, M.B.; Riederer, P.; Szökő, É. Selegiline: A molecule with innovative potential. *J. Neural Transm.* **2020**, *127*, 831–842. [CrossRef]
37. Zheng, Q.Y.; Johnson, K.R.; Erway, L.C. Assessment of hearing in 80 inbred strains of mice by ABR threshold analyses. *Hear. Res.* **1999**, *130*, 94–107. [CrossRef]
38. Bespalov, A.; Michel, M.C.; Steckler, T. (Eds.) *Handbook of Experimental Pharmacology: Good Research Practice in Non-Clinical Pharmacology and Biomedicine*; Springer International Publishing: Cham, Switzerland, 2020; Volume 257, ISBN 978-3-030-33655-4.
39. Ehret, G. Age-dependent hearing loss in normal hearing mice. *Naturwissenschaften* **1974**, *61*, 506–507. [CrossRef] [PubMed]
40. Johnson, K.R.; Longo-Guess, C.; Gagnon, L.H.; Yu, H.; Zheng, Q.Y. A locus on distal chromosome 11 (ahl8) and its interaction with Cdh23ahl underlie the early onset, age-related hearing loss of DBA/2J mice. *Genomics* **2008**, *92*, 219–225. [CrossRef]
41. Nagtegaal, A.P.; Spijker, S.; Crins, T.T.H.; Neuro-Bsik Mouse Phenomics Consortium; Borst, J.G.G. A novel QTL underlying early-onset, low-frequency hearing loss in BXD recombinant inbred strains. *Genes. Brain. Behav.* **2012**, *11*, 911–920. [CrossRef]
42. Wang, Q.; Zhao, H.; Zheng, T.; Wang, W.; Zhang, X.; Wang, A.; Li, B.; Wang, Y.; Zheng, Q. Otoprotective effects of mouse nerve growth factor in DBA/2J mice with early-onset progressive hearing loss. *J. Neurosci. Res.* **2017**, *95*, 1937–1950. [CrossRef]
43. Fetoni, A.R.; Picciotti, P.M.; Paludetti, G.; Troiani, D. Pathogenesis of presbycusis in animal models: A review. *Exp. Gerontol.* **2011**, *46*, 413–425. [CrossRef]
44. Ohlemiller, K.K.; Gagnon, P.M. Apical-to-basal gradients in age-related cochlear degeneration and their relationship to "primary" loss of cochlear neurons. *J. Comp. Neurol.* **2004**, *479*, 103–116. [CrossRef]

45. Duan, M.; Agerman, K.; Ernfors, P.; Canlon, B. Complementary roles of neurotrophin 3 and a N-methyl-D-aspartate antagonist in the protection of noise and aminoglycoside-induced ototoxicity. *Proc. Natl. Acad. Sci. USA* **2000**, *97*, 7597–7602. [CrossRef] [PubMed]
46. Tabuchi, K.; Nishimura, B.; Tanaka, S.; Hayashi, K.; Hirose, Y.; Hara, A. Ischemia-reperfusion injury of the cochlea: Pharmacological strategies for cochlear protection and implications of glutamate and reactive oxygen species. *Curr. Neuropharmacol.* **2010**, *8*, 128–134. [CrossRef]
47. Ruel, J.; Wang, J.; Rebillard, G.; Eybalin, M.; Lloyd, R.; Pujol, R.; Puel, J.-L. Physiology, pharmacology and plasticity at the inner hair cell synaptic complex. *Hear. Res.* **2007**, *227*, 19–27. [CrossRef]
48. Lendvai, B.; Halmos, G.B.; Polony, G.; Kapocsi, J.; Horváth, T.; Aller, M.; Sylvester Vizi, E.; Zelles, T. Chemical neuroprotection in the cochlea: The modulation of dopamine release from lateral olivocochlear efferents. *Neurochem. Int.* **2011**, *59*, 150–158. [CrossRef]
49. Halmos, G.; Doleviczényi, Z.; Répássy, G.; Kittel, A.; Vizi, E.S.; Lendvai, B.; Zelles, T. D2 autoreceptor inhibition reveals oxygen-glucose deprivation-induced release of dopamine in guinea-pig cochlea. *Neuroscience* **2005**, *132*, 801–809. [CrossRef]
50. Halmos, G.; Gáborján, A.; Lendvai, B.; Répássy, G.; Szabó, L.Z.; Vizi, E.S. Veratridine-evoked release of dopamine from guinea pig isolated cochlea. *Hear. Res.* **2000**, *144*, 89–96. [CrossRef]
51. Polony, G.; Humli, V.; Andó, R.; Aller, M.; Horváth, T.; Harnos, A.; Tamás, L.; Vizi, E.S.; Zelles, T. Protective effect of rasagiline in aminoglycoside ototoxicity. *Neuroscience* **2014**, *265*, 263–273. [CrossRef]
52. Vicente-Torres, M.A.; Dávila, D.; Muñoz, E.; Gil-Loyzaga, P. Effects of aging on cochlear monoamine turnover. *Adv. Otorhinolaryngol.* **2002**, *59*, 112–115.
53. Kujawa, S.G.; Liberman, M.C. Synaptopathy in the noise-exposed and aging cochlea: Primary neural degeneration in acquired sensorineural hearing loss. *Hear. Res.* **2015**, *330*, 191–199. [CrossRef] [PubMed]
54. Doleviczényi, Z.; Vizi, E.S.; Gacsályi, I.; Pallagi, K.; Volk, B.; Hársing, L.G.; Halmos, G.; Lendvai, B.; Zelles, T. 5-HT6/7 Receptor Antagonists Facilitate Dopamine Release in the Cochlea via a GABAergic Disinhibitory Mechanism. *Neurochem. Res.* **2008**, *33*, 2364–2372. [CrossRef]
55. Hársing, L.G.; Vizi, E.S. Release of endogenous dopamine from rat isolated striatum: Effect of clorgyline and (-)-deprenyl. *Br. J. Pharmacol.* **1984**, *83*, 741–749. [CrossRef]
56. Timar, J.; Knoll, B.; Knoll, J. Long-term administration of (-)deprenyl (selegiline), a compound which facilitates dopaminergic tone in the brain, leaves the sensitivity of dopamine receptors to apomorphine unchanged. *Arch. Int. Pharmacodyn. Ther.* **1986**, *284*, 255–266.
57. Walsh, T.; Pierce, S.B.; Lenz, D.R.; Brownstein, Z.; Dagan-Rosenfeld, O.; Shahin, H.; Roeb, W.; McCarthy, S.; Nord, A.S.; Gordon, C.R.; et al. Genomic duplication and overexpression of TJP2/ZO-2 leads to altered expression of apoptosis genes in progressive nonsyndromic hearing loss DFNA51. *Am. J. Hum. Genet.* **2010**, *87*, 101–109. [CrossRef]
58. Hertzano, R; Dror, A.A.; Montcouquiol, M.; Ahmed, Z.M.; Ellsworth, B.; Camper, S.; Friedman, T.B.; Kelley, M.W.; Avraham, K.B. Lhx3, a LIM domain transcription factor, is regulated by Pou4f3 in the auditory but not in the vestibular system. *Eur. J. Neurosci.* **2007**, *25*, 999–1005. [CrossRef]
59. Ahituv, N.; Avraham, K.B. Auditory and vestibular mouse mutants: Models for human deafness. *J. Basic Clin. Physiol. Pharmacol.* **2000**, *11*, 181–191. [CrossRef] [PubMed]
60. Boucher, S.; Tai, F.W.J.; Delmaghani, S.; Lelli, A.; Singh-Estivalet, A.; Dupont, T.; Niasme-Grare, M.; Michel, V.; Wolff, N.; Bahloul, A.; et al. Ultrarare heterozygous pathogenic variants of genes causing dominant forms of early-onset deafness underlie severe presbycusis. *Proc. Natl. Acad. Sci. USA* **2020**, *117*, 31278–31289. [CrossRef] [PubMed]
61. Brozoski, T.J.; Spires, T.J.D.; Bauer, C.A. Vigabatrin, a GABA transaminase inhibitor, reversibly eliminates tinnitus in an animal model. *J. Assoc. Res. Otolaryngol.* **2007**, *8*, 105–118. [CrossRef] [PubMed]
62. Bauer, C.A.; Brozoski, T.J. Assessing tinnitus and prospective tinnitus therapeutics using a psychophysical animal model. *J. Assoc. Res. Otolaryngol.* **2001**, *2*, 54–64. [CrossRef]
63. Bickford, P.C.; Adams, C.E.; Boyson, S.J.; Curella, P.; Gerhardt, G.A.; Heron, C.; Ivy, G.O.; Lin, A.M.L.Y.; Murphy, M.P.; Poth, K.; et al. Long-term treatment of male F344 rats with deprenyl: Assessment of effects on longevity, behavior, and brain function. *Neurobiol. Aging* **1997**, *18*, 309–318. [CrossRef]
64. Speiser, Z.; Fine, T.; Litinetsky, L.; Eliash, S.; Blaugrund, E.; Cohen, S. Differential behavioral syndrome evoked in the rats after multiple doses of SSRI fluoxetine with selective MAO inhibitors rasagiline or selegiline. *J. Neural Transm.* **2008**, *115*, 107–116. [CrossRef] [PubMed]
65. Bekesi, G.; Tulassay, Z.; Lengyel, G.; Schaff, Z.; Szombath, D.; Stark, J.; Marczell, I.; Nagy-Repas, P.; Adler, I.; Dinya, E.; et al. The effect of selegiline on total scavenger capacity and liver fat content: A preliminary study in an animal model. *J. Neural Transm.* **2012**, *119*, 25–30. [CrossRef]
66. Boughter, J.D.; Bachmanov, A.A. Behavioral genetics and taste. *BMC Neurosci.* **2007**, *8* (Suppl. 3), S3. [CrossRef]
67. Bucher, J.R. NTP Technical Report on the Toxicity Studies of Sodium Dichromate Dihydrate Administered in Drinking Water to Male and Female F344/N Rats and B6C3F 1 Mice and Male BALB/c and am3-C57BL/6 Mice. *Toxic Rep Ser.* **2007**, *72*, 1–G4.
68. Hamilton, L.W.; Flaherty, C.F. Interactive effects of deprivation in the albino rat. *Learn. Motiv.* **1973**, *4*, 148–162. [CrossRef]
69. Seidman, M.D. Effects of dietary restriction and antioxidants on presbycusis. *Laryngoscope* **2000**, *110*, 727–738. [CrossRef]

70. Someya, S.; Yamasoba, T.; Weindruch, R.; Prolla, T.A.; Tanokura, M. Caloric restriction suppresses apoptotic cell death in the mammalian cochlea and leads to prevention of presbycusis. *Neurobiol. Aging* **2007**, *28*, 1613–1622. [CrossRef] [PubMed]
71. Sweet, R.J.; Price, J.M.; Henry, K.R. Dietary restriction and presbyacusis: Periods of restriction and auditory threshold losses in the CBA/j mouse. *Audiology* **1988**, *27*, 305–312. [CrossRef]
72. Henry, K.R. Effects of dietary restriction on presbyacusis in the mouse. *Audiology* **1986**, *25*, 329–337. [CrossRef]
73. Willott, J.F.; Erway, L.C.; Archer, J.R.; Harrison, D.E. Genetics of age-related hearing loss in mice. II. Strain differences and effects of caloric restriction on cochlear pathology and evoked response thresholds. *Hear. Res.* **1995**, *88*, 143–155. [CrossRef]
74. Stoll, S.; Hafner, U.; Pohl, O.; Müller, W.E. Age-related memory decline and longevity under treatment with selegiline. *Life Sci.* **1994**, *55*, 2155–2163. [CrossRef]
75. Yen, T.T.; Knoll, J. Extension of lifespan in mice treated with Dinh lang (*Policias fruticosum* L.) and (-)deprenyl. *Acta Physiol. Hung.* **1992**, *79*, 119–124.
76. Milgram, N.W.; Racine, R.J.; Nellis, P.; Mendonca, A.; Ivy, G.O. Maintenance on L-deprenyl prolongs life in aged male rats. *Life Sci.* **1990**, *47*, 415–420. [CrossRef]
77. Kitani, K.; Kanai, S.; Ivy, G.O.; Carrillo, M.C. Assessing the effects of deprenyl on longevity and antioxidant defenses in different animal models. *Ann. N. Y. Acad. Sci.* **1998**, *854*, 291–306. [CrossRef] [PubMed]
78. Suzuki, S.; Ishikawa, M.; Ueda, T.; Ohshiba, Y.; Miyasaka, Y.; Okumura, K.; Yokohama, M.; Taya, C.; Matsuoka, K.; Kikkawa, Y. Quantitative trait loci on chromosome 5 for susceptibility to frequency-specific effects on hearing in DBA/2J mice. *Exp. Anim.* **2015**, *64*, 241–251. [CrossRef]
79. Spiby, J. Screening for Hearing Loss in Older Adults. In *External Review against Programme Appraisal Criteria for the UK National Screening Committee (UK NSC)*; The UK National Screening Committee: Waterloo Road, London, UK, 2014.
80. Bagai, A.; Thavendiranathan, P.; Detsky, A.S. Does this patient have hearing impairment? *J. Am. Med. Assoc.* **2006**, *295*, 416–428. [CrossRef]
81. Lycke, M.; Lefebvre, T.; Cool, L.; Van Eygen, K.; Boterberg, T.; Schofield, P.; Debruyne, P.R. Screening methods for age-related hearing loss in older patients with cancer: A review of the literature. *Geriatr.* **2018**, *3*, 48. [CrossRef]
82. Zahnert, T. The Differential Diagnosis of Hearing Loss. *Dtsch. Arztebl.* **2011**, *108*, 433–444. [CrossRef]
83. Olusanya, B.O.; Davis, A.C.; Hoffman, H.J. Hearing loss grades and the international classification of functioning, disability and health. *Bull. World Health Organ.* **2019**, *97*, 725–728. [CrossRef]
84. World Health Organization. Guidelines for Hearing Aids and Services for Developing Countries. Available online: https://www.who.int/publications/i/item/guidelines-for-hearing-aids-and-services-for-developing-countries (accessed on 18 September 2019).

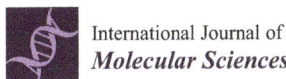 

Article

Constant Light Dysregulates Cochlear Circadian Clock and Exacerbates Noise-Induced Hearing Loss

Chao-Hui Yang [1,2], Chung-Feng Hwang [1,*], Jiin-Haur Chuang [2,3], Wei-Shiung Lian [4], Feng-Sheng Wang [2,4], Ethan I. Huang [5] and Ming-Yu Yang [1,2,*]

1. Department of Otolaryngology, Kaohsiung Chang Gung Memorial Hospital and Chang Gung University College of Medicine, Kaohsiung 83301, Taiwan; chouwhay@gmail.com
2. Graduate Institute of Clinical Medical Sciences, College of Medicine, Chang Gung University, Tao-Yuan 33302, Taiwan; jhchuang@adm.cgmh.org.tw (J.-H.C.); wangfs@ms33.hinet.net (F.-S.W.)
3. Division of Pediatric Surgery, Kaohsiung Chang Gung Memorial Hospital and Chang Gung University College of Medicine, Kaohsiung 83301, Taiwan
4. Core Laboratory for Phenomics & Diagnostics, Department of Medical Research, Kaohsiung Chang Gung Memorial Hospital and Chang Gung University College of Medicine, Kaohsiung 83301, Taiwan; lianws@gmail.com
5. Department of Otolaryngology, Chang Gung Memorial Hospital, Chiayi 61363, Taiwan; ehuang@alumni.pitt.edu
* Correspondence: cfhwang@hotmail.com (C.-F.H.); yangmy@mail.cgu.edu.tw (M.-Y.Y.); Tel.: +886-7-731-7123 (ext. 2533) (C.-F.H.); +886-7-731-7123 (ext. 8865) (M.-Y.Y.); Fax: +886-7-731-3855 (C.-F.H.)

Received: 8 September 2020; Accepted: 9 October 2020; Published: 13 October 2020

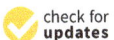

Abstract: Noise-induced hearing loss is one of the major causes of acquired sensorineural hearing loss in modern society. While people with excessive exposure to noise are frequently the population with a lifestyle of irregular circadian rhythms, the effects of circadian dysregulation on the auditory system are still little known. Here, we disturbed the circadian clock in the cochlea of male CBA/CaJ mice by constant light (LL) or constant dark. LL significantly repressed circadian rhythmicity of circadian clock genes *Per1*, *Per2*, *Rev-erbα*, *Bmal1*, and *Clock* in the cochlea, whereas the auditory brainstem response thresholds were unaffected. After exposure to low-intensity (92 dB) noise, mice under LL condition initially showed similar temporary threshold shifts to mice under normal light–dark cycle, and mice under both conditions returned to normal thresholds after 3 weeks. However, LL augmented high-intensity (106 dB) noise-induced permanent threshold shifts, particularly at 32 kHz. The loss of outer hair cells (OHCs) and the reduction of synaptic ribbons were also higher in mice under LL after noise exposure. Additionally, LL enhanced high-intensity noise-induced 4-hydroxynonenal in the OHCs. Our findings convey new insight into the deleterious effect of an irregular biological clock on the auditory system.

Keywords: circadian dysregulation; clock genes; noise-induced hearing loss; sensory hair cells; synaptic ribbons

1. Introduction

The circadian clock and rhythm are important for the regulation of tissue homeostasis and function. Expanding evidence has revealed that daily rhythmic changes modulate a plethora of physiological activities, like sleep, appetite, and hormone production, affecting metabolism and gene expression in various tissues [1]. The suprachiasmatic nucleus (SCN) of the anterior hypothalamus plays an important role in maintaining the internal clock to control physiological activities in a regular 24 h cycle. Increasing reports have uncovered that circadian oscillators are also present in peripheral tissues, including liver, heart, kidney, and peripheral blood leukocytes [2]. More than nine core circadian clock genes control circadian oscillation through the transcriptional and translational feedback loop [1,3,4], and sustain the circadian rhythm of mammalian central and peripheral tissues [5].

Although circadian oscillation is found in several peripheral tissues of the human body, circadian regulation in the auditory system is only beginning to be understood from animal models. Earlier studies indicated that rats living in a constant dark condition showed a poor acoustic startle response [6,7]. The severity of kanamycin-mediated ototoxicity is correlated with diurnal sensitivity of rats [8]. Recently, it was reported that mice receiving noise exposure at night suffered permanent hearing loss while the same exposure during the day resulted in temporary hearing loss only [9]. Park et al. demonstrated a circadian clock in the cochlea and inferior colliculus of adult mice [10] as well as a differential phase arrangement of cellular clocks along the tonotopic axis (base to apex) of mouse cochlear explants [11]. These findings imply a possible role of circadian regulation in auditory function [12,13].

In modern society, social activities and working demands increase the chances of humans staying active at night. Changing a diurnal lifestyle to a nocturnal one prolongs wakefulness in the night and disturbs the circadian rhythm throughout the body. Circadian disruption leads to the interruption of physiological oscillation networks and ultimately escalates tissue dysfunction that increases the risk of disease development [14]. Disrupted circadian rhythm or dysregulated circadian clock genes have been correlated with the development of depression [15], diabetes [16], cancer [17], cardiovascular diseases [18], and degenerative neurologic disorders [19,20]. We previously revealed that alteration of circadian clock genes was present in patients with sudden sensorineural hearing loss [21]. In addition to the irregular circadian lifestyle in modern humans, excess sound in workplaces and entertainment also increases the risk of noise overexposure, which makes noise-induced hearing loss one of the most common causes of acquired hearing loss today [22]. Since people with a lifestyle of irregular circadian rhythms (such as factory shift workers and musicians in clubs) are frequently also populations with excessive exposure to noise, it would be interesting to investigate if circadian dysregulation could impair cochlear function or affect the consequences of noise exposure.

This study aimed to utilize male CBA/CaJ mice in constant light (LL) or constant dark (DD) conditions to dysregulate the circadian clock in the cochlea. We then investigated the impact of circadian dysregulation on auditory thresholds and cochlea after low- or high-intensity noise exposure.

2. Results

2.1. Circadian Oscillation Was Present in the Cochlea

We first characterized circadian oscillation profiles in the cochlea of mice living in a normal light–dark (LD) cycle (12 h/12 h LD cycle with the light intensity kept at about 270–320 lux (lm/m^2) during light-on and darkness during light-off). Cochlear mRNA expression of circadian clock genes was analyzed at six different ZTs (zeitgeber times) every 4 h. Circadian expression of *Per1*, *Per2*, and *Rev-erbα* were present through the study, whereas *Bmal1* and *Clock* expression was changed in antiphase circadian fashion (Figure 1 and Table 1, LD group). In the cochlea, the localization of PER2 was mainly observed in the organ of Corti, with strong PER2 immunofluorescence at zeitgeber time 12 (ZT12) and weak immunoreaction at ZT4 (Supplementary Figure S1). These findings confirmed the presence of circadian oscillation in the cochlea.

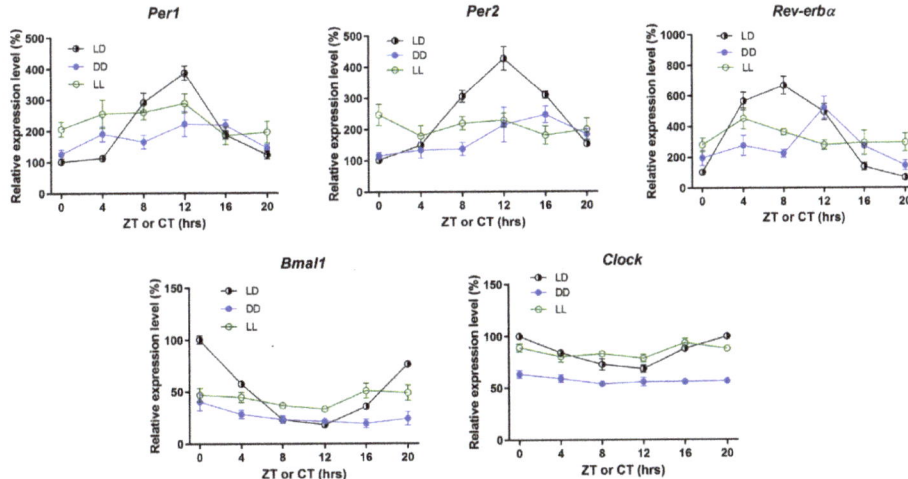

Figure 1. Relative transcript profiles of circadian clock genes in the cochlea at 6 zeitgeber times (ZTs) in the LD (light–dark), and at 6 circadian times (CTs) in constant dark (DD) and constant light (LL) groups. Each value represents the percentage change relative to ZT0 of the LD group, which was normalized to 100%. Data are mean ± SEM. n = 8–10 for each time point in each condition.

Table 1. p-value of F test to detect the circadian rhythmicity of mRNA transcripts of circadian clock genes in the cochlea by CircWave software.

	LD Group	DD Group	LL Group
Per1	0.000012	0.023638	ns
Per2	<0.000001	0.001643	ns
Rev-erbα	<0.000001	0.008508	ns
Bmal1	0.000035	ns	ns
Clock	<0.000001	ns	ns

$p < 0.05$ indicates circadian rhythmicity, ns (not significant) means loss of circadian rhythm.

2.2. LL Dysregulated Cochlear Circadian Oscillation

To evaluate whether constant light (LL) or constant dark (DD) could affect the circadian rhythm in the cochlea, we checked the circadian clock genes' mRNA transcripts in the cochlea of mice under LL or DD condition for 4 weeks (Figure 1). In the DD group, loss of circadian rhythm was evident in *Bmal1* and *Clock*, whereas circadian oscillations were still present in *Per1*, *Per2*, and *Rev-erbα*. In contrast, the circadian expression of *Per1*, *Per2*, *Rev-erbα*, *Bmal1*, and *Clock* were all dampened under the LL condition (Table 1). These results showed that LL disrupted circadian oscillation more in the cochlea. Therefore, LL was used as the model for succeeding experiments to test the impact of circadian dysregulation on the cochlear physiology and the effects of noise exposure.

2.3. LL Did Not Affect Baseline Auditory Thresholds and Neural Response Amplitudes

We examined if LL condition affected auditory thresholds of mice, which were detected by auditory brainstem responses (ABRs). In normal CBA/CaJ mice, the baseline auditory thresholds were less than 25 dB SPL. Mean ABR thresholds after the 4-week LL were around 20 dB SPL, which were not significantly different from the LD group at 8, 16 and 32 kHz (Figure 2a). Likewise, wave I amplitudes, which reflected neural responses of the auditory nerve, were similar at sound intensities of 40 to 80 dB stimulus between LD and LL groups (Figure 2b). The results suggest that LL for 4 weeks did not affect baseline cochlear thresholds and auditory nerve activity.

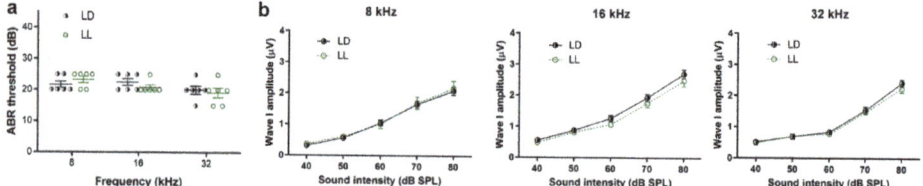

Figure 2. The ABR (auditory brainstem response) thresholds and wave I amplitudes in the LD and LL groups. (**a**). The ABR thresholds in the LD and LL groups. (**b**). Wave I amplitudes at sound intensities of 40 to 80 dB in the LD and LL groups at 8, 16, and 32 kHz. There were no significant differences in ABR thresholds and wave I amplitudes between the LD and LL groups. Data are mean ± SEM (n = 6 for each group).

2.4. LL Did Not Affect Low-Intensity Noise-Induced Temporary Threshold Shift (TTS) and ABR Wave I Amplitudes Changes

To investigate whether LL affected the auditory thresholds during noise-induced hearing loss, we used two models, low-intensity noise (92 dB) or high-intensity noise (106 dB), to induce temporary or permanent threshold shift in CBA/CaJ mice respectively [23] (Figure 3). Animals exposed to no noise were designated in the sham group. In the LD group, 92 dB noise resulted in threshold shifts at 3 h after noise exposure and returned to baseline 3 weeks later, which represented TTS (temporary threshold shift) (Figure 4a). Likewise, exposure to 92 dB noise in the LL group also caused similar threshold shifts initially, and finally returned to baseline thresholds. These results indicated that low-intensity noise in both the LD and LL group caused TTS only.

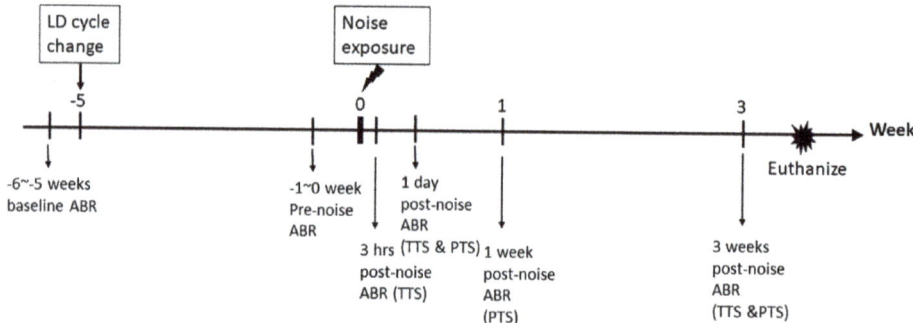

Figure 3. Timeline of experiments for testing the auditory brainstem response (ABR). The ABRs were tested before normal light–dark cycle change, and before noise exposure. Post-noise ABRs were tested at 3 h, 1 day, and 3 weeks after noise exposure in the TTS (temporary threshold shift) experiments, and at 1 day, 1 week, and 3 weeks after noise exposure in the PTS (permanent threshold shift) experiments.

Since decreased ABR wave I amplitudes and loss of synaptic ribbons (cochlear synaptopathy) persist for several weeks at high frequency after low-intensity noise even while ABR has recovered [24], we measured ABR wave I amplitudes over 32 kHz at 3 h, 1 week and 3 weeks after 92 dB noise exposure. Wave I amplitudes decreased significantly at 32 kHz by 3 h after noise exposure and recovered to about 60% 3 weeks later both in the LD and LL groups, while the differences between the two groups were not significant (Figure 4b). The densities of synaptic ribbons per IHC (inner hair cell) were decreased in the noise groups at three weeks after 92 dB noise over 16, 22.6, and 32 kHz, while synaptic ribbon counts were similar in LL and LD groups without significant difference (p = 0.315) (Figure 4c). These results suggested that LL did not affect low-intensity noise-induced synaptopathy.

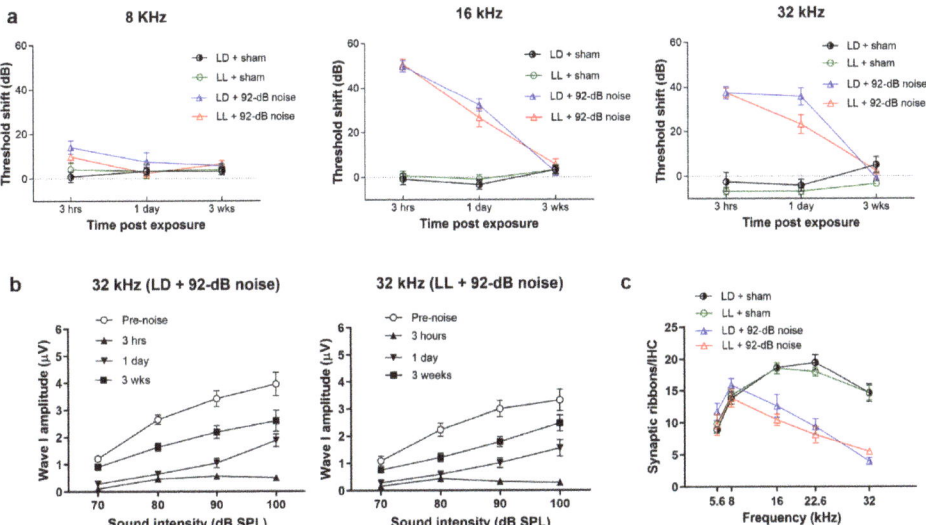

Figure 4. The ABR threshold shifts, wave I amplitudes, and synaptic ribbon counts in the LD and LL groups after 92 dB noise exposure. (**a**) No significant differences in the threshold shifts were observed between the LD and LL groups at 8, 16, and 32 kHz after the 92 dB noise exposure. Data are mean ± SEM ($n = 6$ for each group). (**b**) ABR wave I amplitudes at 32 kHz were mostly attenuated at 3 h after the 92 dB noise exposure and increased later both in the LD and LL groups. There were no differences in wave I amplitudes between LD + 92 dB and LL + 92 dB groups. (**c**) A decreased number of synaptic ribbons were found over 16, 22.6, and 32 kHz at 3 weeks after the 92 dB noise. No significant difference in synaptic ribbon counts was observed between the LD and LL groups postexposure. Data are mean ± SEM ($n = 5$ for each group).

2.5. LL Augmented High-Intensity Noise-Induced Permanent Threshold Shift (PTS) and Outer Hair Cell (OHC) Loss

We next investigated whether LL affected ABR thresholds shift after high-intensity (106 dB) noise exposure. In contrast to the sham groups, threshold shifts in 106 dB noise groups persisted for up to 3 weeks at all tested frequencies of 8, 16, and 32 kHz, which showed PTS (permanent threshold shift) (Figure 5a). Compared to the LD group, the LL group had significantly higher threshold shifts over 8 kHz ($p < 0.001$), 16 kHz ($p < 0.001$), and 32 kHz ($p < 0.001$) at one day after 106 dB noise exposure. The significantly increased thresholds shift in the LL group persisted up to 3 weeks after exposure over 32 kHz ($p = 0.005$). These results revealed that LL augmented high-intensity noise-induced PTS, particularly over high frequency.

Loss of OHCs (outer hair cells) is one of the major cochlear pathologies in permanent noise-induced hearing loss [23]. We therefore checked OHCs at 3 weeks after a 106 dB exposure in cochlear surface preparations. OHC loss was present in a base-to-apex progression in the noise-exposed groups. LL resulted in significant increases in OHC death over basal segment at 4 mm ($p = 0.02$) and 4.75 mm ($p = 0.046$) from the apex (Figure 5b,c). We further investigated the OHC function at 16 kHz, the region without OHC loss (about 2.83 mm from the apex) by distortion product otoacoustic emissions (DPOAEs). DPOAE 2F1-F2 emission amplitudes were significantly different between the four groups in the 16 kHz-region ($p < 0.001$), while post-hoc test revealed that noise exposure significantly reduced DPOAE amplitudes in the LL group ($p = 0.02$) (Figure 5d). These results demonstrate that LL renders OHC vulnerable to high-intensity noise.

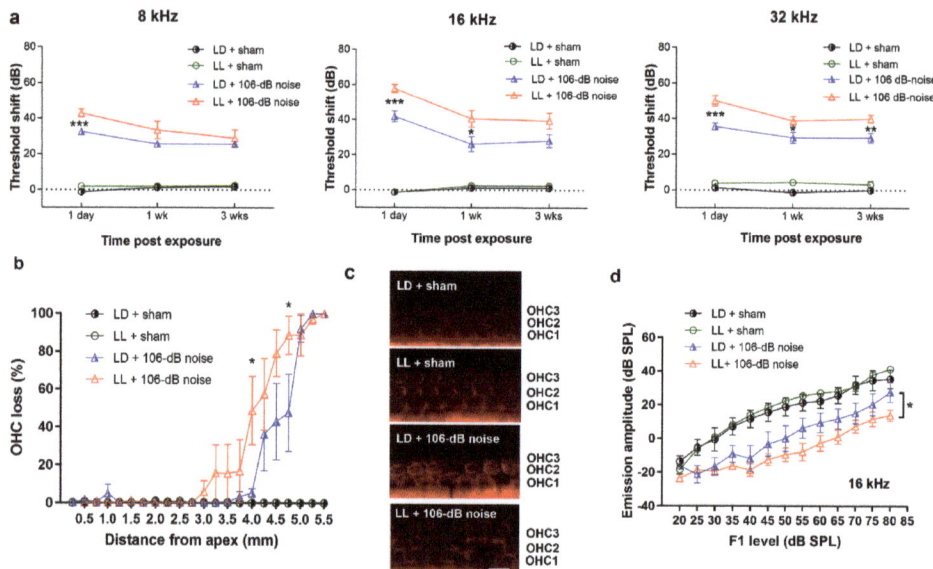

Figure 5. The ABR threshold shifts, OHC (outer hair cell) counts, and DPOAE 2F1-F2 amplitudes in the LD and LL groups after 106 dB noise exposure. (**a**) Significantly higher threshold shifts in the LL group were found over 8 kHz at 1 day postexposure, over 16 kHz at 1 day and 1 week postexposure, and over 32 kHz at 1 day, 1 week, and 3 weeks postexposure. Data are mean ± SEM (n = 8–9 for each group). * $p < 0.05$, ** $p < 0.01$, *** $p < 0.001$ for LD + 106 dB noise vs. LL + 106 dB noise. (**b**) The LL group showed a higher percentage of outer hair cell (OHC) loss in the basal segment than the LD group after exposure to the 106 dB noise. Data are mean ± SEM (LD + sham, n = 7; LL + sham, n = 6; LD + 106 dB noise, n = 5; LL+ 106 dB noise, n = 6). * $p < 0.05$ for LD + 106 dB noise vs. LL + 106 dB noise. (**c**). Representative images of OHCs in the basal segment (about 4 mm from apex) after different treatments. OHC 1, 2, and 3 indicate three rows of OHCs. Scale bar = 10 μm (**d**) DPOAE 2F1-F2 amplitudes were decreased in the LL group after exposure to the 106 dB noise at 16 kHz. Data are mean ± SEM. * $p < 0.05$ for LL + 106 dB noise vs. LD + 106 dB.

2.6. LL Increased High-Intensity Noise-Induced Reduction of Synaptic Ribbons

Since cochlear synaptopathy can also occur after high-intensity noise exposure [25], we further checked the synaptic ribbons over inner hair cells (IHCs) at 3 weeks after exposure. High-intensity noise significantly reduced synaptic ribbons at 16 kHz ($p < 0.001$), 22.6 kHz ($p < 0.001$), and 32 kHz ($p < 0.001$) regions (Figure 6a). Further analysis showed that noise exposure significantly reduced the synaptic ribbon in the LD group at 32 kHz ($p = 0.005$) and LL group at 16 ($p = 0.003$), 22.6 ($p = 0.001$) and 32 kHz ($p < 0.001$). LL increased more high-intensity noise-induced reduction of synaptic ribbons, particularly over 22.6 kHz ($p = 0.04$) (Figure 6a,b). This result suggested that LL augmented cochlear synaptopathy by high-intensity noise.

2.7. LL Increased High-Intensity Noise-Induced 4-Hydroxynonenal (4-HNE) in OHCs

The markers of oxidative stress, such as 4-HNE (the product of lipid oxidation), increase in OHCs after high-intensity noise exposure [23,26]. So, we further evaluated the 4-HNE levels in the OHCs at 1 h after 106 dB noise in cochlear surface preparations (Figure 7a). Immunoreactivity for 4-HNE was significantly different between the four groups in OHCs ($p < 0.001$). Post-hoc quantification analysis of 4-HNE immunolabeling revealed that 106 dB noise significantly increased 4-HNE in the LD ($p = 0.02$) and LL ($p < 0.001$) groups, while a significantly stronger immunoreactivity for 4-HNE was observed in the LL group compared to the LD group after noise exposure ($p = 0.02$) (Figure 7b). These results suggest that high-intensity noise augmented more oxidative stress in OHCs of the LL mice.

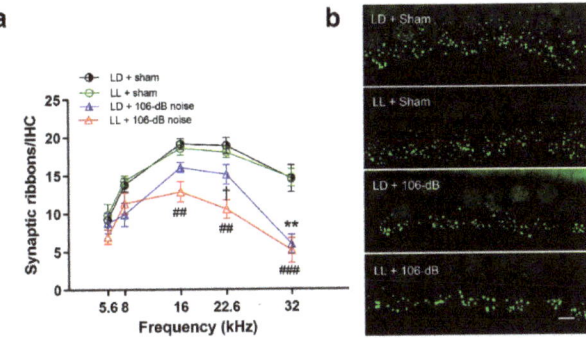

Figure 6. Synaptic ribbon counts in the LD and LL groups after 106 dB noise exposure. (**a**) The number of synaptic ribbons decreased significantly in the LD group at 32 kHz and the LL group at 16, 22.6, and 32 kHz after 106 dB noise exposure, while the significant difference between LD and LL groups was observed at 22.6 kHz. Data are mean ± SEM (n = 5–6 for each group). ** $p < 0.01$ for LD + 106 dB noise vs. LD + sham, ## $p < 0.01$, ### $p < 0.001$ for LL + 106 dB noise vs. LL + sham, † $p < 0.05$ for LD + 106 dB noise vs. LL + 106 dB noise. (**b**) Representative images of synaptic ribbons stained by CTBP2 (green dots) over the 22.6 kHz region. Scale bar = 5 µm.

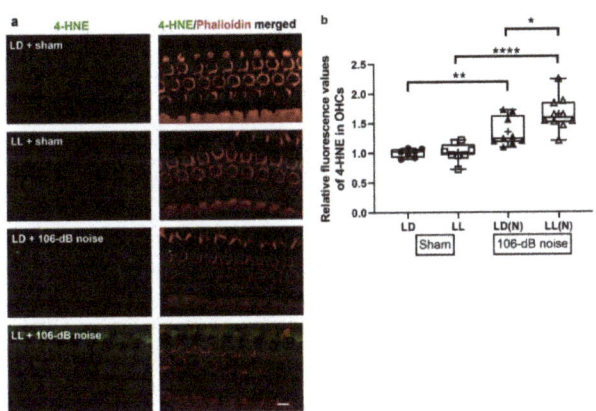

Figure 7. 4-HNE immunolabeling in cochlear surface preparations. (**a**) Representative images of immunoreactivity for 4-HNE in different treatments. Scale bar = 5 µm. (**b**) Quantification of 4-HNE fluorescence in OHCs revealed significantly increased 4-HNE in LD and LL groups after 106 dB noise exposure, while stronger immunolabeling for 4-HNE was observed in the LL(N) group compared to the LD(N) group. Boxplots indicate median and interquartile. + indicates mean value. * $p < 0.05$, ** $p < 0.01$, **** $p < 0.0001$.

3. Discussion

In agreement with the groundbreaking studies of Canlon and colleagues [9], we demonstrated the oscillated expression of circadian clock genes in the cochlea of CBA/CaJ mice. We further showed that cochlear circadian dysregulation by LL is detrimental to the inner ear, causing greater damage of hair cells and synaptic ribbons during high-intensity noise exposure. The effects were most predominant over the higher frequency region of the cochlea, the region mainly affected in noise-induced hearing loss. Our results clarify that the dysregulation of the cochlear circadian clock can influence auditory function and sensitivity of the inner ear during acoustic trauma.

Light is the most important zeitgeber and central modulator for circadian clocks [27]. The manipulation of environmental light has frequently been used to test the effect of circadian disruption on the physiology and behavior of animals [28–30] and prolonged exposure to LL or DD is one of the common models [30–35]. We demonstrate here that exposure of mice to LL resulted in the loss of rhythms in five cochlear circadian clock genes, which is in line with previous studies showing a dampened amplitude of circadian clock gene expression under LL condition in the SCN [36] and peripheral clocks [35].

Change of the LD cycle also impacts the complexity of neurons and behavior in mice [29,37]. Therefore, we tested the cochlear physiology and pathophysiology of mice undergoing circadian dysregulation by prolonged exposure to LL. There were no significant differences in ABR thresholds or neural response amplitudes between LL and LD groups. Even with the severe dampening of cochlear circadian rhythm by LL, the cochlear physiology seems normal. If any alterations of neurotransmitter signaling [38] or desynchronization of neuronal population [37] occur after LL, they are not sufficient to affect threshold sensitivity.

In view of the diurnal sensitivity to noise trauma [9], we further hypothesized that circadian dysregulation by LL may affect the recovery of cochlear threshold shifts in mice following noise exposure. Surprisingly, the ABR thresholds in the LL group completely recovered to pre-exposure levels at three weeks after a low-intensity noise exposure. Moreover, acute cochlear nerve denervation in the LL group, demonstrated by the reduction of suprathreshold wave I amplitude [24], recovered to a similar extent three weeks later in the LD group, suggesting similar decrements of synaptic ribbons in both groups. In contrast, LL augmented high-intensity noise-induced PTS, which is characterized by the death of cochlear sensory cells. These results suggested that circadian dysregulation has different impacts on the pathologic processes underlying temporary and permanent threshold shift [39,40].

As a consequence, the link of LL-induced circadian dysregulation to hair cell pathology in PTS may be explained by the featured molecular oscillators in the neurosensory damage after high-intensity noise. A well-documented hypothesis of traumatic permanent noise-induced hearing loss is oxidative stress in OHCs, characterized by excess reactive oxygen species (ROS) production induced by intense noise exposure [26,41] overwhelming the intrinsic antioxidant defense system. Previous literature has demonstrated the rhythmicity of the cellular antioxidant system, including superoxide dismutase, peroxiredoxin, and glutathione [42,43], which are also important defense systems in hair cells in response to acoustic insults [44,45]. In the cochlea, we observed that PER2 protein was most expressed in the organ of Corti (Supplementary Figure S1a), so the presence of circadian PER2 and antioxidant oscillation in OHCs is possible. Additionally, LL decreased amplitudes of cochlear circadian clock gene mRNA expression and increased 4-HNE in OHCs in response to noise, which is in line with a previous publication showing that LL influences the circadian oscillation of antioxidants [46] and induces oxidative stress [47]. Although the detailed mechanisms need to be investigated further, it is likely that LL attenuated the amplitude of antioxidant oscillation in OHCs, which resulted in increased noise vulnerability. The circadian effects of LL condition on all the longitudinal regions of cochlear sensory epithelium can be revealed by the elevated ABR threshold shifts at one day after 106 dB noise exposure at 8 k, 16 k, and 32 kHz (Figure 5a). However, because the basal OHCs have lower levels of antioxidants and are more vulnerable to ROS damage [48,49], the increased thresholds shifts were more salient in the high frequency at 3 weeks after noise.

Another possibility of circadian perturbation on acoustic trauma is the dysregulation of inflammatory responses [50,51]. Impaired circadian rhythm has been linked to pathological responses that are associated with the development of inflammatory and metabolic diseases [30,52]. In response to noise, a large influx of inflammation cells can be observed in the cochlea [53], causing upregulation of cochlear innate immunity [54] and proinflammatory molecules [55,56]. Since the chronic circadian disruption exaggerates the immune and inflammatory responses to external stimuli [57,58], it is reasonable to speculate that the dysregulation of the cochlear circadian clock may also increase the vulnerability of the cochlea to environmental stressors, such as noise. Particularly, glucocorticoids are well-known oscillators and are important in the modulation of auditory sensitivity to acoustic trauma [59,60]. LL affects the circadian rhythm of the hypothalamic–pituitary–adrenal (HPA) axis [61] and reduces the circadian amplitude of circulating corticosterone levels in C57BL/6J and Swiss Webster mice [34,57,62]. This may link the detrimental effect of LL in our study to increased noise-induced OHC loss, while glucocorticoids were thought as protective against acoustic trauma [60,63]. Of note, the LL-induced circadian plasma corticosterone change seems to vary among strains and animals [64], and the circadian effects of glucocorticoids and the receptors in CBA/CaJ mice are still unknown. Future investigation of the impact of circadian dysregulation on the molecular levels of proinflammatory cytokines and glucocorticoid receptors in the cochlea of CBA/CaJ mice after noise exposure will be helpful for our understanding of underlying mechanisms.

The results of our study could have important clinical implications. Physicians generally educate their patients to adjust their lifestyle to a regular sleep pattern. However, the habit of "to rise with the lark and go to bed with the lamb" is not easy in modern society since too many artificial illuminations from different sources, such as LED lamps and mobile devices (for example, cellphones and tablets), have deeply disrupted the circadian rhythm of the human body. Prolonged work hours throughout the evening, not uncommon in modern society, add to exposure to artificial light that can aggravate circadian disruption. Fortunately, circadian disturbance by LL does not affect the cochlear thresholds in the physiological state or with exposure to low-intensity noise. Our results, however, raise a red flag in regards to circadian dysregulation in excessively noisy environments, be it work or leisure, and emphasizes the need for adequate hearing protection. Alternatively, a compromised circadian clock can be re-adjusted by scheduled light exposure, feeding, or exercise [35], or pharmacological interventions such as melatonin [65]. As a note of caution, we have to consider that our model used LL to dysregulate the cochlear circadian clock, similar to the prolonged light environment in, for example, an intensive care unit. The use of animal models to mimic more common circadian-dysregulated situations such as shift work and jet lag [66] will be helpful in exploring the impact of circadian dysregulation on noise-induced hearing loss.

In summary, we observed that cochlear circadian dysregulation by LL leads to elevated PTS induced by high-intensity noise. Likewise, loss of OHCs and the reduction of synaptic ribbons were larger in the circadian-dysregulated mice exposed to high-intensity noise. In contrast, the deleterious effect of LL was not seen in TTS after low-intensity noise exposure. Our results suggest the importance of the normal circadian clock in the inner ear, particularly in the environment of high-intensity noise.

4. Materials and Methods

4.1. Animals

All animal research protocols and procedures were approved by the Institutional Animal Care and Use Committee, Kaohsiung Chang Gung Memorial Hospital (IACUC Affidavit #2015091901, approved 4 November 2015 and #2017121305, approved 15 March 2018). Male CBA/CaJ mice (4 weeks of age) were procured from National Laboratory Animal Center, Taiwan. Animals were provided with water and rodent chow at libitum. They were housed in an air-conditioned vivarium with 22 ± 1 °C and 12 h/12 h light–dark cycle (lights on: 5:00 (Zeitgeber time 0, ZT0); lights off: 17:00 (ZT12)) to acclimate for 2 weeks before the experiments. During lights-on, the light intensity was kept at about 270–320 lux (lm/m^2).

4.2. Control and Alteration of the Light–Dark Cycle

Two weeks upon acclimating to the normal LD cycle, the mice were randomly divided into 3 groups. In the LD group, mice were housed in the 12 h/12 h LD cycle. In the DD group, animals were accommodated in a light-off condition. In the LL group, mice were housed in a light-on condition. The handling of mice held in the dark was performed under red light.

4.3. Noise Exposure

Three awake CBA/CaJ mice in the same group were placed in a sound chamber, with one mouse per stainless steel cage. The sound produced by a CD player (CD5001; Marantz, Kanagawa, Japan) was amplified using an amplifier (YS-150MP3; Yuan-Sin, Taiwan). The sound chamber was fitted with a loudspeaker (NSD 2005S-8; Eminence Speaker, LLC, Eminence, KY, USA). Broadband noise (BBN) with a frequency of 2 to 20 kHz was compiled onto a CD and equalized with software (CSL4400; Kay, NJ, USA). Before and after the noise exposure, sound levels were calibrated with a sound level meter (type 2250; Brüel & Kjær, Nærum, Denmark) fitted with a microphone (type 4189; Brüel & Kjær, Nærum, Denmark) at the locations of each cage within the sound chamber. For producing temporary or permanent threshold shifts, mice were exposed to 92 dB or 106 dB BBN noise for 2 h (from 8:00 am (ZT3) to 10:00 am (ZT5)). In the sham group, mice were placed in the sound chamber without noise.

4.4. Assessment of Auditory Brainstem Response (ABR) and Distortion Product Otoacoustic Emission (DPOAE)

Mice were anesthetized via an intramuscular injection of xylazine (Bayer) (10 mg/kg) and Zoletil 50 (Virbac) (25 mg/kg) and then placed on a heating pad to maintain their body temperature at around 37 °C. Acoustic stimuli were delivered monaurally to a Beyer earphone attached to a customized plastic speculum inserted in the ear canal. For the measurement of ABRs, electrodes were inserted at the subdermal vertex of the skull under the left and right ears (ground). ABRs were detected at 8, 16, and 32 kHz. Up to 1024 responses were averaged for each stimulus level. Thresholds were determined by decreasing the intensity in 10 dB increments, and then in 5 dB steps near the threshold until no responses were detected. Thresholds were estimated between the lowest stimulus level where a response was observed and the level without a response. ABR thresholds were tested before and 4 weeks after the LD cycle change in all mice (pre-noise ABR). Post-noise ABR was tested 3 h, 1 day, and 3 weeks after noise exposure in the temporary threshold shift experiment. Post-noise ABR was tested 1 day, 1 week, and 3 weeks after noise exposure in the permanent threshold shift experiment (see Figure 3). The ABR threshold shift was defined as the difference between the post- and pre-noise ABR thresholds. For the measurement of DPOAEs, the DPOAEs were generated by two simultaneous tones of frequencies F1 and F2, with F2/F1 ratio set as 1.2 and the F2 level 10 dB lower than the F1 level. The DPOAE input/output (I/O) function was plotted by the curve from the 2F1-F2 emission amplitudes at a fixed F2 frequency.

4.5. Real-Time Quantitative Polymerase Chain Reaction (qRT-PCR) Assay of mRNA Expression

Cochlear tissues were collected to assess the mRNA expression of circadian clock genes at 6 different ZTs or circadian times (CTs). Total RNA was isolated from cochlear tissues using the RNeasy Micro Kits (Qiagen, Valencia, CA, USA). Total RNA (2 μg) was reverse-transcribed to first-strand cDNA using High Capacity cDNA Reverse Transcription Kits (Applied Biosystems, Foster City, CA, USA) according to the manufacturer's protocols. cDNA was diluted (1:10) with ddH$_2$O and stored in aliquots at −20 °C. The expression of the circadian clock genes was analyzed using the TaqMan® system. All TaqMan® gene expression assays were purchased from Applied Biosystems. Expression of the mouse housekeeping gene, *Actb* (*β-actin*), was used to normalize expression of the circadian clock genes in qRT-PCR. All reactions were carried out in a 10 μL final volume containing 25 ng cDNA (as total input RNA), 0.5 μL 20× TaqMan® Gene Expression Assay, and 5 μL 2× TaqMan® Universal PCR Master Mix (Applied Biosystems). Real-time qPCR was performed on an ABI 7500 Fast Real-Time System (Applied Biosystems), and the PCR cycling parameters were set as follows: 95 °C for 10 min followed by 40 cycles of PCR reaction at 95 °C for 20 s and 60 °C for 1 min. The expressions of the circadian clock genes (*Per1*, *Per2*, *Rev-erbα*, *Bmal1*, and *Clock*) were normalized to the internal control *Actb* to obtain the relative threshold cycle (ΔCt). The relative expression levels were calculated by equalizing differences to the ΔCt of ZT0 of the LD group, so the expression level at ZT0 of the LD group equaled 100%. Each data point was the average of three technical replicates.

4.6. Surface Preparation of the Cochlear Sensory Epithelium

The temporal bones of the mice were removed immediately following euthanasia. Scala media was perfused with 4% paraformaldehyde in phosphate-buffered saline (PBS) and fixed at 4 °C overnight. The cochleae were rinsed in PBS and decalcified in 0.12 M sodium ethylenediaminetetraacetic acid (EDTA), which was changed daily for 2 days. Then the cochleae were further dissected by removing the softened otic capsule, stria vascularis, Reissner's membrane, and tectorial membrane.

4.7. Immunocytochemistry for Outer Hair Cell (OHC) Counts

Upon incubating in 3% Triton X-100 in PBS for 30 min and washing 3 times with PBS, the specimens were incubated in rhodamine-phalloidin (1:100; Invitrogen, Carlsbad, CA, USA) for 60 min and followed by PBS rinses. The sections were mounted on glass slides with PermaFluor™ Mountant (Thermo Fisher Scientific, Pittsburgh, PA, USA). Cell populations in the phalloidin-stained stereociliary bundles and circumferential F-actin rings around the cuticular plate of the OHCs were evaluated using an epifluorescence microscope with a 40× oil immersion objective lens. The right objective had a 0.17 mm calibrated scale imposed on the field for reference, and all three rows of OHCs were oriented longitudinally within each 0.17 mm frame. Each successive 0.17 mm field was evaluated beginning from the apex to the base for counting the number of OHCs. Cell counts were entered into a computer program (KHRI Cytocochleogram, version 3.0.7; Kresge Hearing Research Institute, University of Michigan, Ann Arbor, MI, USA) to calculate the percentage of OHC loss from the apical turn to the basal turn of the basal epithelium.

4.8. Immunocytochemistry for Synaptic Ribbon Counts and 4-Hydroxynonenal (4-HNE)

After blocking with 10% donkey anti-mouse serum (Abcam, Cambridge, UK) for 30 min at room temperature (22–24 °C), the basilar membrane was immunostained with primary mouse anti-C-terminal binding protein 2 (CTBP2) IgG1 monoclonal antibody at 1:200 dilution (BD Biosciences, San Diego, CA, USA) or primary rabbit anti-4-HNE polyclonal antibody at 1:50 dilution (Abcam, Inc., Cambridge, MA, USA), and incubated at 37 °C overnight or 4 °C for 72 h, which was co-labeled with donkey anti-mouse AlexaFluor 488-conjugated secondary antibody (Abcam) at 1:1000 dilution at 37 °C for 1 h in the dark. After washing three times with PBS, the tissues were incubated with rhodamine-phalloidin at 1:100 (Invitrogen) at room temperature for 60 min to visualize the structure. CTBP2 or 4-HNE immunostaining was observed by laser confocal microscopy (FV10i; Olympus, Tokyo, Japan) with a 60× magnification lens. For synaptic ribbon counts, regions of interest along the cochlear spiral at 5.6, 8, 16, 22.6, and 32 kHz were examined. The z-stack images were analyzed using the Image J software (NIH, Bethesda, MD, USA) "cell counter" plugin and the mean number of puncta per inner hair cell (IHC) base in the region of interest were counted. For quantification of immunolabeled 4-HNE signals, the immunostaining over each OHC in the basal segment of cochlea was measured. The background fluorescence intensity was subtracted and the average fluorescence of about 60 OHCs was calculated. The relative fluorescence was then quantified by normalizing the ratio of average fluorescence of OHCs in each condition to the LD (sham) group.

4.9. Immunohistochemistry for Cryosections

After the decalcification with 4% EDTA, cochleae were transferred to 30% sucrose and incubated overnight. The cochleae were embedded with OCT for sectioning. Sections of 7 μm thickness were permeabilized with 3% Triton X-100 in PBS for 30 min, washed 3 times with PBS and blocked with 10% donkey anti-mouse serum for 30 min at room temperature. The sections were then immunostained with primary rabbit anti-PER2 IgG1 polyclonal antibody at 1:100 (PER21-A, Alpha Diagnostic, San Antonio, TX, USA), and incubated at 4 °C overnight, which was co-labeled with donkey anti-mouse AlexaFluor 488-conjugated secondary antibody (Abcam) 1:1000 at 37 °C for 1 h in the dark. After washing 3 times with PBS, specimens were incubated with rhodamine-phalloidin (Invitrogen) at 1:100 and

DAPI (Invitrogen) at 1:1000 at room temperature for 60 min to visualize the structure. The cryosections were then observed by laser confocal microscopy.

4.10. Statistical Analysis

GraphPad Prism 8.0 (GraphPad Software, La Jolla, CA, USA) was used for all the statistical analyses. One-way analysis of variance (ANOVA), two-way ANOVA, Tukey's multiple comparisons, and unpaired *t*-tests were utilized to analyze the difference among groups. All tests were two-tailed, and a *p*-value < 0.05 was considered significant. CircWave 1.4 software (www.euclock.org) was used to calculate the waveform and to analyze the circadian rhythmicity of circadian clock gene expression in the LD, LL, and DD groups, using forward linear harmonic regression (F test). CircWave software fits one or more fundamental sinusoidal curves through the individual data points and compares this with a horizontal line through the data mean (a constant). If the fitted circadian clock gene expression pattern follows a sinusoidal curve and differs significantly from the horizontal line, it is considered circadian rhythmic (*p*-value < 0.05).

Supplementary Materials: The following are available online at http://www.mdpi.com/1422-0067/21/20/7535/s1, Figure S1. Representative images of PER2 immunostaining in the cochlea and organ of Corti under normal LD cycle.

Author Contributions: C.-H.Y., hypothesized, designed, carried out the experiments, analyzed the data, and wrote the manuscript. C.-F.H. and M.-Y.Y., planed the experiments, analyzed the data and interpretation. J.-H.C. supervised the study and corrected the manuscript. W.-S.L., F.-S.W. and E.I.H. participated in the result discussion and technical support. All authors have read and agreed to the published version of the manuscript.

Funding: This study was supported by grants from the Ministry of Science and Technology of Taiwan (MOST 107-2314-B-182A-083- & MOST 109-2314-B-182A-016) and Chang Gung Memorial Hospital (CMRPG8E1481, CMRPG8E1482, CMRPG8E1483 & CMRPG8G1101).

Acknowledgments: The authors thank Jochen Schacht for valuable comments and suggestions on the manuscript. We also thank Guoqiang Wan and Ting-Hua Yang for the suggestions about ABR and DPOAE tests. We thank Hsiao-Chuan Chen who provided the broadband noise. We appreciate the molecular imaging core of the Institute for Translational Research in Biomedicine, Kaohsiung Chang Gung Memorial Hospital, Kaohsiung, Taiwan for technical and facility supports on confocal microscope and the Biostatistics Center, Kaohsiung Chang Gung Memorial Hospital for the assistance of statistics work.

Conflicts of Interest: The authors declare no conflict of interest. The funders had no role in the design of the study; in the collection, analyses, or interpretation of data; in the writing of the manuscript, or in the decision to publish the results.

Abbreviations

LD	light/dark
LL	constant light
DD	constant dark
ZT	Zeitgeber time
CT	circadian time
ABR	auditory brainstem response
DPOAE	distortion product otoacoustic emission
TTS	temporary threshold shift
PTS	permanent threshold shift
OHC	outer hair cell
IHC	inner hair cell
SCN	suprachiasmatic nucleus
BBN	broadband noise
qRT-PCR	real-time quantitative polymerase chain reaction
4-HNE	4-hydroxynonenal

References

1. Young, M.W.; Kay, S.A. Time zones: A comparative genetics of circadian clocks. *Nat. Rev. Genet.* **2001**, *2*, 702–715. [CrossRef]
2. Buijs, R.M.; Kalsbeek, A. Hypothalamic integration of central and peripheral clocks. *Nat. Rev. Neurosci.* **2001**, *2*, 521–526. [CrossRef] [PubMed]
3. Balsalobre, A. Clock genes in mammalian peripheral tissues. *Cell Tissue Res.* **2002**, *309*, 193–199. [CrossRef] [PubMed]
4. Ko, C.H.; Takahashi, J.S. Molecular components of the mammalian circadian clock. *Hum. Mol. Genet.* **2006**, *15*, R271–R277. [CrossRef] [PubMed]
5. Zhang, R.; Lahens, N.F.; Ballance, H.I.; Hughes, M.E.; Hogenesch, J.B. A circadian gene expression atlas in mammals: Implications for biology and medicine. *Proc. Natl. Acad. Sci. USA* **2014**, *111*, 16219–16224. [CrossRef] [PubMed]
6. Chabot, C.C.; Taylor, D.H. Circadian modulation of the rat acoustic startle response. *Behav. Neurosci.* **1992**, *106*, 846–852. [CrossRef] [PubMed]
7. Frankland, P.W.; Ralph, M.R. Circadian modulation in the rat acoustic startle circuit. *Behav. Neurosci.* **1995**, *109*, 43–48. [CrossRef]
8. Yonovitz, A.; Fisch, J.E. Circadian rhythm dependent kanamycin-induced hearing loss in rodents assessed by auditory brainstem responses. *Acta Otolaryngol.* **1991**, *111*, 1006–1012. [CrossRef]
9. Meltser, I.; Cederroth, C.R.; Basinou, V.; Savelyev, S.; Lundkvist, G.S.; Canlon, B. TrkB-mediated protection against circadian sensitivity to noise trauma in the murine cochlea. *Curr. Biol.* **2014**, *24*, 658–663. [CrossRef]
10. Park, J.S.; Cederroth, C.R.; Basinou, V.; Meltser, I.; Lundkvist, G.; Canlon, B. Identification of a Circadian Clock in the Inferior Colliculus and Its Dysregulation by Noise Exposure. *J. Neurosci.* **2016**, *36*, 5509–5519. [CrossRef]
11. Park, J.S.; Cederroth, C.R.; Basinou, V.; Sweetapple, L.; Buijink, R.; Lundkvist, G.B.; Michel, S.; Canlon, B. Differential Phase Arrangement of Cellular Clocks along the Tonotopic Axis of the Mouse Cochlea Ex Vivo. *Curr. Biol.* **2017**, *27*, 2623–2629. [CrossRef] [PubMed]
12. Loudon, A.S. Hearing damage and deafness: A role for the circadian clock. *Curr. Biol.* **2014**, *24*, R232–R234. [CrossRef]
13. Basinou, V.; Park, J.S.; Cederroth, C.R.; Canlon, B. Circadian regulation of auditory function. *Hear. Res.* **2017**, *347*, 47–55. [CrossRef]
14. Smolensky, M.H.; Hermida, R.C.; Reinberg, A.; Sackett-Lundeen, L.; Portaluppi, F. Circadian disruption: New clinical perspective of disease pathology and basis for chronotherapeutic intervention. *Chronobiol. Int.* **2016**, *33*, 1101–1119. [CrossRef] [PubMed]
15. Turek, F.W. From circadian rhythms to clock genes in depression. *Int. Clin. Psychopharmacol.* **2007**, *22*, S1–S8. [CrossRef] [PubMed]
16. Marcheva, B.; Ramsey, K.M.; Buhr, E.D.; Kobayashi, Y.; Su, H.; Ko, C.H.; Ivanova, G.; Omura, C.; Mo, S.; Vitaterna, M.H.; et al. Disruption of the clock components CLOCK and BMAL1 leads to hypoinsulinaemia and diabetes. *Nature* **2010**, *466*, 627–631. [CrossRef] [PubMed]
17. Hsu, C.M.; Lin, S.F.; Lu, C.T.; Lin, P.M.; Yang, M.Y. Altered expression of circadian clock genes in head and neck squamous cell carcinoma. *Tumour Biol.* **2012**, *33*, 149–155. [CrossRef] [PubMed]
18. Portaluppi, F.; Tiseo, R.; Smolensky, M.H.; Hermida, R.C.; Ayala, D.E.; Fabbian, F. Circadian rhythms and cardiovascular health. *Sleep Med. Rev.* **2012**, *16*, 151–166. [CrossRef]
19. Wulff, K.; Gatti, S.; Wettstein, J.G.; Foster, R.G. Sleep and circadian rhythm disruption in psychiatric and neurodegenerative disease. *Nat. Rev. Neurosci.* **2010**, *11*, 589–599. [CrossRef]
20. Logan, R.W.; McClung, C.A. Rhythms of life: Circadian disruption and brain disorders across the lifespan. *Nat. Rev. Neurosci.* **2019**, *20*, 49–65. [CrossRef]
21. Yang, C.H.; Hwang, C.F.; Lin, P.M.; Chuang, J.H.; Hsu, C.M.; Lin, S.F.; Yang, M.Y. Sleep Disturbance and Altered Expression of Circadian Clock Genes in Patients with Sudden Sensorineural Hearing Loss. *Medicine* **2015**, *94*, e978. [CrossRef] [PubMed]
22. Yang, C.H.; Schrepfer, T.; Schacht, J. Age-related hearing impairment and the triad of acquired hearing loss. *Front. Cell. Neurosci.* **2015**, *9*, 276. [CrossRef] [PubMed]

23. Yuan, H.; Wang, X.; Hill, K.; Chen, J.; Lemasters, J.; Yang, S.M.; Sha, S.H. Autophagy attenuates noise-induced hearing loss by reducing oxidative stress. *Antioxid. Redox Signal.* **2015**, *22*, 1308–1324. [CrossRef] [PubMed]
24. Kujawa, S.G.; Liberman, M.C. Adding insult to injury: Cochlear nerve degeneration after "temporary" noise-induced hearing loss. *J. Neurosci.* **2009**, *29*, 14077–14085. [CrossRef]
25. Hill, K.; Yuan, H.; Wang, X.; Sha, S.H. Noise-Induced Loss of Hair Cells and Cochlear Synaptopathy Are Mediated by the Activation of AMPK. *J. Neurosci.* **2016**, *36*, 7497–7510. [CrossRef]
26. Yamashita, D.; Jiang, H.Y.; Schacht, J.; Miller, J.M. Delayed production of free radicals following noise exposure. *Brain Res.* **2004**, *1019*, 201–209. [CrossRef]
27. LeGates, T.A.; Fernandez, D.C.; Hattar, S. Light as a central modulator of circadian rhythms, sleep and affect. *Nat. Rev. Neurosci.* **2014**, *15*, 443–454. [CrossRef]
28. Yan, L. Expression of clock genes in the suprachiasmatic nucleus: Effect of environmental lighting conditions. *Rev. Endocr. Metab. Disord.* **2009**, *10*, 301–310. [CrossRef]
29. Karatsoreos, I.N.; Bhagat, S.; Bloss, E.B.; Morrison, J.H.; McEwen, B.S. Disruption of circadian clocks has ramifications for metabolism, brain, and behavior. *Proc. Natl. Acad. Sci. USA* **2011**, *108*, 1657–1662. [CrossRef]
30. Hand, L.E.; Hopwood, T.W.; Dickson, S.H.; Walker, A.L.; Loudon, A.S.; Ray, D.W.; Bechtold, D.A.; Gibbs, J.E. The circadian clock regulates inflammatory arthritis. *FASEB J.* **2016**, *30*, 3759–3770. [CrossRef]
31. Ebling, F.J.; Lincoln, G.A.; Wollnik, F.; Anderson, N. Effects of constant darkness and constant light on circadian organization and reproductive responses in the ram. *J. Biol. Rhythms* **1988**, *3*, 365–384. [CrossRef] [PubMed]
32. Chen, R.; Seo, D.O.; Bell, E.; von Gall, C.; Lee, C. Strong resetting of the mammalian clock by constant light followed by constant darkness. *J. Neurosci.* **2008**, *28*, 11839–11847. [CrossRef] [PubMed]
33. Chabot, C.C.; Connolly, D.M.; Waring, B.B. The effects of lighting conditions and food restriction paradigms on locomotor activity of common spiny mice, Acomys cahirinus. *J. Circadian Rhythms* **2012**, *10*, 6. [CrossRef] [PubMed]
34. Coomans, C.P.; van den Berg, S.A.; Houben, T.; van Klinken, J.B.; van den Berg, R.; Pronk, A.C.; Havekes, L.M.; Romijn, J.A.; van Dijk, K.W.; Biermasz, N.R.; et al. Detrimental effects of constant light exposure and high-fat diet on circadian energy metabolism and insulin sensitivity. *FASEB J.* **2013**, *27*, 1721–1732. [CrossRef]
35. Hamaguchi, Y.; Tahara, Y.; Hitosugi, M.; Shibata, S. Impairment of Circadian Rhythms in Peripheral Clocks by Constant Light Is Partially Reversed by Scheduled Feeding or Exercise. *J. Biol. Rhythms* **2015**, *30*, 533–542. [CrossRef]
36. Sudo, M.; Sasahara, K.; Moriya, T.; Akiyama, M.; Hamada, T.; Shibata, S. Constant light housing attenuates circadian rhythms of mPer2 mRNA and mPER2 protein expression in the suprachiasmatic nucleus of mice. *Neuroscience* **2003**, *121*, 493–499. [CrossRef]
37. Ohta, H.; Yamazaki, S.; McMahon, D.G. Constant light desynchronizes mammalian clock neurons. *Nat. Neurosci.* **2005**, *8*, 267–269. [CrossRef]
38. Matsumura, T.; Nakagawa, H.; Suzuki, K.; Ninomiya, C.; Ishiwata, T. Influence of circadian disruption on neurotransmitter levels, physiological indexes, and behaviour in rats. *Chronobiol. Int.* **2015**, *32*, 1449–1457. [CrossRef]
39. Nordmann, A.S.; Bohne, B.A.; Harding, G.W. Histopathological differences between temporary and permanent threshold shift. *Hear. Res.* **2000**, *139*, 13–30. [CrossRef]
40. Kurabi, A.; Keithley, E.M.; Housley, G.D.; Ryan, A.F.; Wong, A.C. Cellular mechanisms of noise-induced hearing loss. *Hear. Res.* **2017**, *349*, 129–137. [CrossRef]
41. Ohinata, Y.; Miller, J.M.; Altschuler, R.A.; Schacht, J. Intense noise induces formation of vasoactive lipid peroxidation products in the cochlea. *Brain Res.* **2000**, *878*, 163–173. [CrossRef]
42. Wilking, M.; Ndiaye, M.; Mukhtar, H.; Ahmad, N. Circadian rhythm connections to oxidative stress: Implications for human health. *Antioxid. Redox Signal.* **2013**, *19*, 192–208. [CrossRef] [PubMed]
43. Patel, S.A.; Velingkaar, N.S.; Kondratov, R.V. Transcriptional control of antioxidant defense by the circadian clock. *Antioxid. Redox Signal.* **2014**, *20*, 2997–3006. [CrossRef] [PubMed]
44. Le Prell, C.G.; Yamashita, D.; Minami, S.B.; Yamasoba, T.; Miller, J.M. Mechanisms of noise-induced hearing loss indicate multiple methods of prevention. *Hear. Res.* **2007**, *226*, 22–43. [CrossRef]
45. Chen, F.Q.; Zheng, H.W.; Schacht, J.; Sha, S.H. Mitochondrial peroxiredoxin 3 regulates sensory cell survival in the cochlea. *PLoS ONE* **2013**, *8*, e61999. [CrossRef]

46. Subash, S.; Subramanian, P.; Sivaperumal, R.; Manivasagam, T.; Essa, M.M. Constant light influences the circadian oscillations of circulatory lipid peroxidation, antioxidants and some biochemical variables in rats. *Biol. Rhythm Res.* **2006**, *37*, 471–477. [CrossRef]
47. Sharma, A.; Goyal, R. Long-term exposure to constant light induces dementia, oxidative stress and promotes aggregation of sub-pathological Aβ42 in Wistar rats. *Pharmacol. Biochem. Behav.* **2020**, *192*, 172892. [CrossRef]
48. Sha, S.H.; Taylor, R.; Forge, A.; Schacht, J. Differential vulnerability of basal and apical hair cells is based on intrinsic susceptibility to free radicals. *Hear. Res.* **2001**, *155*, 1–8. [CrossRef]
49. Choung, Y.; Taura, A.; Pak, K.; Choi, S.; Masuda, M.; Ryan, A. Generation of highly-reactive oxygen species is closely related to hair cell damage in rat organ of Corti treated with gentamicin. *Neuroscience* **2009**, *161*, 214–226. [CrossRef]
50. Castanon-Cervantes, O.; Wu, M.; Ehlen, J.C.; Paul, K.; Gamble, K.L.; Johnson, R.L.; Besing, R.C.; Menaker, M.; Gewirtz, A.T.; Davidson, A.J. Dysregulation of inflammatory responses by chronic circadian disruption. *J. Immunol.* **2010**, *185*, 5796–5805. [CrossRef]
51. Sarlus, H.; Fontana, J.M.; Tserga, E.; Meltser, I.; Cederroth, C.R.; Canlon, B. Circadian integration of inflammation and glucocorticoid actions: Implications for the cochlea. *Hear. Res.* **2019**, *377*, 53–60. [CrossRef] [PubMed]
52. Voigt, R.M.; Forsyth, C.B.; Keshavarzian, A. Circadian disruption: Potential implications in inflammatory and metabolic diseases associated with alcohol. *Alcohol Res.* **2013**, *35*, 87–96. [PubMed]
53. Hirose, K.; Discolo, C.M.; Keasler, J.R.; Ransohoff, R. Mononuclear phagocytes migrate into the murine cochlea after acoustic trauma. *J. Comp. Neurol.* **2005**, *489*, 180–194. [CrossRef] [PubMed]
54. Vethanayagam, R.R.; Yang, W.; Dong, Y.; Hu, B.H. Toll-like receptor 4 modulates the cochlear immune response to acoustic injury. *Cell Death Dis.* **2016**, *7*, e2245. [CrossRef] [PubMed]
55. Fujioka, M.; Kanzaki, S.; Okano, H.J.; Masuda, M.; Ogawa, K.; Okano, H. Proinflammatory cytokines expression in noise-induced damaged cochlea. *J. Neurosci. Res.* **2006**, *83*, 575–583. [CrossRef] [PubMed]
56. Wakabayashi, K.; Fujioka, M.; Kanzaki, S.; Okano, H.J.; Shibata, S.; Yamashita, D.; Masuda, M.; Mihara, M.; Ohsugi, Y.; Ogawa, K.; et al. Blockade of interleukin-6 signaling suppressed cochlear inflammatory response and improved hearing impairment in noise-damaged mice cochlea. *Neurosci. Res.* **2010**, *66*, 345–352. [CrossRef] [PubMed]
57. Fonken, L.K.; Lieberman, R.A.; Weil, Z.M.; Nelson, R.J. Dim light at night exaggerates weight gain and inflammation associated with a high-fat diet in male mice. *Endocrinology* **2013**, *154*, 3817–3825. [CrossRef]
58. Phillips, D.J.; Savenkova, M.I.; Karatsoreos, I.N. Environmental disruption of the circadian clock leads to altered sleep and immune responses in mouse. *Brain Behav. Immun.* **2015**, *47*, 14–23. [CrossRef]
59. Cederroth, C.R.; Park, J.S.; Basinou, V.; Weger, B.D.; Tserga, E.; Sarlus, H.; Magnusson, A.K.; Kadri, N.; Gachon, F.; Canlon, B. Circadian Regulation of Cochlear Sensitivity to Noise by Circulating Glucocorticoids. *Curr. Biol.* **2019**, *29*, 2477–2487. [CrossRef]
60. Canlon, B.; Meltser, I.; Johansson, P.; Tahera, Y. Glucocorticoid receptors modulate auditory sensitivity to acoustic trauma. *Hear. Res.* **2007**, *226*, 61–69. [CrossRef]
61. Fischman, A.J.; Kastin, A.J.; Graf, M.V.; Moldow, R.L. Constant light and dark affect the circadian rhythm of the hypothalamic-pituitary-adrenal axis. *Neuroendocrinology* **1988**, *47*, 309–316. [CrossRef] [PubMed]
62. Fonken, L.K.; Workman, J.L.; Walton, J.C.; Weil, Z.M.; Morris, J.S.; Haim, A.; Nelson, R.J. Light at night increases body mass by shifting the time of food intake. *Proc. Natl. Acad. Sci. USA* **2010**, *107*, 18664–18669. [CrossRef] [PubMed]
63. Meltser, I.; Canlon, B. Protecting the auditory system with glucocorticoids. *Hear. Res.* **2011**, *281*, 47–55. [CrossRef]
64. Rumanova, V.S.; Okuliarova, M.; Zeman, M. Differential Effects of Constant Light and Dim Light at Night on the Circadian Control of Metabolism and Behavior. *Int. J. Mol. Sci.* **2020**, *21*, 5478. [CrossRef] [PubMed]

65. Schroeder, A.M.; Colwell, C.S. How to fix a broken clock. *Trends Pharmacol. Sci.* **2013**, *34*, 605–619. [CrossRef] [PubMed]
66. Arble, D.M.; Ramsey, K.M.; Bass, J.; Turek, F.W. Circadian disruption and metabolic disease: Findings from animal models. *Best Pract. Res. Clin. Endocrinol. Metab.* **2010**, *24*, 785–800. [CrossRef] [PubMed]

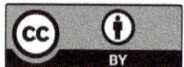

© 2020 by the authors. Licensee MDPI, Basel, Switzerland. This article is an open access article distributed under the terms and conditions of the Creative Commons Attribution (CC BY) license (http://creativecommons.org/licenses/by/4.0/).

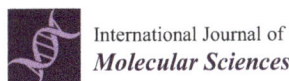 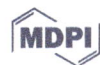

Article

Changes in microRNA Expression in the Cochlear Nucleus and Inferior Colliculus after Acute Noise-Induced Hearing Loss

Sohyeon Park [1,2], Seung Hee Han [2], Byeong-Gon Kim [2,3], Myung-Whan Suh [2], Jun Ho Lee [2,3], Seung Ha Oh [2,3] and Moo Kyun Park [2,3,4,*]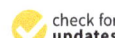

1. Interdisciplinary Program in Neuroscience, Seoul National University College of Natural Sciences, Seoul 08826, Korea; 5liviapark@snu.ac.kr
2. Department of Otorhinolaryngology-Head and Neck Surgery, Seoul National University College of Medicine, Seoul 03080, Korea; hee92h@nate.com (S.H.H.); byeonggone@naver.com (B.-G.K.); drmung@naver.com (M.-W.S.); junlee@snu.ac.kr (J.H.L.); shaoh@snu.ac.kr (S.H.O.)
3. Sensory Organ Research Institute, Seoul National University Medical Research Center, Seoul 03080, Korea
4. Seoul Wide River Institute of Immunology, Seoul National University, Gangwon 25159, Korea
* Correspondence: aseptic@snu.ac.kr

Received: 27 October 2020; Accepted: 19 November 2020; Published: 20 November 2020

Abstract: Noise-induced hearing loss (NIHL) can lead to secondary changes that induce neural plasticity in the central auditory pathway. These changes include decreases in the number of synapses, the degeneration of auditory nerve fibers, and reorganization of the cochlear nucleus (CN) and inferior colliculus (IC) in the brain. This study investigated the role of microRNAs (miRNAs) in the neural plasticity of the central auditory pathway after acute NIHL. Male Sprague–Dawley rats were exposed to white band noise at 115 dB for 2 h, and the auditory brainstem response (ABR) and morphology of the organ of Corti were evaluated on days 1 and 3. Following noise exposure, the ABR threshold shift was significantly smaller in the day 3 group, while wave II amplitudes were significantly larger in the day 3 group compared to the day 1 group. The organ of Corti on the basal turn showed evidence of damage and the number of surviving outer hair cells was significantly lower in the basal and middle turn areas of the hearing loss groups relative to controls. Five and three candidate miRNAs for each CN and IC were selected based on microarray analysis and quantitative reverse transcription PCR (RT-qPCR). The data confirmed that even short-term acoustic stimulation can lead to changes in neuroplasticity. Further studies are needed to validate the role of these candidate miRNAs. Such miRNAs may be used in the early diagnosis and treatment of neural plasticity of the central auditory pathway after acute NIHL.

Keywords: noise-induced hearing loss; microRNAs; cochlear nucleus; inferior colliculus; neuroplasticity

1. Introduction

According to the World Health Organization, 466 million people—more than 5% of the world's population—are affected by hearing loss [1]. Loss of hearing makes communication difficult and can lead to psychosocial problems, such as depression and feelings of loneliness [2]. Therefore, losing the ability to hear can affect people's lives in many ways.

NIHL is a type of acquired hearing loss that is due to a sudden excessively loud sound or continuous moderately loud sounds. Depending on the duration and intensity of the sounds, hearing loss can be temporary or permanent [3]. Threshold sensitivity loss after exposure to a loud noise can be recovered to baseline levels after a few hours to weeks and that is called temporary threshold shift

(TTS). Permanent threshold shift (PTS) occurs when the noise is too loud to recover to its baseline level or the noise takes place repeatedly or continuously, impeding recovery.

Even though hearing thresholds may return to normal, the changes in the synapse may affect auditory processing and hearing upon noise [4]. Exposure to noise not only targets the hair cells (HCs) in the cochlea, but also the neuronal cells in the auditory pathway. Noise exposure can also alter the synaptic transmission and ion channel function, distort sensory maps, and cause abnormal neuronal firing patterns. These cellular and physiological changes can cause another disorder, such as loudness recruitment or tinnitus [5].

NIHL usually progresses slowly over a period of years, making it difficult to recognize. Initial symptoms include difficulty in differentiating conversations against background noise. Later, listening becomes difficult, even in ordinary circumstances. Since NIHL progresses gradually and prevention is so crucial, it is important to diagnose NIHL at an early stage [6].

MicroRNAs (MiRNAs) are small non-coding single-stranded endogenous RNAs that regulate posttranscriptional gene expression. Mature miRNAs are 18–22 nucleotides in length and can repress and degrade target mRNAs by binding to their 3′ or 5′ untranslated regions. MiRNAs are involved in a number of physiological processes and play key roles in neural development and plasticity. MiRNAs are abundant in the brain, due to its complexity [7,8], and are also found in body fluids such as the cerebrospinal fluid, whole blood, plasma, and serum [9]. Consequently, miRNAs can be detected and analyzed non-surgically and may provide the basis for a new generation of therapeutic agents [10]. In fact, there are some miRNA-based therapeutics for cancer and other diseases and several miRNAs are currently being studied in Phase I/II clinical trials, with promising outcomes [11].

Electrical signals from the HCs in the inner ear flow to primary sensory neurons, which are called spiral ganglion neurons. These cochlear nerves combine with vestibular nerves to become branch VIII of the cranial nerve [12], which transfers the converted acoustic information to the cochlear nucleus (CN), developing the neural pathway [13]. The superior olivary complex (SOC) in the ventral auditory brainstem receives auditory information from the CN and sends the signal to the inferior colliculus (IC). The IC plays a crucial role in the auditory pathway and is the first location where parallel auditory signals from both sides of the cochlea are integrated. Most of the auditory information is processed in the IC and sent to the auditory cortex through the medial geniculate body [14].

Noise exposure is one of the most common causes of hearing loss. Exposure to loud noise leads to secondary changes, such as decreases in the number of synapses, the degeneration of auditory nerve fibers, and reorganization of the CN and IC, which may induce neural plasticity in the central auditory pathway. However, little is known about the role of miRNAs in the central auditory pathway. Therefore, this study investigated the role of miRNAs in the neural plasticity of the central auditory pathway after NIHL.

2. Results

2.1. Hearing Changes after Noise Exposure

Tone-burst acoustic stimuli were measured at three different frequencies of 4, 8, and 16 kHz. Our noise-control model ($n = 4$) showed that the auditory brainstem response (ABR) threshold started to decrease at day 1 after the noise exposure. By day 3 after the exposure to noise at 4 and 8 kHz, the ABR thresholds had returned to normal (Figure 1a). The mean ABR thresholds observed for the day 1 control group (4 kHz, 20.6 ± 2.2 dB; 8 kHz, 21.3 ± 2.7 dB; 16 kHz, 25.4 ± 3.6 dB), day 1 group (4 kHz, 20.0 ± 0.0 dB; 8 kHz, 20.8 ± 1.9 dB; 16 kHz, 27.1 ± 3.6 dB), day 3 control group (4 kHz, 20.8 ± 2.4 dB; 8 kHz, 21.9 ± 3.2 dB; 16 kHz, 25.6 ± 4.3 dB), and day 3 group (4 kHz, 24.2 ± 4.8 dB; 8 kHz, 25.8 ± 4.6 dB; 16 kHz, 26.9 ± 3.6 dB) confirmed that hearing levels at all three frequencies were normal before the experiment (Figure 1b–d). After 2 h of noise exposure, both the day 1 group (4 kHz, 81.9 ± 11.6 dB; 8 kHz, 87.1 ± 3.3 dB; 16 kHz, 88.3 ± 2.4 dB) and the day 3 group (4 kHz, 78.8 ± 11.8 dB; 8 kHz, 84.6 ± 2.9 dB; 16 kHz, 86.7 ± 3.8 dB) exhibited significant increases in ABR thresholds compared to the day 1 control group (4 kHz, 20.2 ± 1.0 dB; 8 kHz, 20.4 ± 1.4 dB; 16 kHz, 23.5 ± 3.8 dB) and the day 3 control group (4 kHz, 20.4 ± 1.4 dB; 8 kHz, 21.0 ± 2.5 dB; 16 kHz, 24.4 ± 3.7 dB), respectively (Figure 1b–d). At 4 kHz, the mean ABR threshold of the day 1 group (65.6 ± 19.5 dB) was slightly lower than that of the day 1 control group (81.9 ± 11.6 dB). Moreover, the mean ABR threshold of the day 3 group (42.7 ± 17.1 dB) was lower than that of the day 1 group. The differences between these groups were significant ($p < 0.001$; Figure 1b,e). At 8 kHz, the mean ABR thresholds of both the day 1 (73.3 ± 10.7 dB) and day 3 (51.9 ± 13.7 dB) groups were significantly lower than those of the control groups (87.1 ± 3.3 dB; $p < 0.001$; Figure 1c,f). The mean ABR thresholds of the day 1 (79.4 ± 8.5 dB) and day 3 (63.5 ± 12.6 dB) groups were also significantly lower than those of the control groups (88.3 ± 2.4 dB) at 16 kHz ($p < 0.001$; Figure 1d,g). The day 3 group exhibited significantly better hearing than the day 1 group at all three frequencies ($p < 0.001$; Figure 1e–g).

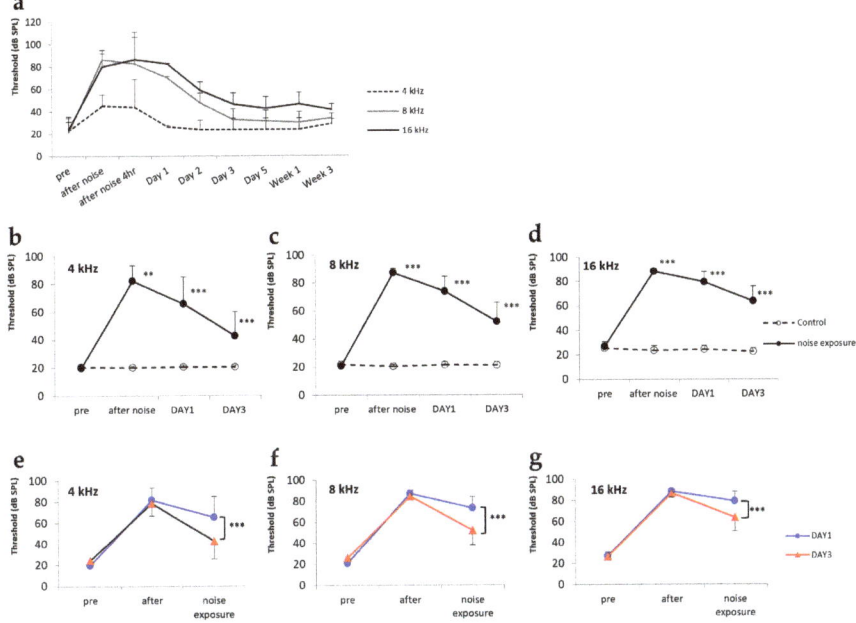

Figure 1. Hearing changes after noise exposure. (**a**) Long-term auditory brainstem response (ABR) data of the noise-control model obtained over a period of 3 weeks. (**b–d**) Line graphs showing differences between control and treatment groups at frequencies of 4, 8, and 16 kHz. *** $p < 0.001$. (**e–g**) Line graphs comparing ABR thresholds at days 1 and 3 after noise exposure at frequencies of 4, 8, and 16 kHz. *** $p < 0.001$.

2.2. ABR Amplitudes

The amplitudes of waves II and IV were calculated based on ABR waveforms. The wave II amplitudes observed in the day 1 treatment group (4 kHz, 0.61 ± 0.28 µV; 8 kHz, 0.62 ± 0.25 µV; 16 kHz, 0.39 ± 0.23 µV) were significantly smaller than those observed in the day 3 treatment group, at all frequencies (4 kHz, 1.56 ± 0.90 µV; 8 kHz, 1.45 ± 0.84 µV; 16 kHz, 1.08 ± 0.0 µV; $p < 0.001$; Figure 2a). At 4 kHz, the mean wave IV amplitude observed in the day 1 treatment group (0.44 ± 0.39 µV) was significantly smaller than that in the day 3 treatment group (0.93 ± 0.22 µV). However, at the other frequencies, the amplitudes observed in the day 1 treatment group (8 kHz, 0.36 ± 0.22 µV; 16 kHz, 0.26 ± 0.18 µV) did not differ significantly from those observed on day 3 (8 kHz, 0.43 ± 0.40 µV; 16 kHz, 0.26 ± 0.26; Figure 2b).

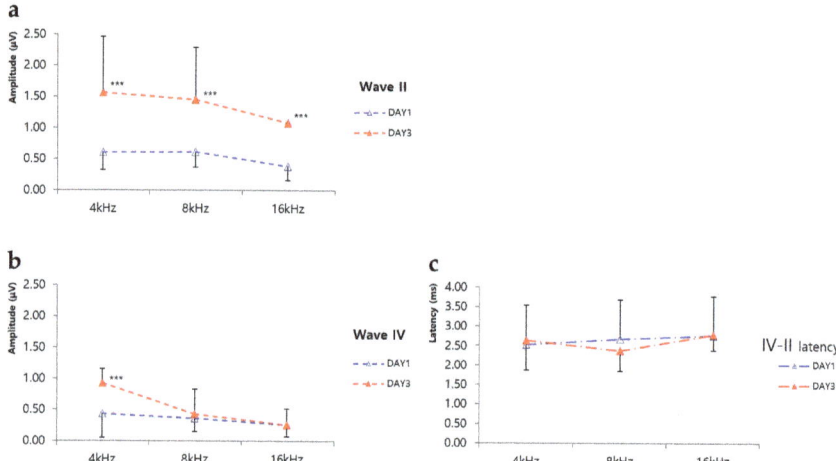

Figure 2. Amplitudes of waves II and IV and latencies of waves IV–II. (**a**) Comparison of the amplitude of wave II at different frequencies. The wave II amplitude for rats assayed at day 3 after noise exposure was significantly larger than that for rats assayed at day 1 after noise exposure, at all frequencies. *** $p < 0.001$. (**b**) Comparison of the amplitude of wave IV among different frequencies. The wave IV amplitude for rats assayed at day 3 after noise exposure was significantly larger than that for rats assayed at day 1 after noise exposure at 4 kHz. *** $p < 0.001$. No significant differences were observed at the other frequencies. (**c**) The latencies of waves IV–II at each frequency. No significant differences were observed at any frequency.

2.3. ABR Latencies

Latencies between waves IV and II were calculated based on ABR waveforms. At 4 kHz, there was no difference in latencies between the day 1 (2.54 ± 0.50 ms) and day 3 treatment groups (2.64 ± 0.77 ms). Similar results were seen at 16 kHz, with no difference in latencies being evident between the day 1 (2.77 ± 0.15 ms) and day 3 treatment groups (2.80 ± 0.41 ms). Conversely, at 8 kHz, the latency observed in the day 3 treatment group (2.38 ± 0.54 ms) was slightly reduced compared to that of the day 1 treatment group (2.68 ± 0.71 ms); however, this difference was not statistically significant (Figure 2c).

2.4. Histology of the Organ of Corti

A series of sagittal sections from decalcified cochleae were stained with hematoxylin and eosin (H&E) to investigate the structure of the organ of Corti. These structures were intact in both the day 1 and day 3 control groups. The apical turn and middle turn sections of the organ of Corti from the day 1 and day 3 treatment groups were also normal, with intact HCs and other non-sensory cells, such as Deiter and pillar cells. However, the basal turn sections of the organs of Corti exhibited abnormalities. The degree of damage differed among cochleae, with some exhibiting only a loss of HCs, and others also exhibiting a loss of supporting cells (Figure 3).

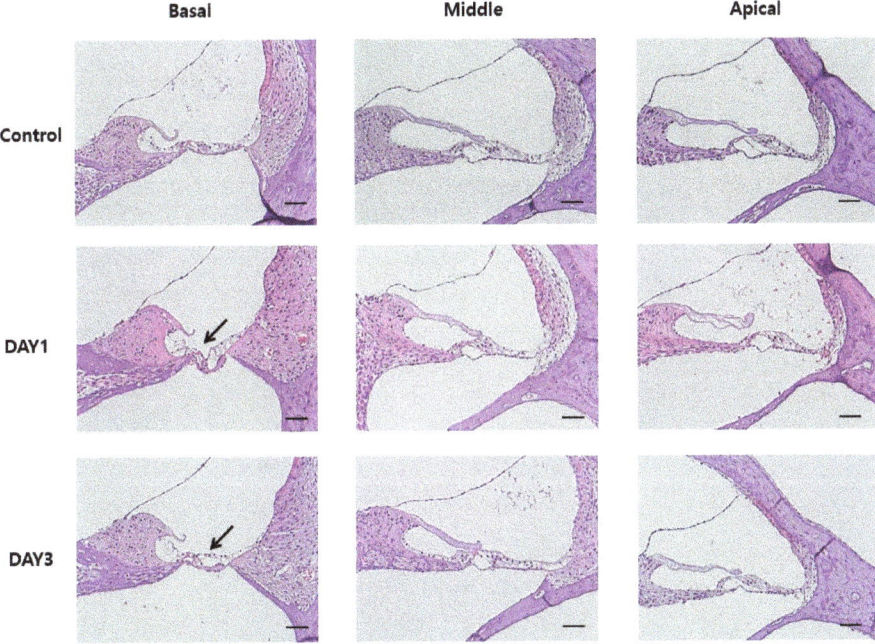

Figure 3. Hematoxylin and eosin (H&E) staining of the basal, middle, and apical turn sections of the organ of Corti. Damage (indicated by black arrows) was only observed in the basal turn section in rats assayed at days 1 and 3 after noise exposure. All scale bars represent 50 μm.

2.5. *Phalloidin Staining of Outer HCs*

Following completion of the whole mount surface preparation procedure, phalloidin was used to stain the outer HCs. Two 200-μm-long segments were selected from each turn section of the organ of Corti, and the mean number of surviving outer HCs was determined. All three rows of outer HCs from all control samples were normal, with no evidence of missing HCs. However, significant HC loss was observed in the basal turn sections in both the day 1 (85% ± 7%; $p = 0.001$) and day 3 (93% ± 6%; $p = 0.019$) treatment groups. Some HCs were also lost from the middle turn sections of samples from the day 1 (99% ± 1%; $p = 0.008$) and day 3 (99% ± 1%; $p < 0.001$) treatment groups. In contrast, outer HCs in the apical turn sections of samples from both the day 1 and day 3 treatment groups were largely intact (both, 100% ± 0%). For the basal turn sections, significantly fewer HCs were lost from the day 3 treatment group compared to the day 1 treatment group ($p = 0.039$). No statistically significant difference in HC loss was observed between the day 1 and day 3 groups for the middle or apical turn sections of the organ of Corti (Figure 4).

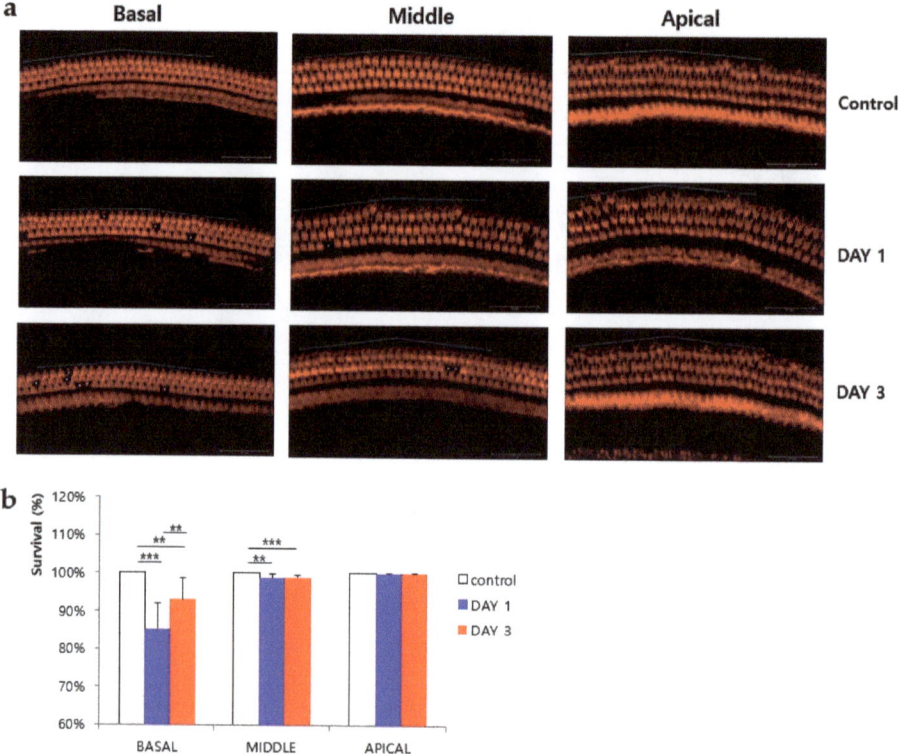

Figure 4. Phalloidin staining of outer hair cells (HCs) and HC survival. (**a**) Fluorescence staining of outer HCs from each turn section of the cochlea. Scale bars represent 50 μm. Asterisks indicate the positions of lost HCs. The blue line along the hair cell line indicates the length of 200 μm. (**b**) Survival rates of outer HCs in each turn section. The surviving HCs per 200 μm along the length of the cochlea in the basal, middle, and apical turn sections were counted. ** $p < 0.05$ and *** $p < 0.001$.

2.6. Selection of Candidate miRNAs

2.6.1. The CN

Microarray analysis of the CN identified 1228 candidate miRNAs. Changes in miRNA expression were assessed via three pair-wise comparisons: Between the day 1 treatment and control groups; between the day 3 treatment and control groups; and between the day 1 and day 3 groups. For each comparison, miRNAs with normalized expression changes ≥1.5-fold ($p < 0.1$) were excluded. Then, the miRNAs from each set were combined and those found in more than one dataset were eliminated. miRNAs that exhibited differences in expression between the day 1 and day 3 groups were also excluded. A hierarchical clustering heat map was created using Multiple Experiment Viewer (http://mev.tm4.org) to visualize the remaining 33 miRNAs (Figure 5a). Then, miRNAs with ≥1.5-fold differences in expression between the day 1 and day 3 control groups were excluded. Of the 21 miRNAs that remained, only those expressed in humans were considered for further analysis, resulting in a final list of 10 candidate miRNAs, including *miR-411-3p*, *miR-183-5p*, *miR-377-3p*, *miR-20b-5p*, *miR-137-5p*, *miR-211-3p*, *miR-483-5p*, *miR-92a-1-5p*, *miR-187-5p*, and *miR-200b-3p* (Table 1).

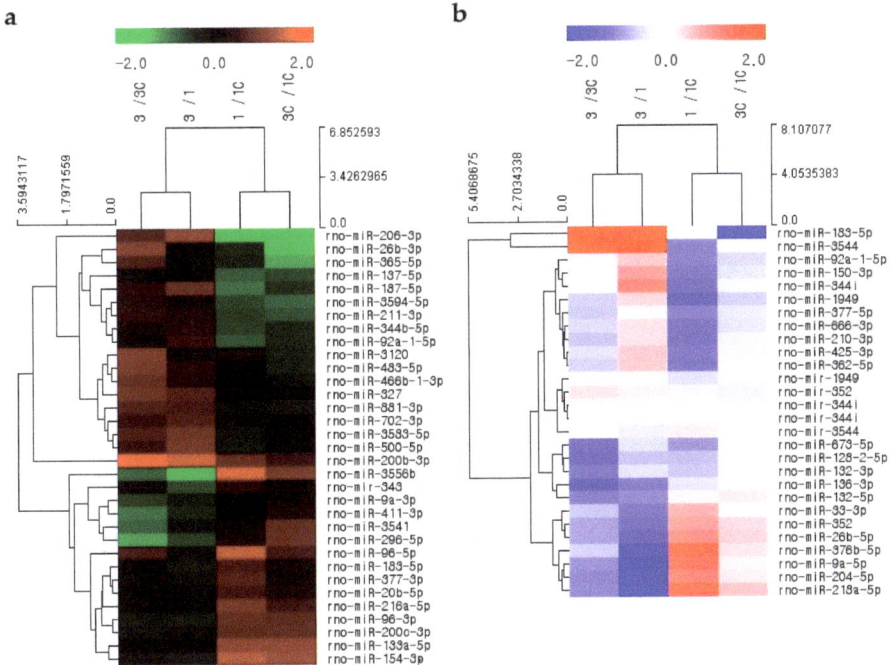

Figure 5. Heat maps of the CN and IC. Heat maps of (**a**) 33 miRNAs from the CN and (**b**) 27 miRNAs from the IC selected based on ≥1.5-fold changes in normalized expression ($p < 0.1$).

Table 1. Candidate microRNAs (miRNAs) of the cochlear nucleus (CN).

Gene Symbol	Chromosome	Sequence Length	Sequence	1/1C [1]	3/3C [2]	3/1 [3]	3C/1C [4]
rno-miR-411-3p	6	20	UAUGUAACACGGUCCACUAA	0.977	0.529	0.712	1.315
rno-miR-183-5p	4	22	UAUGGCACUGGUAGAAUUCACU	1.542	0.957	0.759	1.222
rno-miR-377-3p	6	23	UGAAUCACACAAAGGCAACUUUU	1.652	1.154	0.839	1.201
rno-miR-20b-5p	X	23	CAAAGUGCUCAUAGUGCAGGUAG	1.522	1.029	0.870	1.288
rno-miR-137-5p	2	22	ACGGGUAUUCUUGGGUGGAUAA	0.576	0.871	0.968	0.640
rno-miR-211-3p	1	20	GGCAAGGACAGCAAAGGGGG	0.649	1.420	1.334	0.610
rno-miR-483-5p	1	22	AAGACGGGAGAAGAGAAGGGAG	1.072	2.025	1.393	0.737
rno-miR-92a-1-5p	15	23	AGGUUGGGAUUUGUCGCAAUGCU	0.588	1.194	1.468	0.724
rno-miR-187-5p	18	18	AGGCUACAACACAGGACC	0.529	1.404	1.827	0.688
rno-miR-200b-3p	5	23	UAAUACUGCCUGGUAAUGAUGAC	1.826	3.587	2.895	1.474

[1] Fold change of day 1 treatment vs. control, [2] fold change of the day 3 treatment group vs. control, [3] fold change of the day 1 and day 3 treatment groups, and [4] fold change of the day 1 vs. day 3 control groups. A color index chart for of the fold change data is provided in Supplementary Figure S1.

2.6.2. The IC

Microarray analysis of the IC identified 1200 miRNAs. Changes in miRNA expression were assessed in three pair-wise comparisons: Between the day 1 treatment and control groups; between the day 3 treatment and control groups; and between the day 1 and day 3 groups. For each comparison, miRNAs with ≥1.5-fold normalized expression changes ($p < 0.1$) were excluded. Then, the miRNAs from each set were combined, and those found in more than one dataset were eliminated. miRNAs that exhibited differences in expression between the day 1 and day 3 groups were also excluded. A hierarchical clustering heat map was created using Multiple Experiment Viewer to assess the remaining 27 miRNAs (Figure 5b). Then, miRNAs with expression differences changes >1.5-fold or <0.5-fold between the day 3 and day 1 control groups were excluded. Of the 26 miRNAs that remained, only those expressed in humans were considered for further analysis, resulting in a final list of 13 candidate miRNAs, including *miR-204-5p*, *miR-376b-5p*, *miR-26b-5p*, *miR-136-3p*, miR-132-5p, miR-128-2-5p, miR-132-3p, miR-377-5p, miR-210-3p, miR-92a-1-5p, miR-425-3p, miR-362-5p, and miR-150-3p (Table 2).

Table 2. Candidate miRNAs of the inferior colliculus (IC).

Gene Symbol	Chromosome	Sequence Length	Sequence	1/1C [1]	3/3C [2]	3/1 [3]	3C/1C [4]
rno-miR-204-5p	1	22	UUCCCUUUGUCAUCCUAUGCCU	2.020	0.511	0.299	1.181
rno-miR-376b-5p	6	22	GUGGAUAUUCCUUCUAUGGUUA	2.606	0.712	0.332	1.215
rno-miR-26b-5p	9	21	UUCAAGUAAUUCAGGAUAGGU	1.842	0.585	0.413	1.301
rno-miR-136-3p	6	22	CAUCAUCGUCUCAAAUGAGUCU	0.777	0.357	0.484	1.055
rno-miR-132-5p	10	22	ACCGUGGCUUUCGAUUGUUACU	1.085	0.491	0.534	1.180
rno-miR-128-2-5p	8	21	GGGGGCCGAUGCACUGUAAGA	0.650	0.412	0.658	1.039
rno-miR-132-3p	10	22	UAACAGUCUACAGCCAUGGUCG	0.670	0.472	0.782	1.109
rno-miR-377-5p	6	22	AGAGGUUGCCCUUGGUGAAUUC	0.499	0.676	1.066	0.786
rno-miR-210-3p	1	22	CUGUGCGUGUGACAGCGGCUGA	0.452	0.659	1.217	0.834
rno-miR-92a-1-5p	15	23	AGGUUGGGAUUUGUCGCAAUGCU	0.498	0.918	1.333	0.723
rno-miR-425-3p	8	21	AUCGGGAAUAUCGUGUCCGCC	0.479	0.749	1.352	0.865
rno-miR-362-5p	X	24	AAUCCUUGGAACCUAGGUGUGAAU	0.464	0.699	1.353	0.898
rno-miR-150-3p	1	19	CUGGUACAGGCCUGGGGGA	0.474	1.023	1.669	0.774

[1] Fold change of day 1 treatment group vs. control, [2] fold change of the day 3 treatment group vs. control, [3] fold change of the day 1 vs. day 3 treatment groups, and [4] fold change of the day 1 vs. day 3 control groups. A color index chart for the fold change data is provided in Supplementary Figure S1.

2.7. Validation of Candidate miRNAs Using qRT-PCR

2.7.1. The CN

Based on the results of the microarray analysis of the CN, 10 candidate miRNAs were selected for further analysis, including *miR-411-3p*, *miR-183-5p*, *miR-377-3p*, *miR-20b-5p*, *miR-137-5p*, *miR-211-3p*, *miR-483-5p*, *miR-92a-1-5p*, *miR-187-5p*, and *miR-200b-3p* (Figure 6a). Microarray data of the day 3 and day 1 treatment groups are compared in Figure 6b, along with the accompanying qRT-PCR results. Based on these data, five miRNAs were selected due to their consistent expression patterns, including *miR-411-3p*, *miR-183-5p*, *miR-377-3p*, *miR-20b-5p*, and *miR-200b-3p*. The expression of *miR-200b-3p* increased after noise exposure, whereas that of the other miRNAs decreased.

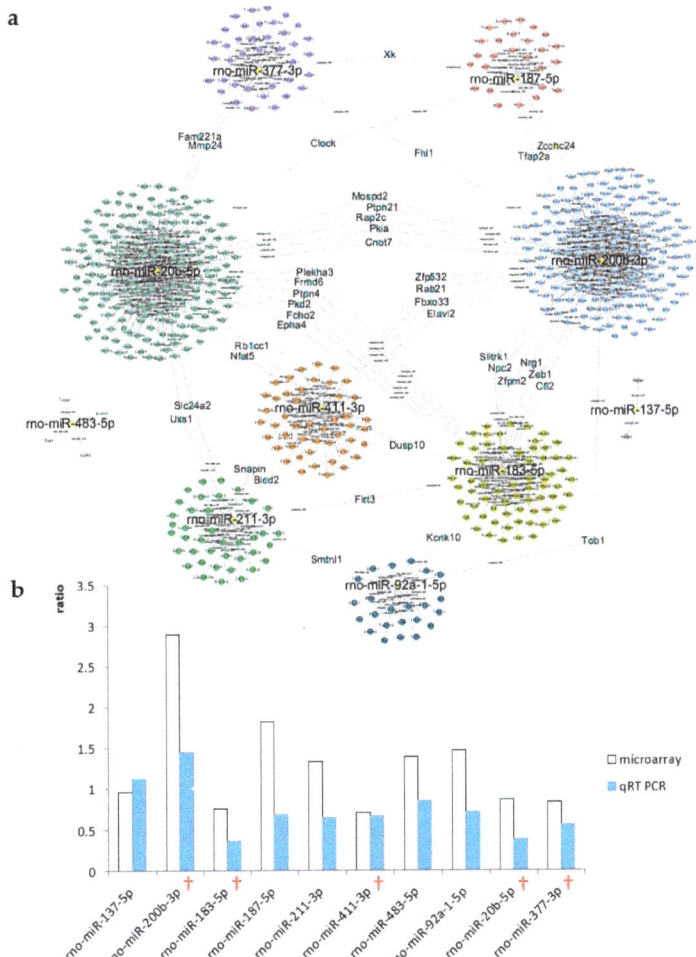

Figure 6. A Cytoscape map of the CN and validation of candidate miRNAs. Cytoscape was used to visualize networks among candidate miRNAs. Only miRNAs that were connected to other miRNAs were selected for validation by quantitative reverse transcription polymerase chain reaction (qRT-PCR). (**a**) A total of 10 miRNAs were selected as CN candidate miRNAs. (**b**) Ratio of expression of each candidate miRNA in the CN between the day 3 and day 1 treatment groups. Expression levels were measured using microarray analysis (open bars) and qRT-PCR (filled bars). Crosses indicate validated candidate miRNAs.

2.7.2. The IC

Based on the results of the microarray analysis of the IC, 13 candidate miRNAs were selected for further analysis, including *miR-204-5p*, *miR-376b-5p*, *miR-26b-5p*, *miR-136-3p*, *miR-132-5p*, *miR-128-2-5p*, *miR-132-3p*, *miR-377-5p*, *miR-210-3p*, *miR-92a-1-5p*, *miR-425-3p*, *miR-362-5p*, and *miR-150-3p* (Figure 7a). Microarray data of the day 3 and day 1 treatment groups are compared in Figure 7b, along with the accompanying qRT-PCR results. Three miRNAs were selected due to their consistent expression patterns, including *miR-92a-1-5p*, *miR-136-3p*, and *miR-26b-5p*. The expression of *miR-92a-1-5p* increased after noise exposure, whereas that of the other miRNAs decreased.

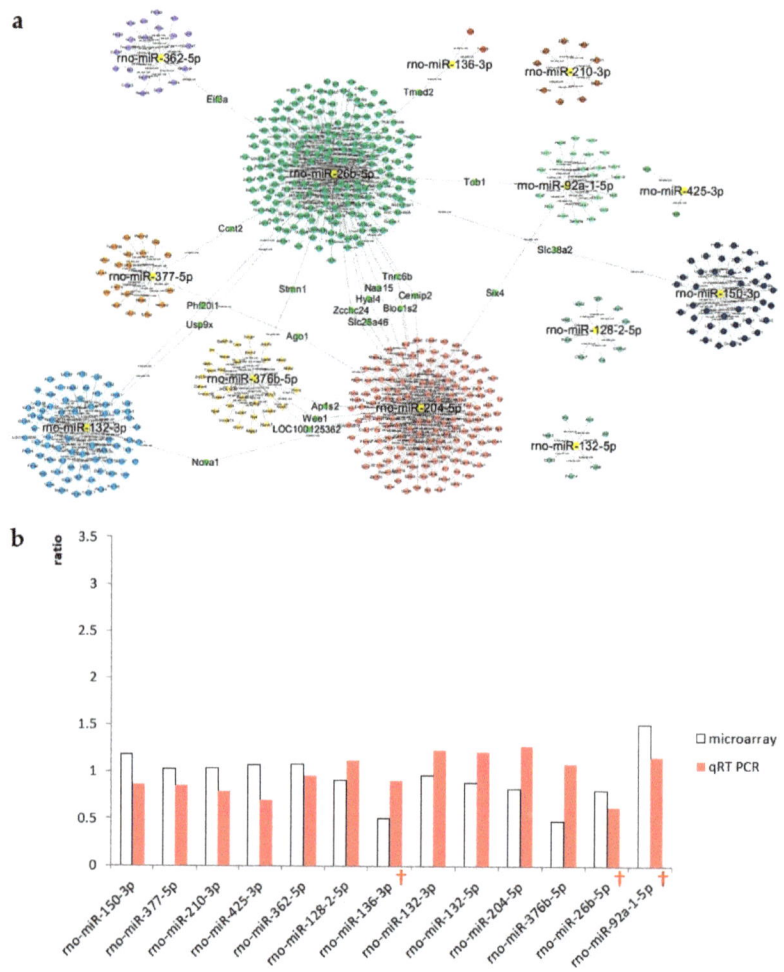

Figure 7. A Cytoscape map of the IC and validation of candidate miRNAs. Cytoscape was used to visualize networks among the candidate miRNAs. Only miRNAs that were connected to other miRNAs were selected for validation by qRT-PCR. (**a**) A total of 13 miRNAs were selected as IC candidate miRNAs. (**b**) Ratio of expression of each candidate miRNA in the IC between the day 3 and day 1 treatment groups. Expression levels were measured using microarray analysis (open bars) and qRT-PCR (filled bars). Crosses indicate validated candidate miRNAs.

2.8. Target Pathway Analysis of Candidate miRNAs

2.8.1. The CN

Five candidate miRNAs expressed in the CN were validated using qRT-PCR, including *miR-411-3p, miR-183-5p, miR-377-3p, miR-20b-5p,* and *miR-200b-3p*. DIANA-miRPath software (ver. 3.0; http://www.microrna.gr/miRPathv3) was used to investigate the regulation of biological pathways by miRNAs in the CN. A Kyoto Encyclopedia of Genes and Genomes (KEGG) analysis identified 12 significantly overrepresented pathways. The most relevant pathways for these miRNAs involved mitogen-activated protein kinase (MAPK) signaling, axon guidance, and transforming growth factor-beta (TGF-β) signaling (Figure 8a).

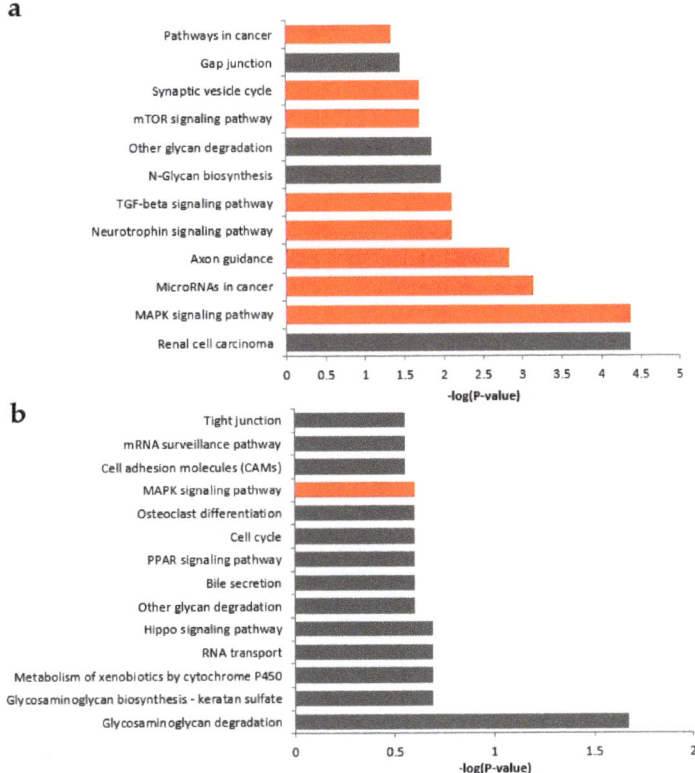

Figure 8. Kyoto Encyclopedia of Genes and Genomes (KEGG) pathway analysis of candidate miRNAs. (**a**) KEGG pathway analysis for the CN. Of the 12 possible in silico pathways identified, eight (marked in red) were highlighted based on their relevance to the five candidate miRNAs. (**b**) KEGG pathway analysis for the IC. Of the 14 possible in silico pathways identified, only the mitogen-activated protein kinase (MAPK) signaling pathway (marked in red) was identified as a relevant target for the three candidate miRNAs. Abbreviations: mTOR, mammalian target of rapamycin; TGF, transforming growth factor; PPAR, peroxisome proliferator-activated receptor.

2.8.2. The IC

Three candidate miRNAs expressed in the IC were validated using qRT-PCR, including *miR-92a-1-5p*, *miR-136-3p*, and *miR-26b-5p*. DIANA-miRPath software (ver. 3.0; DIANA TOOLS, http://www.microrna.gr/miRPathv3) was used to investigate the regulation of biological pathways by miRNAs in the IC. A KEGG analysis identified 14 significantly overrepresented pathways. The most relevant pathway for these three miRNAs was the MAPK signaling pathway (Figure 8b).

3. Discussion

Our results demonstrated that even short-term acoustic stimulation can cause changes in miRNA expression in the CN and IC, and that these changes may also induce plasticity in the central auditory pathway. Microarray analysis and qRT-PCR suggested that miRNAs play a key role in neural plasticity after noise exposure in both the CN (i.e., *miR-411-3p*, *miR-183-5p*, *miR-377-3p*, *miR-20b-5p*, and *miR-200b-3p*) and IC (i.e., *miR-92a-1-5p*, *miR-136-3p*, and *miR-26b-5p*). Further research is necessary to understand the specific roles of these candidate miRNAs, with preliminary evidence suggesting that they may be involved in regulating the MAPK signaling pathway, axon guidance, and the TGF-β signaling pathway. Numerous studies have investigated NIHL without identifying a reliable tool for early diagnosis or a treatment that results in complete recovery. Currently, hearing aids and cochlear implants are used to treat patients with severe hearing loss, but more effective methods for diagnosing and treating NIHL are required. Since miRNAs are stable over long periods of time and can be detected in the blood, as well as in brain tissue, these sequences may represent a viable diagnostic target for blood tests, enabling earlier diagnosis of NIHL and potentially protecting people against tinnitus. Moreover, gene therapy involving the transfer of miRNAs to target cells using viral vectors or siRNAs could be used to treat NIHL in the future.

Consecutive ABR tests were performed in this study, with evidence of ABR threshold recovery beginning as early as day 1 after noise exposure. The shift in the ABR threshold decreased significantly on days 2 and 3 after noise exposure, and was insignificant after day 3. Based on these observations, we hypothesized that significant changes may occur within this time frame. We therefore chose day 1 and 3 after noise exposure as our two major time points.

We focused on the CN and IC, because the latter is the origin of the central auditory pathway and the IC forms its core. The central auditory pathway receives the bilateral auditory signal, with waves II and IV corresponding to the CN and IC, respectively [15]. Therefore, we evaluated the latency between waves IV and II, and the height of these waves relative to their resting points. The latency between waves IV and II was slightly reduced at 8 kHz in the day 3 treatment group; however, the difference was not statistically significant. Changes in the latency of wave I might be expected because the auditory nerve is the primary region affected by HC loss [16]. An increased latency of wave I may indicate dysfunction in action potential propagation along the auditory nerve [17]. However, it is difficult to measure wave I using the ABR [18]. Moreover, short-term noise exposure may affect auditory nerve fibers, but not the CN or IC.

We observed a statistically significant difference in the amplitude of wave II between the day 1 and day 3 treatment groups. The amplitude of wave II was greater in the day 3 treatment group at all frequencies. In general, the ABR amplitude of wave I is reduced by overexpressed sound stimuli [19,20], while the amplitudes of later ABR waves (i.e., II–V) should increase due to compensatory hyperactivity of the central auditory pathway. A reduced sensory input from both ears triggers an increase in excitatory activity and/or a decrease in inhibitory activity [21]. Regarding interpretation of the ABR wave, latency represents the speed of transmission and amplitude represents the number of neurons that fire together [22]. One possible explanation for our observations is that the number of neurons in the CN decreased. However, either the damaged neurons recovered, or axonal sprouting from the original neurons must have occurred, because the measured amplitudes were large. Moreover, with the exception of the 4 kHz frequency measurements, there was no difference in the amplitude of wave IV between the two noise exposure groups. This suggests that the levels of noise used in this study were insufficient for affecting the IC, or that neuronal activity in the CN was able to compensate for the damage.

All three rows of outer HCs in the control groups were normal, and there were no missing HCs. Only a few HCs were missing in the middle and basal turn sections in the day 1 and day 3 treatment groups. The minimum survival rates of outer HCs in the basal turn and apical turn sections were 78% and 99%, respectively. This suggests that outer HC loss was mild in general. The confirmation of outer HC loss indicates that our noise-exposure protocol can cause a PTS, while also providing evidence that as little as 2 h of noise exposure can permanently damage the cochlea [23]. When a TTS occurs, the ABR threshold returns to its normal level, but long-term damage to the synapses may exist, even in the absence of HC loss. The disruption of signaling between the inner HCs and type-1 afferent auditory nerve fibers causes degeneration of the auditory nerve fibers and spiral ganglia. In particular, if synapses connecting low-spontaneous-rate auditory nerve fibers deteriorate, communication may be disrupted due to the signals being less distinct from background noise [24]. Therefore, it is important to protect the auditory canals from noise, regardless of its intensity and duration.

Loss of HCs after noise exposure can lead to secondary damage, including auditory synaptopathy. Noise exposure not only damages the cochlea, but also triggers extensive changes in the central auditory pathway. Sensory deprivation due to a decrease in the number of HCs can induce a reduction in the cell density in the upper auditory structures. For example, after overstimulation, the cell population in the ventral CN (VCN) has been shown to decrease due to apoptosis [25].

It is important to understand the molecular events that occur after acoustic trauma, in order to minimize damage to the central auditory pathway. A bioinformatics analysis by Alagramam et al. showed that exposure to both 116 and 110 dB noise could induce genes related to the MAPK signaling pathway For example, the Fos gene, which has a putative role in neuronal apoptosis and cell death, was induced in response to both treatments [26].

Acoustic overstimulation, unlike ablation, can lead to widespread axon degeneration and death. A study of cats with acoustic trauma demonstrated that new axons are able to grow in the VCN. Following noise exposure, cochlear nerve endings in the VCN degenerated over a period of several months and disappeared completely after 3 years. However, other small axons subsequently began to appear throughout the VCN, suggesting that degenerated neurons can reorganize the structure of the CN by generating new axons [27].

The CN is the primary point of convergence between auditory and somatosensory inputs. The balance of auditory sensory inputs can be disrupted by a decrease therein due to peripheral hearing loss. This imbalance, caused by increased excitatory activity and/or decreased inhibitory activity, enhances central neural receptivity and leads to hyperexcitability [28]. This change in the plasticity of the CN occurs in the form of axonal sprouting, which is regulated by the TGF-β signaling pathway [29]. However, such axonal sprouting can trigger tinnitus, which may itself be problematic for some patients [30]. Therefore, many researchers are trying to develop treatments that prevent axonal sprouting by inhibiting the TGF-β signaling pathway.

Among the potential genes targeted by the miRNAs described here, dual specificity protein phosphatase 10 (DUSP 10; Gene ID, 11221) is co-regulated by *miR-411-3p* and *miR-183-5p*. The expression levels of both *miR-411-3p* and *miR-183-5p* were shown to decrease after acoustic trauma, leading to an increase in the DUSP 10 level. The by-products of DUSP 10 inactivate p38 and stress-activated protein kinase/c-Jun NH(2)-terminal kinase (SAPK/JNK), thereby inhibiting the JNK pathway. As the JNK pathway serves as a major driver of apoptosis, inhibition thereof is likely to protect cells against apoptosis [31].

Profilin2 (PFN2) is also co-regulated by *miR-411-3p* and *miR-183-5p*. The expression levels of both *miR-411-3p* and *miR-183-5p* were shown to decrease after acoustic trauma, leading to an increase in PFN2. PFN2 is an actin binding protein that plays an important role in maintaining the structure of synapses in neural tissues [32]. In the case of TTS, afferent synapses are damaged and an increase in PFN2 expression may promote structural recovery of the damaged synapses [33].

4. Materials and Methods

4.1. Study Design

Noise-induced hearing loss (NIHL) was achieved by exposing subjects to 2 h of noise at a 115 dB sound pressure level (SPL). Tests of the auditory brainstem response (ABR) and histological examinations of the cochleae confirmed loss of hearing. Microarray analysis of the CN and IC tissues was used to identify candidate microRNAs (miRNAs). These miRNAs were validated using quantitative reverse transcription polymerase chain reaction (qRT-PCR) and target pathway analysis.

4.2. Animal Subjects

All of the animal experiments described were approved (8 February 2018) by the Institutional Animal Care and Use Committee of Seoul National University Hospital (Seoul, Korea; 18-0025-C1A0), which is endorsed by the Association for the Assessment and Accreditation of Laboratory Animal Care International. The animals used in these experiments were kept under 12-h/12-h day/light cycle conditions, with free access to food and water. They were acclimated to laboratory conditions 1 week prior to the initiation of these experiments. A total of 48 male Sprague–Dawley rats, aged 6 weeks, were randomly separated into four groups (all, $n = 12$). One group was assayed 1 day after noise exposure (day 1), one group was assayed 3 days after noise exposure (day 3), and the other two groups were used as the day 1 and day 3 controls.

4.3. Noise-Exposure Protocol

Animals were anesthetized using a mixture of 40 mg/kg Zoletil (Zoletil 50; Virbac, Bogotá, Colombia) and 10 mg/kg xylazine (Rumpun; Bayer-Korea, Seoul, Korea) via an intramuscular injection before noise exposure. Each animal was placed in a separate wire cage to avoid unequal noise exposure, and each experiment was performed in a customized acrylic box in a sound-attenuating laboratory booth (900 mm × 900 mm × 1720 mm) with an electromagnetic shield. The animals were exposed to 2 h of broadband white noise at 115 dB SPL using a 2446-J compression driver (JBL Professional, Los Angeles, CA, USA) with an MA-620 power amplifier (Inkel, Incheon, Korea), in order to create the bilateral NIHL animal model (Supplementary Figure S2a,b). The sound intensity within the acrylic box was measured every hour using a CR152B sound level meter (Cirrus Research plc, Hunmanby, UK) to confirm that there were no alterations in the sound level during the noise-exposure treatments. The control animals were injected with the same dose of anesthetic and kept in the sound attenuating booth for the same period of time, without noise exposure [34]. Audiometry was performed at 4 h after noise-exposure treatments, to allow stable measurements to be recorded.

4.4. Auditory Brainstem Response (ABR) Recordings

The hearing function of all animals was evaluated before noise exposure using the ABR. Animals were anesthetized and placed in sound-attenuating booths. Subdermal needle electrodes were positioned at the nape of the neck as the vertex, the ipsilateral mastoid as the negative, and the contralateral mastoid as the ground (Supplementary Figure S2c) [35]. Sound stimuli tone-bursts of 4, 8, and 16 kHz (duration, 1562 μm; CoS shaping, 21 Hz) were applied. High-frequency software (ver. 3.30; Intelligent Hearing Systems, Miami, FL, USA) and high-frequency transducers (HFT9911-20-0035; Intelligent Hearing Systems) were used to measure the ABR. Before obtaining the electroencephalography signal, the impedance between the electrodes was assessed to establish whether this was less than 2 kΩ. Responses to the signal were amplified approximately 100,000-fold and band-pass filtered (100–1500 Hz). The intensity of the stimuli ranged from 90 to 20 dB SPL in 5 dB increments. A total of 512 sweeps were averaged at each intensity level. Additional ABR measurements were recorded at 4 h, and on days 1 and 3 after noise exposure. The ABR threshold was defined as the smallest stimulus intensity level that produced a visible waveform for wave II or IV.

4.5. Cochlear Whole-Mount Surface Preparation

Both control ($n = 8$) and noise-exposed ($n = 8$) animals were sacrificed under anesthesia. For each sample, the cochlea was detached from the temporal bone and fixed in 4% paraformaldehyde solution for 24 h at 4 °C. Fixed ears were washed three times in 1× phosphate-buffered saline (PBS) [36]. The thin layer of laminar bone covering the cochlea was trimmed under a SZ2-ILST stereomicroscope (Olympus Corporation, Tokyo, Japan) using a drill (Strong 90; Saeshin Precision, Daegu, Korea) with a 2 mm-diameter diamond burr attachment (Supplementary Figure S3a). A hole was created by breaking the bone between the oval and round windows using very fine forceps (Supplementary Figure S3b,c). The laminar bone was removed using a conventional 1-mm syringe needle (Supplementary Figure S3d–f). The cochlear nerve was cut and the spiral structure of the organ of Corti was isolated. Next, the stria vascularis and Reissner's membrane were removed (Supplementary Figure S3g,h). The first turn from the top of the organ of Corti was removed using scissors. This was called the 'apical turn' section. A second turn was removed and called the 'middle turn' section and a final half-turn section was removed and called the 'basal turn' section

(Supplementary Figure S3i). The sections were placed in 1× PBS solution to prevent them from drying out.

4.6. Outer HC Staining

Phalloidin was used to stain F-actin, and the photostable orange fluorescent Alexa Fluor 546 dye was used to visualize the cuticular plate and stereocilia within the HCs. After surface preparation, the isolated spiral structure of the organ of Corti was incubated in a mixed solution of 0.3% Triton X-100 and Alexa Fluor 546 phalloidin (1:100 dilution; Invitrogen, Carlsbad, CA, USA) for 45 min at room temperature in a lightproof box [37]. The sample was washed three times in 1× PBS and separated into three segments using Vannas capsulotomy scissors (E-3386; Karl Storz SE & Co. KG, Tuttlingen, Germany), consisting of the apical, middle, and basal turn sections. The first complete turn from the apex was the apical turn, the next complete turn was the middle turn, and the final half-turn was the basal turn. Each turn section was mounted on a slide using ProLong™ Gold Antifade mountant (P36930; Invitrogen) to prevent the fluorescent dyes from fading. Images were generated using a STED CW confocal laser scanning system (Leica, Wetzlar, Germany) and HCs within the images were counted.

4.7. Cochlear Histology

Cochleae from both control ($n = 8$) and noise-exposed ($n = 8$) rats were fixed and washed. Samples were decalcified using 10% (w/v) ethylenediaminetetraacetic acid (Santa Cruz Biotechnology, Dallas, TX, USA) in 1× PBS for 4 weeks. A histological examination was performed weekly to determine when the samples were ready for the embedding procedure. The tissues were dehydrated using a series of ethanol washes, and the ethanol was then removed using xylene. After the ethanol was removed, tissues were infiltrated with paraffin wax [38] in a PELORIS II tissue processing system (Leica). The processed cochleae were embedded in a stainless mold and trimmed into 4-μm-thick sagittal sections using a RM2255 microtome (Leica). The sections were deparaffinized for 1 h at 60 °C in a dry oven and cleaned using a series of ethanol washes. Next, the nuclei were stained for 7 min with hematoxylin (DAKO, Jena, Germany) and the cytoplasm was stained for 30 s with eosin Y (Sigma-Aldrich, St. Louis, MO, USA). The stained slides were dehydrated and preserved in 70% ethanol [39]. After mounting, the organ of Corti was examined using a light microscope (ECLIPSE Ci-L; Nikon, Tokyo, Japan).

4.8. RNA Extraction

Whole brain tissue was harvested, and the bilateral CN and IC were dissected out using a brain matrix. The locations of the CN (−9.30 to −11.30 mm from the bregma) and the IC (−8.30 to −9.30 mm from the bregma) were determined according to the rat brain atlas [40] (Supplementary Figure S4a–c). Tissues were frozen in liquid nitrogen immediately after removal and stored at −80 °C. The harvested tissue was lysed in 1 mL QIAzol solution using a TissueLyzerII (Qiagen, Hilden, Germany) and incubated at room temperature for 5 min. The samples were placed on a vortex mixer after adding 200 μL chloroform to each and then incubated at room temperature for 3 min. Next, the samples were centrifuged at 12,000× g for 15 min at 4 °C and the upper aqueous phase containing the RNA was removed to a fresh tube. A total of 500 μL isopropyl alcohol was added to each tube. The tubes were then inverted and incubated at room temperature for 10 min. Thereafter, the tubes were centrifuged at 7500× g for 5 min at 4 °C and the RNA pellets were washed twice with 1 mL 75% ethanol. The pellets were dried for approximately 5 min and redissolved in RNase-free water.

4.9. Analysis of miRNA Arrays

The analysis of miRNAs was performed by Ebiogen Inc. (Seoul, Korea) using the Affymetrix GeneChip miRNA 4.0 array (Affymetrix, Santa Clara, CA, USA). A total of 24 animals were randomly separated into two treatment groups and two corresponding control groups. Treated rats were exposed to noise and assayed after 1 or 3 days. After hearing loss was confirmed, the CN and IC from two animals from the same group were combined and treated as a single sample, and three samples from each group were used for the analysis. Extracted total RNA was assessed for quality and quantity using a Bioanalyzer 2100 system (Agilent, Santa Clara, CA, USA). A total of 250 ng of RNA was analyzed. After ligating biotin-labeled 3DNA dendrimers, each RNA strand was labeled using poly-A polymerase. The biotinylated RNA strands were hybridized for 18 h at 48 °C on an Affymetrix GeneChip miRNA 4.0 array. The hybridized GeneChip was washed and stained using an Affymetrix 450 Fluidics station. Fluorescence signals from the 3DNA dendrimers were detected using an Affymetrix GeneChip 3000 7G scanner.

4.10. Quantitative Reverse Transcription Polymerase Chain Reaction (qRT-PCR)

Using an miScript® II RT kit (Qiagen, Hilden, Germany), 2 µg of RNA was mixed with reverse-transcription master mix and incubated for 60 min at 37 °C. To inactivate the miScript reverse transcriptase, the mixture was incubated for 5 min at 95 °C and then placed on ice. A total of 20 µL of cDNA was diluted to 1:16 and used as template cDNA. The miScript SYBR® Green PCR kit (Qiagen) was used with miScript Primer Assay reagents (Qiagen) for qRT-PCR. U6 small nuclear RNA was used as an endogenous control gene [41]. The miScript Primer Assay reagents and the reaction mix were dispensed into wells containing template cDNA. The PCR plate was sealed with film and centrifuged at 1000× g for 1 min at room temperature. Initial activation was performed for 15 min at 95 °C. The reactions consisted of 40 cycles of denaturation, annealing, and extension, and fluorescence data were collected during the extension phase. The reactions were performed using an ABI 7500 real-time PCR system (Applied Biosystems, Foster City, CA, USA). Relative quantification values were obtained for each of the target genes using the observed cycle threshold (Ct) results and the $2^{-\Delta\Delta Ct}$ method.

4.11. Pathway Analysis of Candidate miRNAs

For the CN and IC, a total of 10 and 13 candidate miRNAs were selected from the microarray analysis based on 1.5-fold changes in normalized intensity values ($p < 0.1$) respectively. Of these, five and three miRNAs, respectively, were selected following qRT-PCR validation. Using DIANA-miRPath software (ver. 3.0), a KEGG pathway analysis was performed using DIANA-microT-CDS (ver. 5.0; DIANA TOOLS, http://diana.imis.athena-innovation.gr/DianaTools/index.php?r=microT_CDS/index) with a threshold of 0.8 and a false discovery rate correction [42,43]. A total of 12 and 14 KEGG pathways were identified for the CN and IC, respectively, using a gene union module and a p-value threshold of 0.05 and 0.3.

4.12. Statistical Analyses

All data are expressed as the means ± standard error of the mean, and all data were analyzed using SPSS software (ver. 25; IBM, Armonk, NY, USA). An F-test was performed to determine whether the levels of variation within the groups were equal. After the F-test, data were analyzed using Student's t-tests to identify significant differences between groups. A p-value of <0.05 was considered statistically significant.

5. Conclusions

Using a noise exposure animal model, we were able to show that even acute short-term noise exposure can lead to hearing loss. Changes in the ABR amplitude of wave II suggest an alteration in either synaptic transmission or the number of neuronal cells. To investigate the role of miRNAs in the central auditory pathway, CN and IC were compared in both the treatment and control groups, with microarray analysis and qRT-PCR results suggesting that *miR-200b-3p*, *miR-183-5p*, *miR-411-3p*, *miR-20b-5p*, *miR-377-3p*, *miR-92a-1-5p*, *miR-136-3p*, and *miR-26b-5p* may play key roles in the neuroplasticity of the central auditory pathway. Using the KEGG database, we found that five of these candidate miRNAs may be involved in the MAPK signaling pathway, axon guidance, and the neurotrophin signaling pathway in the CN, while an additional three candidate miRNAs may influence the MAPK signaling pathway in the IC. Further validation of these candidate miRNAs will be achieved using miRNA oligomers such as mimics and inhibitors, in order to better refine the specific signaling pathways underlying these processes. These target miRNAs, which play crucial roles in the central auditory pathway, can be used for diagnosis in the early stage of NIHL, and for treatment of the damage caused by the cellular and physiological changes after NIHL.

Supplementary Materials: Supplementary Materials can be found at http://www.mdpi.com/1422-0067/21/22/8792/s1.

Author Contributions: Conceptualization, J.H.L. and S.H.O.; methodology, B.-G.K.; validation, B.-G.K. and S.H.H.; formal analysis, B.-G.K. and S.H.H.; investigation, M.-W.S. and S.H.O.; resources, M.-W.S. and J.H.L.; data curation, S.H.H.; writing—original draft preparation, S.P. and M.K.P.; writing—review and editing, S.P. and M.K.P.; visualization, S.P.; supervision, J.H.L. and S.H.O.; project administration, S.H.H. and S.P.; funding acquisition, S.P. and M.K.P. All authors have read and agreed to the published version of the manuscript.

Funding: This research was supported by the Basic Science Research Program through the National Research Foundation of Korea (NRF) funded by the Ministry of Science, ICT & Future Planning (NRF-2017R1D1A 1B03034832) and the SNUH Research Fund (03-2020-0240).

Conflicts of Interest: The authors declare no conflict of interest. The funders had no role in the design of the study; in the collection, analyses, or interpretation of data; in the writing of the manuscript; or in the decision to publish the results.

Abbreviations

ABR	Auditory Brainstem Response
CN	Cochlear Nucleus
HC	Hair Cell
IC	Inferior Colliculus
KEGG	Kyoto Encyclopedia of Genes and Genomics
MAPK	Mitogen-Activated Protein Kinase
MiRNA	MicroRNA
NIHL	Noise-induced Hearing Loss
PFN2	Profilin2
PTS	Permanent Threshold Shift
SAPK/JNK	Stress-Activated Protein Kinase/c-Jun NH(2)-terminal Kinase
SNHL	Sensorineural Hearing Loss
SOC	Superior Olivary Complex
SPL	Sound Pressure Level
TTS	Temporary Threshold Shift
TGF-β	transforming growth factor-beta
VCN	Ventral Cochlear Nucleus

References

1. World Health Organization. *Deafness and Hearing Loss*. 20 March 2019. Available online: https://www.who.int/news-room/fact-sheets/detail/deafness-and-hearing-loss (accessed on 17 February 2019).
2. Barker, A.B.; Leighton, P.; Ferguson, M.A. Coping together with hearing loss: A qualitative meta-synthesis of the psychosocial experiences of people with hearing loss and their communication partners. *Int. J. Audiol.* **2017**, *56*, 297–305. [CrossRef] [PubMed]
3. Le, T.N.; Straatman, L.V.; Lea, J.; Westerberg, B. Current insights in noise-induced hearing loss: A literature review of the underlying mechanism, pathophysiology, asymmetry, and management options. *J. Otolaryngol. Head Neck Surg.* **2017**, *46*, 41. [CrossRef] [PubMed]
4. Ryan, A.F.; Kujawa, S.G.; Hammill, T.; Le Prell, C.; Kil, J. Temporary and Permanent Noise-induced Threshold Shifts: A Review of Basic and Clinical Observations. *Otol. Neurotol.* **2016**, *37*, e271–e275. [CrossRef] [PubMed]
5. Wang, W.; Zhang, L.S.; Zinsmaier, A.K.; Patterson, G.; Leptich, E.J.; Shoemaker, S.L.; Yatskievych, T.A.; Gibboni, R.; Pace, E.; Luo, H.; et al. Neuroinflammation mediates noise-induced synaptic imbalance and tinnitus in rodent models. *PLoS Biol.* **2019**, *17*, e3000307. [CrossRef] [PubMed]

6. Shin, S.-O. Updates in Noise Induced Hearing Loss. *Korean J. Otorhinolaryngol. Head Neck Surg.* **2014**, *57*, 584. [CrossRef]
7. Tang, C.; Wang, H.; Wu, H.; Yan, S.; Han, Z.; Jiang, Z.; Na, M.; Guo, M.; Lu, D.; Lin, Z. The MicroRNA Expression Profiles of Human Temporal Lobe Epilepsy in HS ILAE Type 1. *Cell Mol. Neurobiol.* **2019**, *39*, 461–470. [CrossRef]
8. Minones-Moyano, E.; Porta, S.; Escaramis, G.; Rabionet, R.; Iraola, S.; Kagerbauer, B.; Espinosa-Parrilla, Y.; Ferrer, I.; Estivill, X.; Marti, E. MicroRNA profiling of Parkinson's disease brains identifies early downregulation of miR-34b/c which modulate mitochondrial function. *Hum. Mol. Genet.* **2011**, *20*, 3067–3078. [CrossRef]
9. Maffioletti, E.; Cattaneo, A.; Rosso, G.; Maina, G.; Maj, C.; Gennarelli, M.; Tardito, D.; Bocchio-Chiavetto, L. Peripheral whole blood microRNA alterations in major depression and bipolar disorder. *J. Affect. Disord.* **2016**, *200*, 250–258. [CrossRef]
10. Rupaimoole, R.; Slack, F.J. MicroRNA therapeutics: Towards a new era for the management of cancer and other diseases. *Nat. Rev. Drug Discov.* **2017**, *16*, 203–222. [CrossRef]
11. To, K.K.W.; Fong, W.; Tong, C.W.S.; Wu, M.; Yan, W.; Cho, W.C.S. Advances in the discovery of microRNA-based anticancer therapeutics: Latest tools and developments. *Expert Opin. Drug Discov.* **2020**, *15*, 63–83. [CrossRef]
12. Kandel, E.R. *Principles of Neural Science*, 5th ed.; McGraw-Hill: New York, NY, USA, 2013; p. l. 1709p.
13. Sonntag, M.; Blosa, M.; Schmidt, S.; Rubsamen, R.; Morawski, M. Perineuronal nets in the auditory system. *Hear. Res.* **2015**, *329*, 21–32. [CrossRef] [PubMed]
14. Ono, M.; Ito, T. Functional organization of the mammalian auditory midbrain. *J. Physiol. Sci.* **2015**, *65*, 499–506. [CrossRef] [PubMed]
15. Alvarado, J.C.; Fuentes-Santamaria, V.; Jareno-Flores, T.; Blanco, J.L.; Juiz, J.M. Normal variations in the morphology of auditory brainstem response (ABR) waveforms: A study in Wistar rats. *Neurosci. Res.* **2012**, *73*, 302–311. [CrossRef] [PubMed]
16. Sugawara, M.; Corfas, G.; Liberman, M.C. Influence of supporting cells on neuronal degeneration after hair cell loss. *J. Assoc. Res. Otolaryngol.* **2005**, *6*, 136–147. [CrossRef] [PubMed]
17. Tagoe, T.; Barker, M.; Jones, A.; Allcock, N.; Hamann, M. Auditory nerve perinodal dysmyelination in noise-induced hearing loss. *J. Neurosci.* **2014**, *34*, 2684–2688. [CrossRef] [PubMed]
18. Mehraei, G.; Hickox, A.E.; Bharadwaj, H.M.; Goldberg, H.; Verhulst, S.; Liberman, M.C.; Shinn-Cunningham, B.G. Auditory Brainstem Response Latency in Noise as a Marker of Cochlear Synaptopathy. *J. Neurosci.* **2016**, *36*, 3755–3764. [CrossRef] [PubMed]
19. Liu, H.; Lu, J.; Wang, Z.; Song, L.; Wang, X.; Li, G.L.; Wu, H. Functional alteration of ribbon synapses in inner hair cells by noise exposure causing hidden hearing loss. *Neurosci. Lett.* **2019**, *707*, 134268. [CrossRef]
20. Schrode, K.M.; Muniak, M.A.; Kim, Y.H.; Lauer, A.M. Central Compensation in Auditory Brainstem after Damaging Noise Exposure. *eNeuro* **2018**, *5*. [CrossRef]
21. Shore, S.E.; Koehler, S.; Oldakowski, M.; Hughes, L.F.; Syed, S. Dorsal cochlear nucleus responses to somatosensory stimulation are enhanced after noise-induced hearing loss. *Eur. J. Neurosci.* **2008**, *27*, 155–168. [CrossRef]
22. Abadi, S.P.; Khanbabaee, G.M.; Sheibani, K.M. Auditory Brainstem Response Wave Amplitude Characteristics as a Diagnostic Tool in Children with Speech Delay with Unknown Causes. *Iran. J. Med. Sci.* **2016**, *41*, 415–421.
23. Liberman, M.C. Noise-Induced Hearing Loss: Permanent Versus Temporary Threshold Shifts and the Effects of Hair Cell Versus Neuronal Degeneration. *Adv. Exp. Med. Biol.* **2016**, *875*, 1–7. [CrossRef] [PubMed]
24. Shi, L.; Chang, Y.; Li, X.; Aiken, S.; Liu, L.; Wang, J. Cochlear Synaptopathy and Noise-Induced Hidden Hearing Loss. *Neural Plast.* **2016**, *2016*, 6143164. [CrossRef] [PubMed]
25. Basta, D.; Groschel, M.; Ernst, A. Central and peripheral aspects of noise-induced hearing loss. *HNO* **2018**, *66*, 342–349. [CrossRef] [PubMed]
26. Alagramam, K.N.; Stepanyan, R.; Jamesdaniel, S.; Chen, D.H.; Davis, R.R. Noise exposure immediately activates cochlear mitogen-activated protein kinase signaling. *Noise Health* **2014**, *16*, 400–409. [CrossRef]
27. Schacht, J.; Fay, R.R. *Auditory Trauma, Protection, and Repair*; Springer: New York, NY, USA, 2008.
28. Gerken, G.M. Central tinnitus and lateral inhibition: An auditory brainstem model. *Hear. Res.* **1996**, *97*, 75–83. [CrossRef]
29. Mun, S.K.; Han, K.H.; Baek, J.T.; Ahn, S.W.; Cho, H.S.; Chang, M.Y. Losartan Prevents Maladaptive Auditory-Somatosensory Plasticity After Hearing Loss via Transforming Growth Factor-beta Signaling Suppression. *Clin. Exp. Otorhinolaryngol.* **2019**, *12*, 33–39. [CrossRef]

30. Bartels, H.; Staal, M.J.; Albers, F.W. Tinnitus and neural plasticity of the brain. *Otol. Neurotol.* **2007**, *28*, 178–184. [CrossRef]
31. Kurabi, A.; Keithley, E.M.; Housley, G.D.; Ryan, A.F.; Wong, A.C. Cellular mechanisms of noise-induced hearing loss. *Hear. Res.* **2017**, *349*, 129–137. [CrossRef]
32. Jeong, D.H.; Choi, Y.N.; Seo, T.W.; Lee, J.S.; Yoo, S.J. Ubiquitin-proteasome dependent regulation of Profilin2 (Pfn2) by a cellular inhibitor of apoptotic protein 1 (cIAP1). *Biochem. Biophys. Res. Commun.* **2018**, *506*, 423–428. [CrossRef]
33. Lobarinas, E.; Spankovich, C.; Le Prell, C.G. Evidence of "hidden hearing loss" following noise exposures that produce robust TTS and ABR wave-I amplitude reductions. *Hear. Res.* **2017**, *349*, 155–163. [CrossRef]
34. Shi, Z.T.; Lin, Y.; Wang, J.; Wu, J.; Wang, R.F.; Chen, F.Q.; Mi, W.J.; Qiu, J.H. G-CSF attenuates noise-induced hearing loss. *Neurosci. Lett.* **2014**, *562*, 102–106. [CrossRef] [PubMed]
35. Chang, M.Y.; Rhee, J.; Kim, S.H.; Kim, Y.H. The Protective Effect of Egb 761 Against 3-Nitropropionic Acid-Induced Hearing Loss: The Role of Sirtuin 1. *Clin. Exp. Otorhinolaryngol.* **2018**, *11*, 9–16. [CrossRef] [PubMed]
36. Paciello, F.; Fetoni, A.R.; Rolesi, R.; Wright, M.B.; Grassi, C.; Troiani, D.; Paludetti, G. Pioglitazone Represents an Effective Therapeutic Target in Preventing Oxidative/Inflammatory Cochlear Damage Induced by Noise Exposure. *Front. Pharmacol.* **2018**, *9*, 1103. [CrossRef] [PubMed]
37. Frimmer, M. What We Have Learned from Phalloidin. *Toxicol. Lett.* **1987**, *35*, 169–182. [CrossRef]
38. Zhu, G.J.; Wang, F.; Chen, C.; Xu, L.; Zhang, W.C.; Fan, C.; Peng, Y.J.; Chen, J.; He, W.Q.; Guo, S.Y.; et al. Myosin light-chain kinase is necessary for membrane homeostasis in cochlear inner hair cells. *PLoS ONE* **2012**, *7*, e34894. [CrossRef]
39. Fischer, A.H.; Jacobson, K.A.; Rose, J.; Zeller, R. Hematoxylin and eosin staining of tissue and cell sections. *CSH Protoc.* **2008**, *2008*, pdb prot4986. [CrossRef] [PubMed]
40. Paxinos, G.; Watson, C. *The Rat Brain in Stereotaxic Coordinates*; Elsevier/Academic: Amsterdam, The Netherlands, 2009.
41. Luo, M.; Gao, Z.; Li, H.; Li, Q.; Zhang, C.; Xu, W.; Song, S.; Ma, C.; Wang, S. Selection of reference genes for miRNA qRT-PCR under abiotic stress in grapevine. *Sci. Rep.* **2018**, *8*, 4444. [CrossRef]
42. Vlachos, I.S.; Zagganas, K.; Paraskevopoulou, M.D.; Georgakilas, G.; Karagkouni, D.; Vergoulis, T.; Dalamagas, T.; Hatzigeorgiou, A.G. DIANA-miRPath v3.0: Deciphering microRNA function with experimental support. *Nucleic Acids Res.* **2015**, *43*, W460–W466. [CrossRef]
43. Paraskevopoulou, M.D.; Georgakilas, G.; Kostoulas, N.; Vlachos, I.S.; Vergoulis, T.; Reczko, M.; Filippidis, C.; Dalamagas, T.; Hatzigeorgiou, A.G. DIANA-microT web server v5.0: Service integration into miRNA functional analysis workflows. *Nucleic Acids Res.* **2013**, *41*, W169–W173. [CrossRef]

Publisher's Note: MDPI stays neutral with regard to jurisdictional claims in published maps and institutional affiliations.

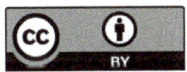

© 2020 by the authors. Licensee MDPI, Basel, Switzerland. This article is an open access article distributed under the terms and conditions of the Creative Commons Attribution (CC BY) license (http://creativecommons.org/licenses/by/4.0/).

Regulator of G Protein Signalling 4 (RGS4) as a Novel Target for the Treatment of Sensorineural Hearing Loss

Christine Fok, Milan Bogosanovic, Madhavi Pandya, Ravindra Telang, Peter R. Thorne and Srdjan M. Vlajkovic *

Department of Physiology and The Eisdell Moore Centre, Faculty of Medical and Health Sciences, The University of Auckland, Private Bag 92019, Auckland 1142, New Zealand; c.fok@auckland.ac.nz (C.F.); milan.bogosanovic@uq.net.au (M.B.); m.pandya@auckland.ac.nz (M.P.); r.telang@auckland.ac.nz (R.T.); pr.thorne@auckland.ac.nz (P.R.T.)
* Correspondence: s.vlajkovic@auckland.ac.nz; Tel.: +64-9-9239782

Abstract: We and others have previously identified signalling pathways associated with the adenosine A_1 receptor (A_1R) as important regulators of cellular responses to injury in the cochlea. We have shown that the "post-exposure" treatment with adenosine A_1R agonists confers partial protection against acoustic trauma and other forms of sensorineural hearing loss (SNHL). The aim of this study was to determine if increasing A_1R responsiveness to endogenous adenosine would have the same otoprotective effect. This was achieved by pharmacological targeting of the Regulator of G protein Signalling 4 (RGS4). RGS proteins inhibit signal transduction pathways initiated by G protein-coupled receptors (GPCR) by enhancing GPCR deactivation and receptor desensitisation. A molecular complex between RGS4 and neurabin, an intracellular scaffolding protein expressed in neural and cochlear tissues, is the key negative regulator of A_1R activity in the brain. In this study, Wistar rats (6–8 weeks) were exposed to traumatic noise (110 dBSPL, 8–16 kHz) for 2 h and a small molecule RGS4 inhibitor CCG-4986 was delivered intratympanically in a Poloxamer-407 gel formulation for sustained drug release 24 or 48 h after noise exposure. Intratympanic administration of CCG-4986 48 h after noise exposure attenuated noise-induced permanent auditory threshold shifts by up to 19 dB, whilst the earlier drug administration (24 h) led to even better preservation of auditory thresholds (up to 32 dB). Significant improvement of auditory thresholds and suprathreshold responses was linked to improved survival of sensorineural tissues and afferent synapses in the cochlea. Our studies thus demonstrate that intratympanic administration of CCG-4986 can rescue cochlear injury and hearing loss induced by acoustic overexposure. This research represents a novel paradigm for the treatment of various forms of SNHL based on regulation of GPCR.

Keywords: sensorineural hearing loss; noise-induced cochlear injury; cochlear rescue; otoprotection; adenosine A_1 receptor; regulator of G protein signalling 4; CCG-4986; intratympanic drug delivery

1. Introduction

Hearing loss is the most prevalent form of sensory impairment, affecting about 466 million people worldwide including 34 million children [1]. Most of the hearing loss is sensorineural due to disease, degeneration, or trauma to the cochlea of the inner ear [2]. Treatment options for sensorineural hearing loss (SNHL) are currently limited to prosthetic devices such as hearing aids and cochlear implants. Both devices can partly restore auditory function, but these have limitations because the ear remains damaged. There is thus a significant need for the development of effective therapies to prevent cochlear damage and hearing loss or restore cochlear sensorineural structure and hearing. We have identified that signalling pathways activated by adenosine receptors are important regulators of cellular responses to injury in cochlear tissues. Animal studies reveal that stimulation of the A_1 adenosine receptor (A_1R) is particularly promising for the treatment of acute noise-induced cochlear injury [3,4] and other forms of SNHL such as from cytotoxic drugs, including cisplatin and aminoglycoside antibiotics [5,6]. The principal advantage of this approach is that the A_1R stimulation affects multiple mechanisms of cochlear injury (e.g., oxidative stress, glutamate excitotoxicity, activation of apoptotic pathways), thus providing comprehensive protection from SNHL [7]. One of the issues with advancing these approaches to clinical applicability is the delivery of receptor agonists to the inner ear and their suitability for long-term therapy.

As an alternative to the use of exogenous A_1R agonists, we have previously considered other strategies that would regulate the action of endogenous adenosine, for example by manipulating intracellular adenosine metabolism [8]. Recently, we have identified a novel otoprotective paradigm based on increasing A_1R responsiveness to endogenous adenosine, which can be achieved by inhibiting the Regulator of G protein Signalling 4 (RGS4). RGS is a large family of proteins that inhibit signal transduction pathways initiated by G protein-coupled receptors (GPCR) including A_1R [9–11]. RGS increase the intrinsic GTPase activity of G proteins and thus enhance G protein inactivation and promote receptor desensitisation [9].

In the past two decades, RGS proteins have received increasing interest as potential drug targets in cardiovascular disease, CNS disorders and several types of cancer [12–15]. Targeted inhibition of RGS proteins could potentially provide a way to fine-tune GPCR signalling by potentiating or prolonging the effect of receptor agonists. This approach could also be used to enhance endogenous ligand effects on GPCR. A few small molecule RGS inhibitors have been identified, particularly in the well-studied RGS4 family [16,17]. The selectivity of RGS proteins is mediated either through direct interaction with target receptors, or through selective interactions with accessory proteins [16]. For example, the neurabin-RGS4 molecular complex regulates A_1R signalling events in the brain. Neurabin is an intracellular scaffolding protein (protein phosphatase 1 regulatory inhibitor subunit 9a, PPP1R9A) expressed in neural tissues which facilitates interactions of RGS4 with the A_1R [18]. After A_1R stimulation by endogenous or exogenous ligands, neurabin forms a complex with RGS4 and recruits it to the cell surface to the A_1R [18]. Disruption of the neurabin-RGS4 complex, either by genetic deletion of neurabin or by selective inhibitors of RGS4, enhances A_1R signalling even without administration of exogenous A_1R ligands. Mice with genetic deletion of neurabin are protected against kainate-induced seizures, evidenced by reduced severity and occurrence of seizures, improved neuronal survival and overall lower mortality [18]. Similarly, this anticonvulsant and neuroprotective effect is also conferred by CCG-4986, a small molecule inhibitor of RGS4 [18]. The neurabin/RGS4 complex thus appears to be the key regulator of A_1R activity in the brain and a promising neuroprotective target.

Here, we investigated an otoprotective strategy based on inhibition of the neurabin/RGS4 complex in the cochlea, with the aim to increase A_1R responsiveness to endogenous adenosine released from cochlear tissues during acoustic stress. This novel otoprotective strategy is based on intratympanic injection of a small molecule RGS4 inhibitor to the round window membrane (RWM) of the cochlea.

2. Results

2.1. Expression and Immunolocalisation of RGS4 and Neurabin I in the Cochlea

RT-PCR demonstrated the expression of neurabin isoforms I and II in the rat cochlea (Figure 1A). Generated PCR products corresponded to the predicted sizes of DNA fragments (Table 1). Omitting reverse transcriptase (-RT) in control reactions resulted in the absence of reaction products (Figure 1A). As only the neurabin I isoform makes complexes with RGS4 and the A_1R, immunolocalisation studies were only performed for this isoform. Neurabin I was immunolocalised in the inner and outer hair cells in the organ of Corti and cell bodies of the spiral ganglion neurons (Figure 1B). Neurabin I distribution in sensory hair cells and spiral ganglion neurons coincided with the RGS4 immunofluorescence pattern (Figure 1C). In addition, RGS4 immunofluorescence was observed in the auditory nerve fibres in the osseous spiral lamina and blood vessels in the spiral limbus (Figure 1C).

No immunofluorescence was detected when the primary antibody was replaced with control mouse IgG (Figure 1D) or control rabbit IgG (not shown).

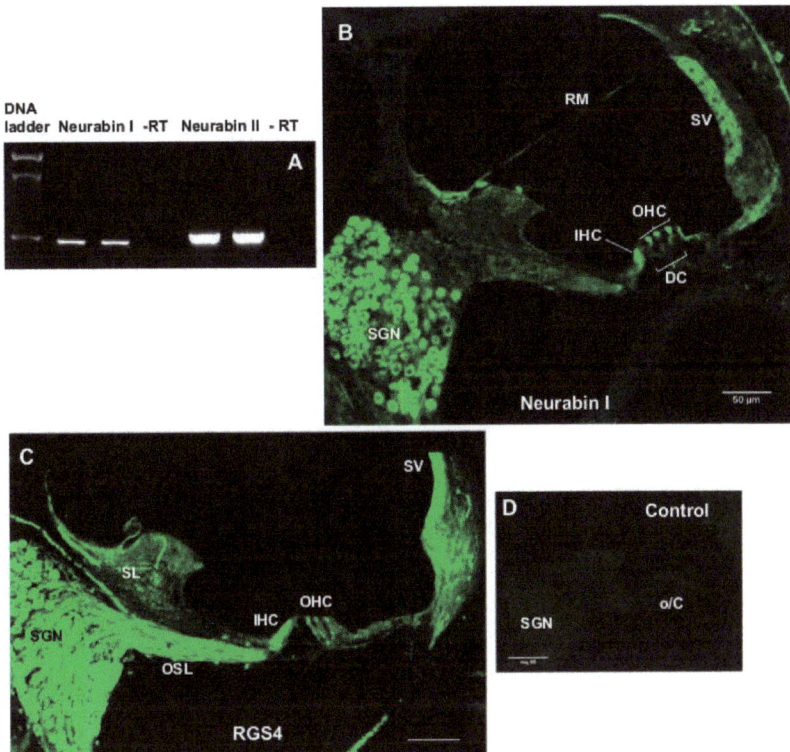

Figure 1. (**A**) Expression of Neurabin I and II isoforms in the rat cochlea. PCR products (shown in duplicates) correspond to the neurabin I (520 bp) and neurabin II (561 bp) isoforms, respectively. In the absence of reverse transcriptase (-RT controls) no amplification was observed. (**B**) The most prominent neurabin I immunostaining was observed in sensory inner hair cells (IHC) and outer hair cells (OHC) in the organ of Corti (o/C) and spiral ganglion neurons (SGN). (**C**) The RGS4 antibody also demonstrated predilection for sensory hair cells (IHC and OHC) and SGN. RGS4 immunofluorescence was also observed in the auditory nerve fibres in the osseous spiral lamina (OSL) and blood vessels in the spiral limbus (SL). (**D**) Control section where the primary antibody was replaced by IgG isotype control. Abbreviations: DC, Deiters' cells; RM, Reissner's membrane; SV, stria vascularis. Scale bars, 50 μM.

Table 1. Primer sequences and positions for neurabin I and II isoforms.

Primer	Forward (Sense)	Reverse (Antisense)
Neurabin I (NM_053473)	5′-GGAGCCGTTAGAAGATGCTG-3′ position: 1247–1266	5′-CCCATCCTCATCTTTCTCCA-3′ position: 1766–1747
Neurabin II (NM_053474)	5′-GAGTGGAGAGGTTGGAGCTG-3′ position: 1976–1995	5′-GGAGCTCCTTGAACTTGTGC-3′ position: 2536–2517

Expected amplicon length: Neurabin I—520 bp, Neurabin II—561 bp.

2.2. Auditory Brainstem Responses and the Effect of Treatment 48 Hours after Noise Exposure

Auditory brainstem responses (ABR) were used to measure auditory thresholds prior to noise exposure (baseline), and 16 days after noise exposure (final) to determine noise-induced threshold shifts.

The baseline auditory thresholds were similar in noise-exposed and non-exposed animals (Figure 2A–C). The control group exposed to ambient noise levels in the animal facility showed no change in ABR thresholds 16 days after initial ABR measurement (Figure 2A). In contrast, exposure to octave band noise (8–16 kHz at 110 dB SPL) for two hours induced a permanent threshold shift (PTS) in both drug- and vehicle-treated animals (Figure 2B–D). In the control vehicle-treated group, the average threshold shift was between 40 and 50 dB at frequencies above 4 kHz (Figure 2B,D). ABR thresholds were still elevated after treatment with CCG-4986 (100 µM), but to a lesser degree than in control drug vehicle-treated animals (Figure 2C). At mid-to-high frequencies (8–28 kHz), CCG-4986 treatment reduced noise-induced PTS by 10–19 dB compared to the vehicle-treated animals (Figure 2D). The greatest improvement of ABR thresholds was observed at 8–16 kHz (Figure 2D), with average threshold shift reductions of 19 dB at 8 kHz ($p = 0.029$), 19 dB at 12 kHz ($p = 0.018$) and 17 dB at 16 kHz ($p = 0.013$).

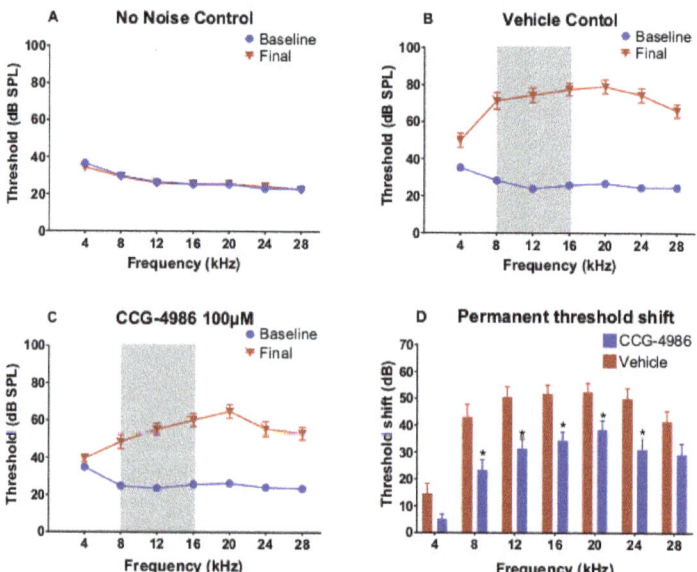

Figure 2. Baseline and final auditory brainstem responses (ABR) thresholds for 4–28 kHz tone pips in animals exposed to octave band noise (8–16 kHz, 110 dB SPL) for 2 h and non-exposed animals. Grey area denotes noise band. (**A**) Controls exposed to ambient noise (55–65 dB SPL) in the animal facility. (**B**) Noise-exposed vehicle-treated control group. (**C**) Animals treated with CCG-4986 (100 µM) 48 h post-exposure. (**D**) Comparison of permanent threshold shifts 16 days post-exposure in drug- and vehicle-treated animals. Data presented as mean ± SEM. No noise control, $n = 10$; Vehicle control, $n = 16$; CCG-4986, $n = 17$. * $p < 0.05$; Two-way ANOVA followed by Holm–Sidak post-hoc test.

2.3. Input–Output Functions

To further investigate the otoprotective effects of CCG-4986 treatment, three frequencies (4 kHz, 16 kHz and 28 kHz), were selected as representative of the low, mid, and high frequency regions of the cochlea, respectively. The amplitudes and latencies of wave I were analysed at suprathreshold intensities (80, 85, and 90 dB; Figure 3A).

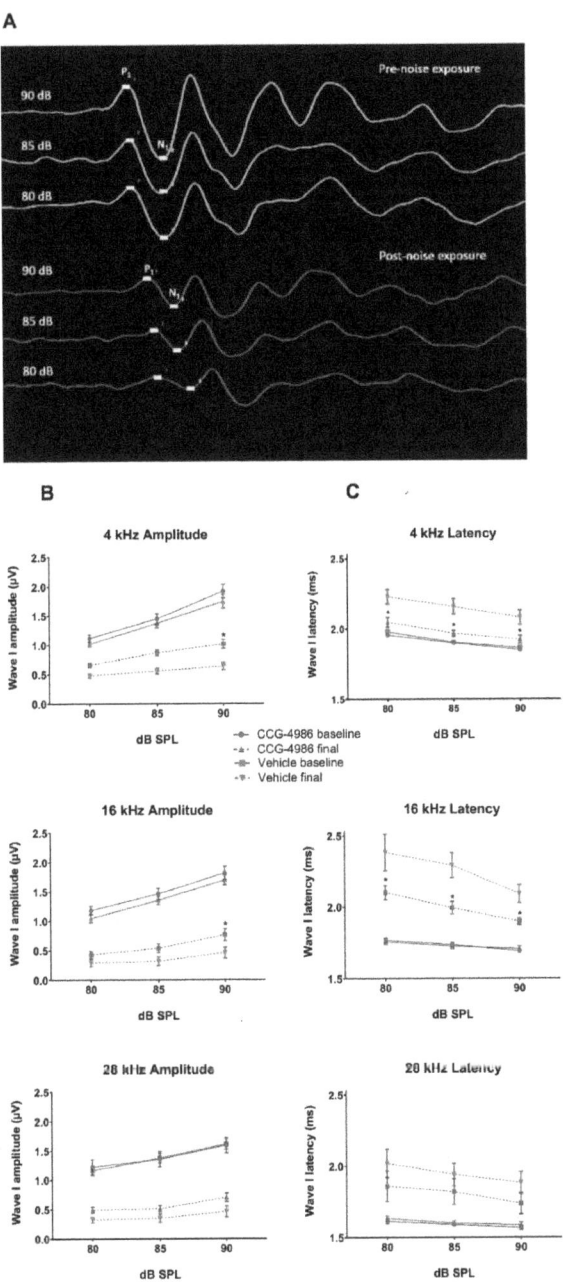

Figure 3. (**A**) Representative traces of ABR Wave I prior to noise exposure (green) and post-exposure (red). P_1 represents a positive peak and N_1 a negative peak. ABR responses were recorded at 16 kHz at suprathreshold intensities (80–90 dB SPL). Average baseline and final ABR wave I amplitudes (**B**) and latencies (**C**) at suprathreshold intensities in noise-exposed animals treated with CCG-4986 (100 μM) or drug vehicle solution 48 h after noise exposure. Solid lines represent baseline amplitudes/latencies and dashed lines represent final amplitudes/latencies. Data presented as mean ± SEM, Vehicle control, $n = 16$; CCG-4986, $n = 17$. * $p < 0.05$; Multivariate ANOVA followed by planned contrast comparisons.

Prior to noise exposure, ABR Wave I amplitudes and latencies were similar in drug- and vehicle-treated rats at each test frequency. As expected, wave I amplitudes decreased, and latencies increased after noise exposure in all animals (Figure 3B,C).

The vehicle-treated control animals showed an average 60–70% reduction in wave I amplitude at 90 dB, with 16 kHz as the most affected frequency (70% reduction). CCG-4986 treatment improved wave I amplitudes compared to vehicle-treated rats, which was significant for 4 kHz ($p = 0.03$) and 16 kHz ($p = 0.05$) at 90 dB (Figure 3B). At 28 kHz the effect of CCG-4986 treatment was not significant ($p = 0.052$).

After noise exposure, wave I latency increased by 10–22% in vehicle-treated animals, with the greatest increase at 16 kHz (Figure 3C). CCG-4986 treatment significantly ($p < 0.05$) reduced wave I latencies 4 kHz and 16 kHz compared to vehicle-treated animals, although the latencies remained elevated relative to pre-noise levels (Figure 3C).

2.4. Hair Cell Survival

As expected from exposure to the octave band noise (8–16 kHz), turn-related differences in hair cell loss were observed in both vehicle- and drug-treated animals. The loss of outer hair cells (OHC; Figure 4A) exceeded the loss of the inner hair cells (IHC; Figure 4C) in both the middle and the basal segment of the cochlea (Figure 4B). The most heavily affected region was the basal segment of the cochlea (Figure 4B), whilst there was virtually no hair cell loss in the apical segment (data not shown).

The average OHC loss in vehicle-treated animals was 38% ± 10.1% and 85% ± 5.7% in the middle and basal segments, respectively (Figure 4B). Treatment with CCG-4986 reduced OHC loss to 8.7% ± 4% ($p = 0.0027$) in the middle segment and to 25% ± 5.4% ($p < 0.001$) in the basal segment (Figure 4B).

The average IHC loss in the middle turn was low (~2%), and there was no difference between the drug- and vehicle-treated animals (Figure 4B). In contrast, the survival of IHC in the basal turn was significantly improved with CCG-4986 treatment (12.0% ± 3.5%) compared to vehicle-treated controls (32% ± 6.4%; $p = 0.0008$).

2.5. Synaptic Ribbon Counts

Confocal imaging of afferent synapses in controls exposed to ambient noise showed turn-related differences in the average number of paired synapses per IHC (Figure 5A–C). The greatest number of synapses was found in the middle turn (Figure 5B), with an average of 24.3 ± 0.4 paired synapses per IHC. In comparison, apical and basal turns had an average of 19.8 ± 0.2 and 22.4 ± 0.6 synapses per IHC respectively (Figure 5A,C). To identify and quantify afferent synapses, whole mounts of the organ of Corti were immunolabelled with antibodies to CtBP2 (component of the presynaptic ribbon), GluA2 subunit (postsynaptic glutamate receptor) and myosin VIIa (IHC) (Figure 5E–H).

Under ambient noise levels (no-noise controls), vast majority of synaptic ribbons were paired with the post-synaptic GluA2 receptor (Figure 5F). Only about 1% of synapses were characterised as orphan synapses (unpaired pre-synaptic ribbon or post-synaptic glutamate receptor). The percentage of orphan synapses, however increases with noise exposure (Figure 5D,E,G,H).

The number of synapses in the apical turn was similar in non-exposed and noise-exposed animals, regardless of the treatment (Figure 5A). At higher frequencies, noise exposure significantly reduced the number of paired synapses. In animals treated with drug vehicle solution, the number of paired synapses decreased to 15.9 ± 2.0 and 17.0 ± 1.8 in the middle and basal turns respectively (Figure 5B,C). There was also a significant increase in the proportion of orphan synapses in these regions (10% and 8% respectively; Figure 5D).

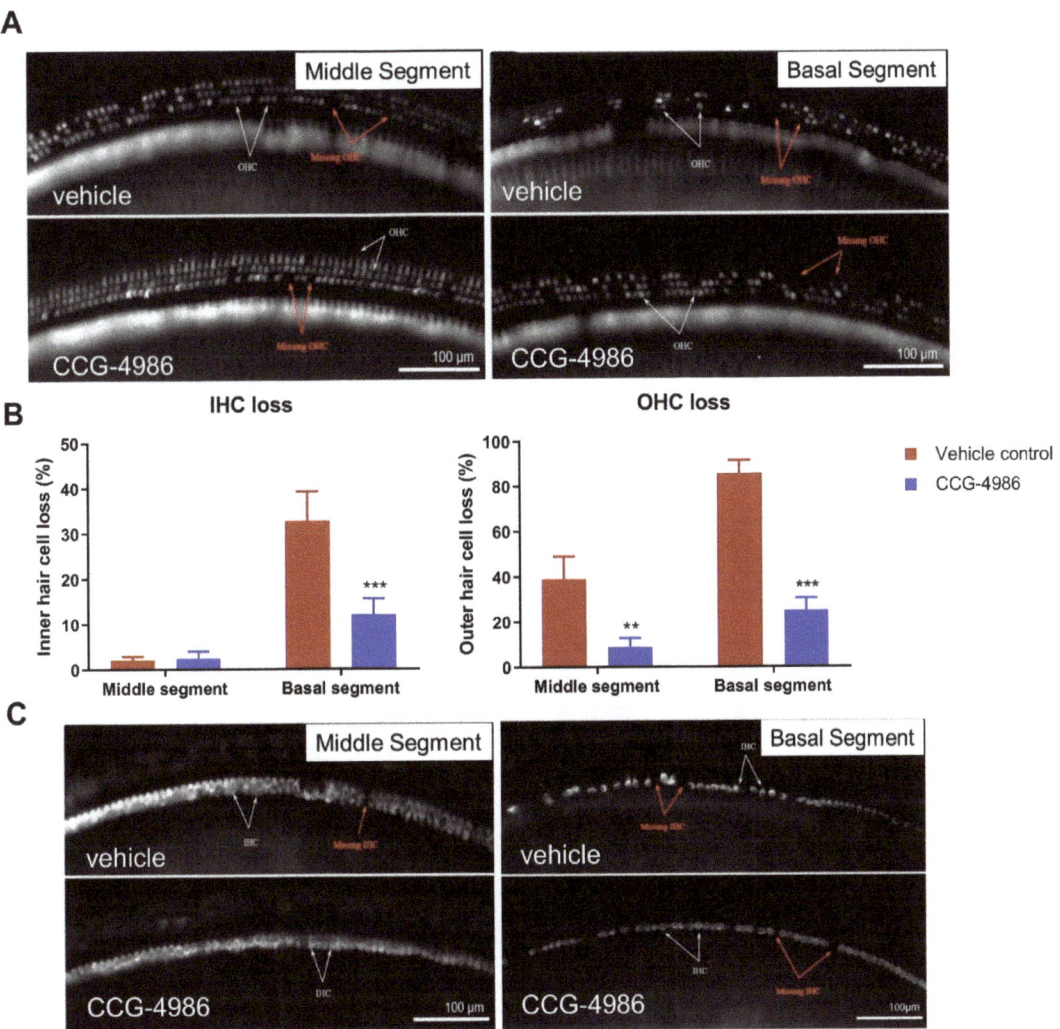

Figure 4. (**A**) Representative images of OHC in the middle and the basal segment of the cochlea in noise-exposed vehicle-treated and CCG-4986 treated animals. (**B**) Percentage of hair cell loss (OHC and IHC) in the middle and basal cochlear segments of vehicle- and CCG-4986 treated animals. Data presented as mean ± SEM, vehicle control n = 16, CCG-4986 n = 17. ** p <0.01, *** p < 0.0001; Two-way ANOVA followed by Holm–Sidak post-hoc test. (**C**) Representative images of IHC in the middle and the basal segment of the cochlea of vehicle-treated and CCG-4986 treated animals. White arrows point at the sensory hair cells and red arrows at spaces with missing hair cells.

Treatment with CCG-4986 significantly (p = 0.0085) reduced the loss of synapses in the middle turn (Figure 5B) but did not improve the survival of afferent synapses in the basal turn (Figure 5C). In the middle turn, the number of paired synapses improved to 21.1 ± 1.3 synapses per IHC in CCG-4986-treated animals, which was similar to the number of synapses in non-noise exposed controls (Figure 5B).

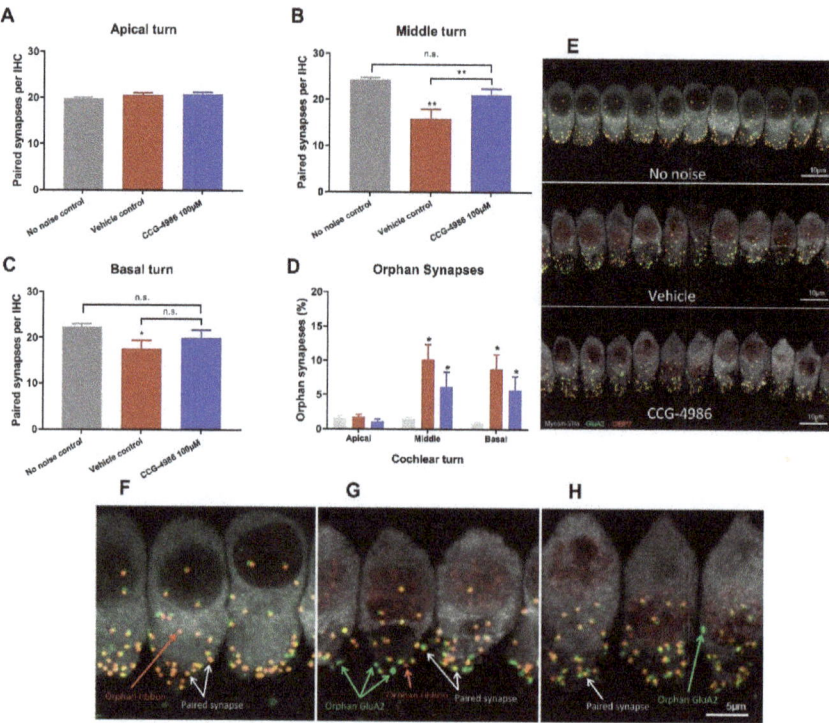

Figure 5. The average number of synapses per IHC at various frequency regions of the cochlea. (**A**) Number of paired synapses in the apical turn (low frequency region), (**B**) Middle turn (mid frequency region) and (**C**) Basal turn (high frequency region). (**D**) Number of orphaned synapses in all turns expressed as a percentage of total synapses per IHC. Data presented as mean ± SEM. No-noise control, $n = 10$, vehicle-treated, $n = 16$, CCG-4986 treated, $n = 17$. * $p < 0.05$, ** $p < 0.01$, n.s. not significant. One-way ANOVA followed by Holm–Sidak post-hoc test. (**E**) Representative images of IHC-auditory nerve synapses in the middle turn for controls exposed to traumatic or ambient noise. Labelling shows IHCs (grey), post-synaptic glutamate receptors (green) and pre-synaptic ribbons (red). (**F–H**) High power projection of IHC synapses in (**F**) No-noise controls, (**G**) Noise-exposed vehicle-treated and (**H**) Noise-exposed CCG-4986-treated animals. White arrows indicate paired ribbon synapses, green arrows orphaned post-synaptic glutamate receptors, and red arrows orphaned pre-synaptic ribbons.

2.6. Spiral Ganglion Neuron Counts

At ambient sound levels (non-exposed controls), the average SGN density in the middle turn of the cochlea was 2530 ± 72 cells/mm^2 (Figure 6A,D). Noise exposure induced a significant ($p < 0.0001$) loss of SGNs in both vehicle- and drug-treated animals (Figure 6B–D). CCG-4986 treatment did not reduce the loss of SGN, and the average cell densities for CCG-4986 treated (2209 ± 97 cells/mm^2) and vehicle controls (2183 ± 161 cells/mm^2) were similar (Figure 6D).

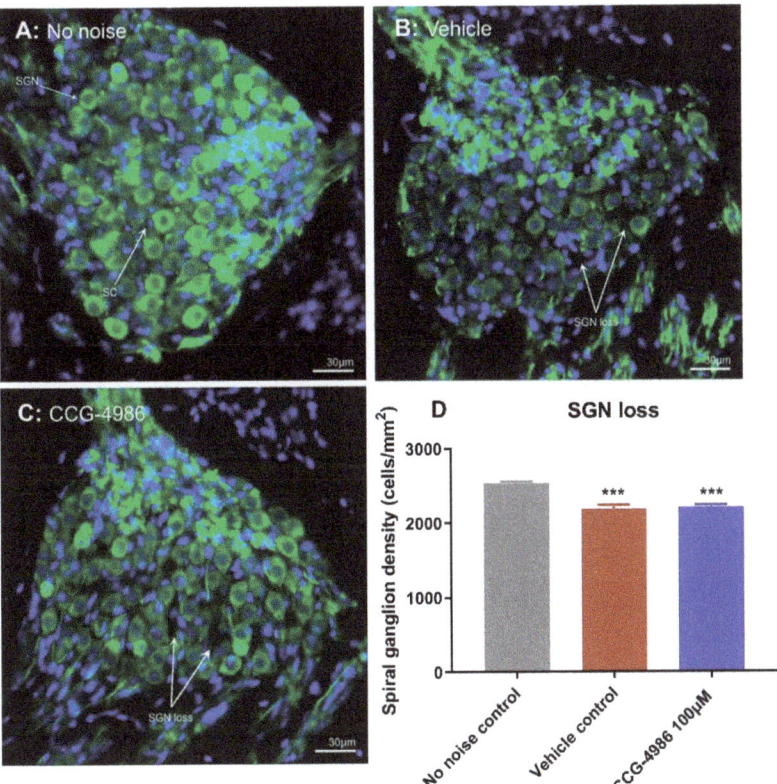

Figure 6. Loss of spiral ganglion neurons (SGN) after noise exposure. (**A–C**) Representative images of Rosenthal's canal in the middle turn of the cochlea. (**A**) Control non-exposed animals, (**B**) Noise-exposed vehicle-treated, (**C**) Noise exposed CCG-4986 treated. SGN were immunostained with the neurofilament antibody (cytoplasm, green) and Hoescht (nucleus, blue). White arrows point at spaces with missing SGN. Abbreviations: SC, satellite cell; SGN, Spiral ganglion neuron. (**D**) Average SGN densities in the middle turn of the cochlea in noise-exposed vs. non-exposed animals. Data presented as mean ± SEM. No noise control, $n = 10$; Vehicle control, $n = 16$; CCG-4986, $n = 17$. *** $p < 0.001$; One-way ANOVA followed by Holm–Sidak post hoc test.

2.7. Auditory Brainstem Responses and the Effect of Treatment 24 Hours after Noise Exposure

We have also investigated the effect of earlier CCG-4986 treatment (24 h after noise exposure) on ABR thresholds and suprathreshold responses. Like the previous study, exposure to octave band noise (8–16 kHz) for 2 h resulted in 40–50 dB PTS in vehicle-treated (control) animals at frequencies above 4 kHz (Figure 7A,C). However, the administration of a small molecule RGS4 inhibitor, CCG-4986 (100 μM), 24 h after noise exposure reduced PTS by up to 32 dB (Figure 7B,C). The greatest effect was observed at mid-frequencies (12–20 kHz), representing the region of the cochlea most damaged by noise exposure. Average threshold shift was reduced by 32 dB at 12 kHz ($p = 0.0025$), 23 dB at 16 kHz ($p = 0.01$), and 28 dB at 20 kHz ($p = 0.001$). A significant improvement (12–18 dB; $p < 0.05$) was also observed at other test frequencies (Figure 7C).

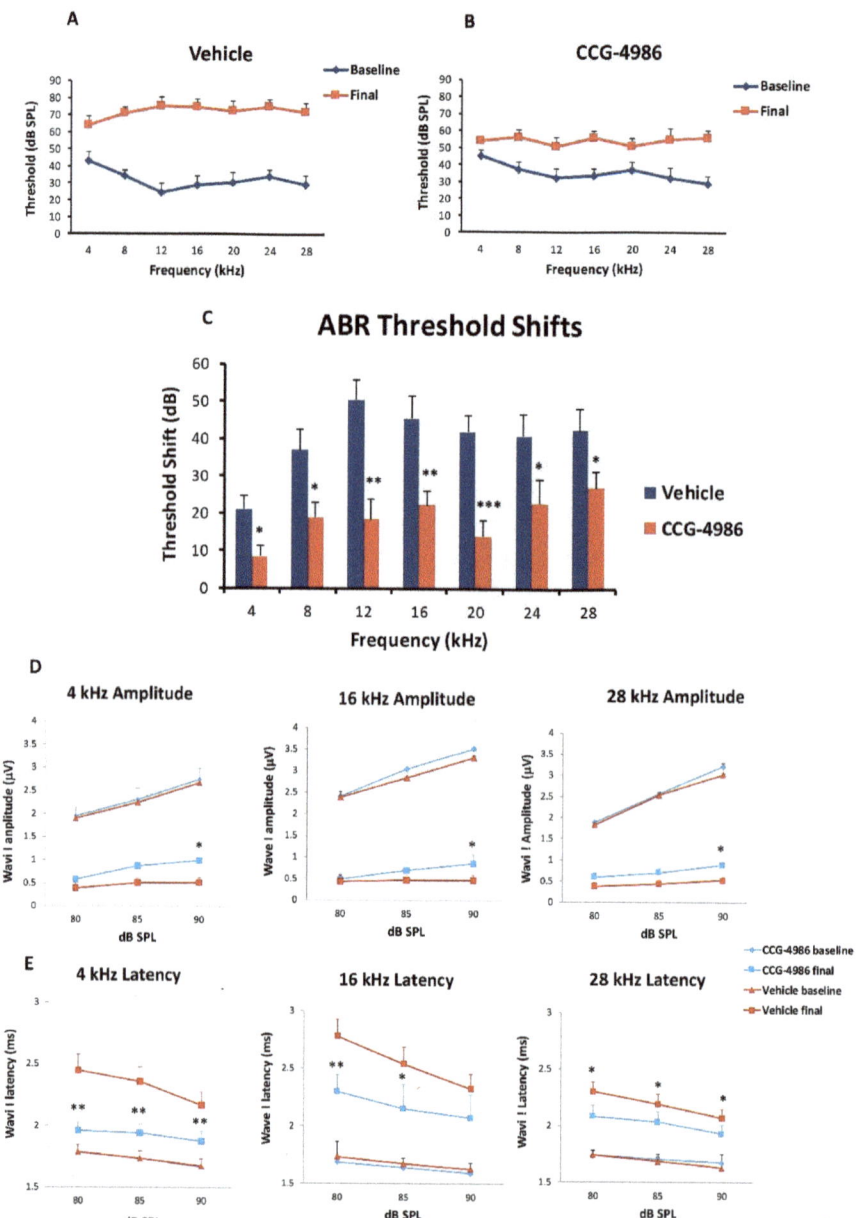

Figure 7. Baseline and final ABR thresholds for 4–28 kHz tone pips in animals exposed to octave band noise (8–16 kHz, 110 dB SPL) for 2 h and non-exposed animals. (**A**) Noise-exposed vehicle-treated animals, (**B**) Animals treated with CCG-4986 (100 µM) 24 h post-exposure. (**C**) Comparison of permanent threshold shifts 15 days after exposure in drug- and vehicle-treated animals. Average baseline and final ABR wave I amplitudes (**D**) and latencies (**E**) at suprathreshold intensities in noise-exposed animals treated with CCG-4986 (100 µM) or drug vehicle solution 24 h after noise exposure. Data presented as mean ± SEM. Vehicle control, $n = 10$; CCG-4986, $n = 9$. * $p < 0.05$ ** $p < 0.01$; *** $p < 0.001$. Two-way ANOVA followed by Holm–Sidak post-hoc test (ABR thresholds), Multivariate ANOVA followed by planned contrast comparisons (ABR suprathreshold responses).

We have also observed improved suprathreshold responses (ABR Wave 1 amplitudes) after treatment with CCG-4986 24 h post-exposure (Figure 7D,E). The amplitudes and latencies of ABR Wave I were analysed at suprathreshold levels (80–90 dB SPL) in different frequency regions of the cochlea (4 kHz, 16 kHz, and 28 kHz) to assess auditory nerve function. Noise exposure reduced ABR Wave I amplitudes by 60–70% and increased latencies by up to 25% (Figure 7D,E).

CCG-4986 treatment slightly improved Wave I amplitudes compared to vehicle-treated rats in all three test frequencies (90 dB; $p < 0.05$; Figure 7D). In addition, Wave I latencies were reduced after treatment with CCG-4986 (Figure 7E), suggesting partial recovery of neural function.

3. Discussion

Our study demonstrates the cochlear rescue effect of CCG-4986 treatment in rats up to 48 h after traumatic noise exposure. This novel treatment is based on enhanced endogenous adenosine A_1R activity in the cochlea. CCG-4986 is a small molecule RGS4 inhibitor which disrupts the signalling complex (RGS4/Neurabin) that regulates A_1R activation [18]. We have shown that immunolocalisation of this molecular complex in sensory hair cells and spiral ganglion neurons corresponds to A_1R distribution in the rat cochlea [19,20]. Local intratympanic administration of CCG-4986 48 h after acoustic overexposure mitigated noise-induced threshold shifts by 10–19 dB, which is considered clinically significant. This otoprotective effect was greater when the CCG-4986 treatment was delivered earlier (24 h after noise exposure), effectively reducing moderate-severe hearing loss to mild hearing loss. CCG-4986 administration also improved suprathreshold responses in noise-exposed animals (increased amplitudes and reduced latencies of ABR wave I), suggesting partial recovery of auditory nerve function. The treatment enhanced the survival of sensory hair cells in the noise-exposed cochlea and mitigated noise-induced loss of afferent synapses in the frequency-specific regions. Noise-induced loss of spiral ganglion neurons was, however, irreversible. The present study thus demonstrates that the RGS4 inhibition is the promising strategy for the treatment of noise-induced cochlear injury and introduces a novel paradigm for the treatment of NIHL and other forms of SNHL based on regulation of GPCR.

3.1. Drug Delivery to the Inner Ear

The intratympanic method of drug delivery to the round window membrane has two principle advantages. Firstly, it precludes off-target effects of A_1R activation in cardiovascular and other tissues, which is an important caveat for systemic administration. Secondly, poloxamer-407 is liquid at low temperatures, but becomes a gel at body temperature which allows slow drug release to the cochlear perilymph [21]. The small size of CCG-4986 (375 g/mol) and its apparent otoprotective effect suggest that this drug readily crosses into cochlear perilymph through the round window membrane. However, further studies are required to establish CCG-4986 concentration in cochlear fluid compartments after intratympanic injection and its pharmacokinetic properties.

3.2. ABR Threshold Shifts and Suprathreshold Responses are Mitigated by CCG-4986

CCG-4986 treatment 48 h post-exposure produced a cochlear rescue effect by reducing PTS at all test frequencies above 4 kHz. The PTS reduction of >10 dB is considered clinically significant [22]. As expected, the earlier treatment 24 h post-exposure enhanced the rescue effect of CCG-4986 (up to 32 dB at 12 kHz). The window of opportunity to treat NIHL was thus reminiscent of our previous study using an A_1R agonist adenosine amine congener [23].

Whilst auditory thresholds are considered a good metric of hair cell function, they are poor indicator of neuronal damage in the cochlea [24]. In this study, the changes in wave I amplitude and latency were used as indicators of afferent neural fibre (ANF) integrity. Noise overstimulation leads to a decrease in suprathreshold Wave 1 amplitudes [25] and prolonged latencies [26] due to reductions in synchronous firing, lower discharge rates, and decreased recruitment of the high threshold ANF [27]. Recent studies postulate that the synaptopathy and the loss of ANF is a primary and mostly irreversible event in noise-induced hearing loss [28]. This loss of cochlear afferents is functionally measured by reduced suprathreshold responses, due to preferential vulnerability of high threshold, low spontaneous rate ANF [29]. The diffuse afferent denervation that cannot be detected by measuring auditory thresholds is thought to contribute to poor performance in complex auditory tasks such as speech discrimination in a noisy environment, and thus has been termed "hidden hearing loss" [30]. In this study, treatment with CCG-4986 24 and 48 h after noise exposure reduced the ABR wave I latencies at all test frequencies, but only a minor improvement of wave I amplitudes was observed, suggesting partial recovery of neural injury.

3.3. CCG-4986 Improves the Survival of Sensory Hair Cells

Auditory threshold shifts are largely determined by the integrity of sensory hair cells; hence, the quantitative histological analysis of hair cell survival was carried out in the apical, middle, and basal turns of the noise-exposed cochleae. The hair cell population in the apical segment was virtually unaffected by noise exposure, but a significant loss of OHC was observed in the middle and basal segments of the cochlea, the latter being most severely affected. There was very little IHC loss in the apical and middle turns, but almost one third of IHC was missing in the basal turn of the cochlea.

The increased vulnerability of OHC to noise, particularly in the basal turn, have been well documented in the past. "Inappropriate" loss of high frequency hair cells has also been observed in previous studies where the noise exposures targeted lower frequencies [31]. Basal OHC are particularly vulnerable to acoustic insult, likely due to their lower antioxidant buffering capacity leading to increased susceptibility to oxidative stress [32].

CCG-4986 treatment conferred a significant protection from noise-induced OHC loss in the middle segment and both IHC and OHC loss in the basal segment of the cochlea. Hair cell death is primarily mediated by oxidative stress and calcium overload leading to caspase-dependent cell death pathways [33]. We postulate that the RGS4 inhibition by CCG-4986 enhanced endogenous adenosine A_1R signalling, which in turn improved antioxidant defences and restored calcium homeostasis [3,18].

3.4. CCG-4986 Partly Restores Afferent Synapses but does not Prevent Neuronal Loss

In the absence of noise exposure, the vast majority of IHC synapses contain a pre-synaptic ribbon paired with a post-synaptic terminal from a single ANF, and only around 1% of synapses appear as orphaned pre-synaptic ribbons or post-synaptic terminals [25]. The survival of IHC-auditory nerve synapses is considered a sensitive metric for quantitative analysis of afferent innervation in the cochlea [25].

Noise exposure affected only synaptic ribbons in the mid and high frequency regions, whilst IHC synapses in the low frequency region were mostly intact. Treatment with CCG-4986 yielded a robust neuroprotective effect in the middle turn, to such extent that the average number of functional (paired) synapses in drug-treated animals was not significantly different from control animals exposed to ambient noise.

IHC synaptic loss is an acute event that is usually complete within 24 h after noise exposure. It is generally considered that the loss of afferent synapses is irreversible [25,34,35] but, more recently, post-exposure regeneration of afferent synapses has also been reported after intratympanic administration of neurotrophin-3 [36]. Given that CCG-4986 was administered 48 h after acoustic trauma, it is unclear how it prevents synaptic loss or regenerates afferent synapses. Further studies are required to investigate the timeline of IHC synaptopathic injury in the rat cochlea and establish the underlying mechanism of the rescue effect by CCG-4986.

CCG-4986 treatment 48 h post-insult, however, did not protect against SGN loss. SGN loss usually progresses at a much slower rate than the loss of afferent synapses after acoustic overexposure [25]. Since SGN loss was measured only at one time point (16 days after insult), further studies investigating SGN survival months after acoustic insult are required to fully assess the neuroprotective effect of CCG-4986.

3.5. Putative Mechanisms of Otoprotection by CCG-4986

CCG-4986 is a small molecule inhibitor of RGS4 which enhances adenosine A_1R signalling by disrupting the molecular complex (Neurabin/RGS4) that terminates A_1R signalling [18]. RGS4 is a GTP-activating protein (GAP) that selectively terminates A_1R signalling at the level of G protein activation, by accelerating the intrinsic GTPase self-mediated hydrolysis and thus reverting $G\alpha$ and $G\beta\gamma$ subunits to an inactive state [37]. This effectively terminates the intracellular response following adenosine A_1R activation.

CCG-4986 blocks RGS4 activity by a dual mode of inhibition, through covalent modification of two different surface-exposed cysteine residues. Firstly, CCG-4986 modifies the Cys132 residue near the binding site of $G\alpha$ protein and competitively prevents $G\alpha$ protein binding to RGS4, which moderately reduces the binding affinity of $G\alpha$ protein to RGS4 [37,38]. The second, more dominant mechanism, involves modification of the Cys148 residue located in an allosteric site that causes a conformational change in RGS4 that prevents $G\alpha$ from interacting with RGS4, subsequently inhibiting GAP activity and thus extending adenosine A_1R signalling [37].

Chen et al. [18] demonstrated that the scaffolding protein neurabin is required to facilitate the interaction between RGS4 and A_1R in the brain. In the absence of A_1R stimulation, RGS4 is localised to the cytosol. After A_1R activation, RGS4 is recruited by neurabin to the cell surface, forming the A_1R/neurabin/RGS4 complex that specifically regulates A_1R signalling.

Our study shows that CCG-4986 can partially rescue the cochlea from noise-induced injury, most likely by enhancing A_1R signalling. Noise exposure can induce the release of adenosine into the cochlear fluids and lead to up-regulation of A_1R expression in cochlear tissues [3,39]. Adenosine A_1R signalling reduces oxidative stress and lipid peroxidation, likely by boosting endogenous antioxidant defences, including superoxide dismutase and glutathione peroxidase activity [3,40]. A_1 receptors in the central nervous system are known to exhibit an inhibitory tone by preventing neuronal excitability and synaptic transmission [41]. A_1R activation thus has a potential to directly counteract the main mechanisms of noise-induced cochlear injury, including oxidative stress, calcium overload, and glutamate excitotoxicity [23,33].

There is a certain advantage of CCG-4986 treatment over adenosine A_1R agonists such as ADAC and R-PIA, which activate A_1R with greater selectivity than adenosine. Our previous study [23] demonstrated a biphasic dose-response relationship effect of ADAC after systemic administration, otoprotective at doses 100–200 µg/kg and less effective at higher doses. This "effect inversion" might be due to overstimulation of A_1R causing their desensitisation and internalisation [42]. In contrast, inhibition of the neurabin/RGS4 complex bolsters the A_1R signalling without causing a change in A_1R number or affinity [18].

4. Materials and Methods

4.1. Animals

For this study, male Wistar rats (6–8 weeks) were sourced from the animal facility at the University of Auckland. Animals were housed in standard cages with ad libitum access to food and water, under controlled conditions (constant humidity and temperature, 12-h light/dark cycle). A minimum of two animals were housed together, up to a maximum of four per cage. Animal welfare was continuously assessed during the study to ensure that animal health was maintained at the highest standard. Noise-exposed animals were randomly assigned into drug treatment or drug vehicle-treated (control) group. All experimental procedures were carried out with the approval of the University of Auckland Animal Ethics Committee (approval # 1631, 8 September 2015), in agreement with the Animal Welfare Act (1999).

4.2. Auditory Brainstem Responses

Auditory brainstem responses (ABR) were used to determine auditory thresholds in rats prior to noise exposure (baseline) and 14 days after intratympanic drug or vehicle injection (final). The ABR is an auditory evoked potential that represents the synchronised summation of neuronal activity in response to auditory clicks and tone pip stimuli. ABR recordings were made in a custom-built sound isolating chamber (Shelberg Acoustics, Sydney, Australia), equipped with internal ventilation and a light source. Animals were anesthetised with a mixture of Ketamine (25 mg/kg) and Domitor (0.5 mg/kg) given intraperitoneally. The tympanic membrane was checked for signs of infection, physical trauma, or scarring before ABR recording. Only the left ear was used for assessment of ABR thresholds in each animal. Animals were placed on a thermostatically controlled electric blanket during recordings to maintain body temperature at 37 °C. The Tucker-Davis Technologies (TDT) System 3 and BioSig digital signal processing software (Alachua, FL, USA) were used to generate the auditory stimuli. A multi-field magnetic speaker (MF1, TDT) with 10 cm plastic tubing was used to deliver auditory stimuli into the ear. Three subdermal needle electrodes connected to a Medusa RA4LI headstage amplifier ($\times 20$ gain) were used to measure ABR responses. The active electrode was placed at the vertex of the scalp, the reference electrode at the mastoid region of the ear of interest, and the ground electrode at the mastoid region of the contralateral ear. Tone pips (5 ms duration, 2 ms rise/fall, presented at a 21/s rate) were used to elicit ABR responses at intensities between 90 dB SPL to 5 dB SPL, presented in decremental 5 dB steps. Tone pip responses were acquired at an alternating polarity sampling rate of 512 and averaged for each sound intensity. A bandpass filter (300–3000 Hz, 50 Hz notch) was applied to all responses. The ABR wave I was used to determine auditory thresholds defined as the lowest sound intensity level capable of eliciting a reproducible waveform. The cut off amplitude was set at ≥ 120 nV, as consistently reproducible waveforms were obtained at and above this amplitude. ABR recordings were repeated at sound intensities 10 dB above and 5 dB below the threshold in 5 dB decrements to confirm threshold intensity. In cases where the threshold ceiling was exceeded (above 90 dB SPL), these thresholds were arbitrarily assigned a value of 95 dB SPL. ABR assessments were carried out one day prior to noise exposure (baseline) and 14 days after intratympanic injection (final).

The amplitudes and latencies of wave I were assessed at suprathreshold intensities for selected frequencies (4, 16, and 28 kHz) to investigate the effect of CCG-4986 treatment on noise-induced neuronal injury. Animals with final auditory thresholds of 80 dB SPL or lower were included for input-output functional analysis. The amplitude of wave I (peak to trough) was measured at 90, 85, and 80 dB SPL intensities, and latency was measured as the time taken to reach the peak (including 0.3 ms signal transduction time from the speaker to the ear).

4.3. Noise Exposure

Twenty-four hours after baseline ABR measurements, animals were exposed to an octave band noise (8–16 kHz) for 2 h at 110 dB SPL. Acoustic overstimulation was carried out in a custom-built sound-attenuating chamber (Shelburg Acoustics, Sydney, Australia), equipped with internal ventilation, light source, and speakers suspended from the ceiling. Frequency and intensity of sound were adjusted by external controls. The speakers were calibrated using a sound level meter (Precision Sound level Meter Type 2235, Brüel & Kjær; Nærum, Denmark) prior to each noise exposure session, with the average sound pressure intensity measuring 110 ± 1.5 dB SPL across the cage floor. Animals exposed to noise were placed inside a conventional rat cage, positioned with a 30 cm distance underneath the speakers, and allowed to acclimatise for 5 min. Sound intensity was gradually increased over a period of 5 min. Control animals were placed in the sound isolating chamber for two hours to control for relocation stress. Afterwards, animals were returned to the animal housing facility and kept at ambient noise levels (55–65 dB SPL) for the remainder of the experimental timeline.

4.4. Intratympanic Injections

RGS4 inhibitor CCG-4986 or drug vehicle solution (control) was delivered by intratympanic injection into the middle ear cavity 24 or 48 h after noise exposure. Drug solution was made by dissolving CCG-4986 (ChemBridge™; San Diego, CA, USA) in 1% DMSO and 0.9% saline with the final 100 µM working dilution for intratympanic injection. Control animals were treated with the drug vehicle solution (1% DMSO in 0.9% saline). Drug and vehicle solutions were mixed with 17% *w/w* poloxamer-407 (Sigma-Aldrich) and placed on ice until fully dissolved. Solutions were then aliquoted and stored at $-20\ °C$ for later use. Poloxamer-407 allows for slow drug delivery to the cochlea as the solution becomes a gel at body temperature [21].

Prior to drug treatment, animals were anaesthetised with a mixture of Ketamine (25 mg/kg) and Domitor (0.5 mg/kg) injected intraperitoneally and administered one dose of Temgesic (Buprenorphine; 0.05 mg/kg, subcutaneously) for analgesia. Intratympanic injections were carried out using a Hamilton syringe mounted on a micromanipulator arm. The needle was inserted through the posterior-superior quadrant of the tympanic membrane to deliver injection solution into the vicinity of the round window membrane of the cochlea. A total solution volume of 27 µL was slowly injected into the middle ear. The animal was then returned to a recovery cage and left on its side for 30 min to allow the solution to settle onto the RWM in a gel form. Then the procedure was repeated for the contralateral ear. Animals were then given a subcutaneous dose of Antisedan (1 mg/kg) to reverse the effects of ketamine/domitor anaesthesia.

4.5. Cochlear Tissue Preparation for Histology and Immunohistochemistry

After the final ABR assessment, animals were euthanized by an anaesthetic overdose (pentobarbitone, 90–100 mg/kg intraperitoneally). The animals were perfused with the flush solution (0.9% NaCl containing 10% $NaNO_2$) and then tissue fixative (4% paraformaldehyde (PFA) in 0.1 M phosphate buffer (PB, pH 7.4) overnight at 4 °C. Cochleae were then decalcified using 5% EDTA in 0.1 M PB for 9 days at 4 °C, cryoprotected overnight in 30% sucrose in 0.1 M PB and embedded in optimal cutting temperature compound (OCT). Cochleae were then snap frozen using N-pentane and stored at $-80\ °C$ for further processing.

4.6. Hair Cell and Ribbon Synapse Counting

The extracted cochleae were decapsulated and micro-dissected into the apical, middle, and basal segments (turns), after removal of the lateral wall, Reissner's membrane and tectorial membrane. Cochlear turns were transferred into a 48 well plate containing 0.1 M PBS (pH 7.4), permeabilised with 1% Triton X-100 and blocked with 10% Normal Goat Serum (NGS) for 2 h at room temperature (RT). Whole mount tissues were then incubated overnight at RT with the following primary antibodies: rabbit polyclonal anti-Myosin-VIIa (Proteus Biosciences, 1:500), mouse anti-C-terminal binding protein 2 (CtBP2; IgG1; BD Biosciences, 1:500) and mouse anti-Glutamate receptor 2 (GluA2; IgG2; Merck Millipore, 1:500) in antibody solution containing 0.1% Triton X-100 in 0.1 M PBS with 5% NGS. The following day, sections were washed three times for 60 min with 0.1 M PBS and then incubated at RT with the following secondary antibodies: goat anti-rabbit (Alexa 568, 1:500; Invitrogen), goat anti-mouse IgG1 (Alexa 647, 1:500; Invitrogen), and goat anti-mouse IgG2 (Alexa 488, 1:500; Invitrogen) in antibody solution containing 0.1% Triton X-100 and 5% NGS in 0.1 M PBS. Whole mounts were then washed for 60 min with 0.1 M PBS and then mounted on glass slides using Citifluor AFI mounting medium, cover slipped, sealed with nail polish, and stored in the dark at 4 °C. Inner hair cell-auditory nerve synapses were imaged and analysed at three frequency regions (4, 16, and 28 kHz) of the cochlea, based on the distance from the cochlear apex [43]. Immunostained synapses were imaged using confocal microscopy (Olympus FV1000 Live Cell System, Tokyo, Japan) with oil immersion 60× objective (1.35 NA) and 2.6× digital zoom. Images were captured as a z-stack, with the z dimension sampled in 0.2 µm steps, imaging frame in the *xy* dimension capturing 10 adjacent inner hair cells. Z-stacks were processed to remove nuclear CtBP2 staining and compiled into a colour composite stack: inner hair cells labelled with Myosin-VIIa (grey), post-synaptic terminals labelled with GluA2 (green), pre-synaptic ribbons labelled with CtBP2 (red). As a max z-projection could potentially obscure juxtaposed paired synapses in the z-dimension, synapses were counted frame by frame in the z-dimension using the cell counter plugin in ImageJ, with markers displayed through the stack to avoid duplicate counts. A paired synapse was defined as a post-synaptic terminal (GluA2) immediately adjacent to a presynaptic ribbon (CtBP2). Any unpaired pre-synaptic ribbons or post-synaptic terminals were defined as orphan synapses. The total number of synapses were counted for 10 inner hair cells and averaged to get the mean number of synapses per IHC. The number of unpaired (orphan) synapses was expressed as a percentage of the total synapse count per IHC.

For hair cell counting, each cochlea was divided into three segments covering the entire length of the cochlea and representing different frequency regions. The apical segment occupied approximately 0–30% from the apex, middle segment 30–75% from the apex, and basal segment 75–100% from the apex. The organ of Corti was imaged with a Zeiss Axioplan 2 epifluorescence microscope (Carl Zeiss, Jena, Germany) with 20× objective (0.6 NA), and captured with a Photometrics Prime sCMOS monochrome camera. Inner and outer hair cells were counted in ImageJ using the CellCounter to mark intact and missing hair cells, with the number of missing cells expressed as a percentage of the total number of hair cells counted. For regions with complete OHC loss, but intact IHC, one IHC was approximated to three missing OHC (one in each row). For regions of absolute hair cell loss, an adjacent length of IHC was measured (3–4 cells) to calculate pixel width per IHC. The distance of the lesion was measured and the number of missing IHC and corresponding missing OHC was estimated.

4.7. Spiral Ganglion Neuron Counting

Cochleae designated for spiral ganglion neuron counts were cryosectioned at 12 μm, and every second mid-modiolar section was placed into 0.1 M PBS (pH 7.4) in a 24 well plate. Cryosections were washed with 0.1 M PBS, permeabilised with 1% Triton X-100 in 0.1 M PBS and blocked with 10% normal donkey serum (NDS) for 1 h at RT. Cochlear sections were then incubated overnight at 4 °C with goat polyclonal Neurofilament (NF-L) antibody (2 μg/mL; Santa Cruz Biotechnology, Inc., Dallas, TX, USA) in antibody solution containing 0.1% Triton X-100 and 10% NDS in 0.1 M PBS. The next day sections were washed (3 × 10 min) with 0.1 M PBS and incubated with donkey anti-goat secondary antibody (Alexa Fluor 488, 1:600 dilution; Invitrogen) for 2 h at RT. Sections were then washed with 0.1 M PBS (10 min), incubated with Hoechst 33342 nuclear stain (1 μg/mL in 0.1 M PBS, pH 7.4; Thermo Fisher Scientific) for 15 min, then washed with 0.1 M PBS for 10 min. Sections were mounted on a glass slide in Citifluor AF1 mounting medium, covered with a coverslip and stored in the dark at 4 °C. Tissues were imaged with a Zeiss Axioplan 2 epifluorescence microscope (Carl Zeiss, Jena, Germany) with 40× objective. Images of the spiral ganglion neurons located in the middle turn were captured at two different wavelengths (UV and 488) using a Photometrics Prime sCMOS monochrome camera and merged to identify individual spiral ganglion neurons. The spiral ganglion area, represented by the bony edge of Rosenthal's canal, was selected using the "free-hand selection tool" in ImageJ. Individual neurons with unambiguous round nuclei in the middle turn of the cochlea were counted in each section and then averaged to determine SGN density for each animal as described previously [44].

4.8. Characterisation of Neurabin Expression in the Rat Cochlea

To determine mRNA expression of the two neurabin isoforms (Neurabin I and II), four intact rat cochleae were extracted, decapsulated, and placed into separate Eppendorf tubes containing cold lysis buffer (100 mM TRIS-HCl pH 7.5, 500 mM LiCl, 10 mM EDTA pH 8.0, 1% LiDS, 5 mM dithiothreitol (DTT) and RNase inhibitors) pre-chilled to 4 °C. Cochleae were then homogenised using sterile Teflon mini-pestles. Polyadenylated RNA (mRNA) was extracted using the magnetic Dynabeads® (Oligo(dT)25 (5 mg/mL)) mRNA DIRECT kit (Invitrogen). First-strand cDNA synthesis was carried out in a 20-µl reverse transcription (RT) reaction with random hexamers, dNTPs and Superscript III reverse transcriptase (Invitrogen). The complementary DNA was amplified by PCR with rat-specific primers for neurabin isoforms (Table 1) designed using OligoPerfect™ (Invitrogen). Negative control without reverse transcriptase was included in each PCR run. RT-PCR with a 40 cycle profile was performed as follows: 94 °C denaturation (1 min), 60 °C annealing (1.5 min), 72 °C extension (2 min) steps using PTC-100™ Programmable Thermal Controller (MJ Research Inc., Waltham, MA, USA). PCR amplicons were separated by agarose gel electrophoresis, and visualised using SYBR safe DNA gel stain (Invitrogen). PCR products were purified by PureLink™ PCR Purification Kit (Invitrogen) and the identity of the amplicons confirmed by DNA sequencing (Centre for Genomics & Proteomics, School of Biological Sciences, the University of Auckland, Auckland, New Zealand).

4.9. RGS4 and Neurabin Immunohistochemistry

The immunolocalisation of RGS4 and neurabin I isoform which forms molecular complexes with RGS4 was demonstrated in the rat cochleae using immunofluorescence. Briefly, rat cochlear tissues were cryosectioned at 30 µm using a CM3050 S cryostat (Leica, Germany) and mid-modiolar sections were placed in a 24 well plate containing 0.1 M PBS (pH 7.4) and washed twice for 20 min. Sections were then incubated in blocking and permeabilisation solution (10% NGS, 1% Triton X-100 in 0.1 M PBS) for 1 h at RT, followed by incubation with a mouse monoclonal RGS4 antibody (Santa Cruz Biotechnologies, sc-398658; 2 µg/mL) or rabbit polyclonal neurabin I antibody (Santa Cruz Biotechnologies; 2 µg/mL) overnight at 4 °C. Control sections were incubated with the normal mouse or rabbit IgG (2 µg/mL) instead of the primary antibody. The next day, sections were washed with 0.1 M PBS three times (60 min), followed by the incubation with the secondary antibody (Alexa Fluor 488 goat anti-mouse or anti-rabbit IgG, dilution 1:500) for 2 h at RT. After a washout with 0.1 M PBS (3 × 10 min), cryosections were mounted on glass slides using Citifluor AF1 Mounting Medium, covered with a coverslip and sealed with nail polish. Images of mid-modiolar cochlear cryosections were acquired using a confocal microscope (Olympus FluoView FV1000) and processed with FluoView software (version 2.0c, Olympus, Tokyo, Japan).

4.10. Data Analysis

The researchers were blinded for all ABR assessments, tissue collections, and histological analyses. Animals were assigned a subject ID by an independent researcher and allocated into the treatment or vehicle control group using a randomly generated number list (https://www.randomizer.org). Aliquoted injection solutions were labelled only by subject ID. All data were tested for normality using the Shapiro–Wilk Test. Auditory thresholds, ribbon synapse and hair cell counts were analysed using a two-way ANOVA with a post-hoc Holm–Sidak test. Spiral ganglion counts were analysed with one-way ANOVA. Suprathreshold data were analysed using multi-level factorial ANOVA with planned orthogonal contrasts to determine differences between groups. Data are presented as mean ± SEM.

5. Conclusions

Intratympanic administration of a small molecule RGS4 inhibitor presents a novel therapeutic strategy that precludes systemic side effects associated with systemic administration of adenosine A_1R agonists, while demonstrating a strong rescue effect against noise-induced cochlear injury. Translational studies are required to determine clinical potential of this treatment for NIHL and other forms of SNHL. Future studies will need to determine pharmacokinetic and pharmacodynamic CCG-4986 profile in the cochlea after intratympanic administration, its effect on adenosine concentrations in cochlear perilymph, metabolism, and toxicity profile, before considering clinical trials.

Author Contributions: S.M.V. designed the experiments and coordinated the study; C.F., M.B., M.P., and R.T. performed the experiments; S.M.V. and C.F. prepared the manuscript; P.R.T. contributed to study design, data interpretation and critically revised the manuscript. All authors have read and agreed to the published version of the manuscript.

Funding: This study was supported by a research grant from the Auckland Medical Research Foundation (New Zealand).

Institutional Review Board Statement: All experimental procedures were carried out with the approval of the University of Auckland Animal Ethics Committee (approval # 1631, 8 September 2015), in agreement with the Animal Welfare Act (1999).

Conflicts of Interest: The authors declare no conflict of interest.

References

1. World Health Organisation: Deafness and Hearing Loss. 2020. Available online: https://www.who.int/news-room/fact-sheets/detail/deafness-and-hearing-loss (accessed on 1 March 2020).
2. Dror, A.A.; Avraham, K.B. Hearing impairment: A panoply of genes and functions. *Neuron* **2010**, *68*, 293–308. [CrossRef]
3. Wong, A.C.Y.; Guo, C.X.; Gupta, R.; Housley, G.D.; Thorne, P.R.; Vlajkovic, S.M. Post-exposure administration of A_1 adenosine receptor agonists attenuates noise-induced hearing loss. *Hear. Res.* **2010**, *260*, 81–88. [CrossRef]
4. Vlajkovic, S.M.; Lee, K.H.; Wong, A.C.Y.; Guo, C.X.; Gupta, R.; Housley, G.D.; Thorne, P.R. Adenosine amine congener mitigates noise-induced cochlear injury. *Purinergic Signal.* **2010**, *6*, 273–281. [CrossRef] [PubMed]
5. Gunewardene, N.; Guo, C.X.; Wong, A.C.Y.; Thorne, P.R.; Vlajkovic, S.M. Adenosine Amine Congener ameliorates cisplatin-induced hearing loss. *World J. Otorhinolaryngol.* **2013**, *3*, 100–107. [CrossRef]
6. Lin, S.C.Y.; Thorne, P.R.; Housley, G.D.; Vlajkovic, S.M. Purinergic signalling and aminoglycoside ototoxicity: The role of P1 (adenosine) and P2 (ATP) receptors. *Front. Cell. Neurosci.* **2019**, *13*, 207. [CrossRef] [PubMed]
7. Vlajkovic, S.M.; Housley, G.D.; Thorne, P.R. Adenosine and the auditory system. *Curr. Neuropharmacol.* **2009**, *7*, 246–256. [CrossRef] [PubMed]
8. Vlajkovic, S.M.; Guo, C.X.; Telang, R.; Wong, A.C.Y.; Paramananthasivam, V.; Boison, D.; Housley, G.D.; Thorne, P.R. Adenosine kinase inhibition in the cochlea delays the progression of age-related hearing loss. *Exp. Gerontol.* **2011**, *46*, 905–914. [CrossRef] [PubMed]
9. Bansal, G.; Druey, K.M.; Xie, Z. R4 RGS proteins: Regulation of G protein signaling and beyond. *Pharmacol. Ther.* **2007**, *116*, 473–495. [CrossRef]
10. Sjögren, B. The evolution of regulators of G protein signalling proteins as drug targets 20 years in the making: IUPHAR Review 21. *Br. J. Pharmacol.* **2017**, *174*, 427–437. [CrossRef]
11. Neubig, R.R. RGS-insensitive G proteins as in vivo probes of RGS function. *Prog. Mol. Biol. Transl. Sci.* **2015**, *133*, 13–30.
12. Mittmann, C.; Chung, C.H.; Hoppner, G.; Michalek, C.; Nose, M.; Schuler, C.; Schuh, A.; Eschenhagen, T.; Weil, J.; Pieske, B.; et al. Expression of ten RGS proteins in human myocardium: Functional characterization of an upregulation of RGS4 in heart failure. *Cardiovasc. Res.* **2002**, *55*, 778–786. [CrossRef]
13. Riddle, E.L.; Schwartzman, R.A.; Bond, M.; Insel, P.A. Multi-tasking RGS proteins in the heart: The next therapeutic target? *Circ. Res.* **2005**, *96*, 401–411. [CrossRef] [PubMed]
14. Hurst, J.H.; Hooks, S.B. Regulator of G-protein signaling (RGS) proteins in cancer biology. *Biochem. Pharmacol.* **2009**, *78*, 1289–1297. [CrossRef]
15. Sjögren, B.; Blazer, L.L.; Neubig, R.R. Regulators of G protein signaling proteins as targets for drug discovery. *Prog. Mol. Biol. Transl. Sci.* **2010**, *91*, 81–119. [PubMed]
16. Hayes, M.P.; Bodle, C.R.; Roman, D.L. Evaluation of the selectivity and cysteine dependence of inhibitors across the Regulator of G Protein signaling family. *Mol Pharmacol.* **2018**, *93*, 25–35. [CrossRef]
17. Blazer, L.L.; Storaska, A.J.; Jutkiewicz, E.M.; Turner, E.M.; Calcagno, M.; Wade, S.M.; Wang, Q.; Huang, X.P.; Traynor, J.R.; Husbands, S.M.; et al. Selectivity and anti-Parkinson's potential of thiadiazolidinone RGS4 inhibitors. *ACS Chem. Neurosci.* **2015**, *6*, 911–919. [CrossRef]
18. Chen, Y.; Liu, Y.; Cottingham, C.; McMahon, L.; Jiao, K.; Greengard, P.; Wang, Q. Neurabin scaffolding of adenosine receptor and RGS4 regulates anti-seizure effect of endogenous adenosine. *J. Neurosci.* **2012**, *32*, 2683–2695. [CrossRef]
19. Vlajkovic, S.M.; Abi, S.; Wang, C.J.H.; Housley, G.D.; Thorne, P.R. Differential distribution of adenosine receptors in rat cochlea. *Cell Tissue Res.* **2007**, *328*, 461–471. [CrossRef]
20. Kaur, T.; Borse, V.; Sheth, S.; Sheehan, K.; Ghosh, S.; Tupal, S.; Jajoo, S.; Mukherjea, D.; Rybak, L.P.; Ramkumar, V. Adenosine A1 receptor protects against cisplatin ototoxicity by suppressing the NOX3/STAT1 inflammatory pathway in the cochlea. *J. Neurosci.* **2016**, *36*, 3962–3977. [CrossRef]
21. Wang, X.; Dellamary, L.; Fernandez, R.; Harrop, A.; Keithley, E.M.; Harris, J.P.; Ye, Q.; Lichter, J.; LeBel, C.; Piu, F. Dose-dependent sustained release of dexamethasone in inner ear cochlear fluids using a novel local delivery approach. *Audiol. Neurootol.* **2009**, *14*, 393–401. [CrossRef]
22. Oishi, N.; Schacht, J. Emerging treatments for noise-induced hearing loss. *Expert Opin. Emerg. Drugs* **2011**, *16*, 235–245. [CrossRef]

23. Vlajkovic, S.M.; Chang, H.; Paek, S.Y.; Chi, H.H.-T.; Sreebhavan, S.; Telang, R.S.; Tingle, M.D.; Housley, G.D.; Thorne, P.R. Adenosine amine congener as a cochlear rescue agent. *BioMed Res. Int.* **2014**, *2014*, 841489. [CrossRef]
24. Schuknecht, H.F.; Woellner, R.C. An experimental and clinical study of deafness from lesions of the cochlear nerve. *J. Laryngol. Otol.* **1955**, *69*, 75–97. [CrossRef]
25. Kujawa, S.G.; Liberman, M.C. Adding insult to injury: Cochlear nerve degeneration after "temporary" noise-induced hearing loss. *J. Neurosci.* **2009**, *29*, 14077–14085. [CrossRef] [PubMed]
26. Sohmer, H.; Kinarti, R.; Gafni, M. The latency of auditory nerve-brainstem responses in sensorineural hearing loss. *Eur. Arch. Oto-Rhino-Laryngol.* **1981**, *230*, 189–199. [CrossRef]
27. Wan, G.; Corfas, G. No longer falling on deaf ears: Mechanisms of degeneration and regeneration of cochlear ribbon synapses. *Hear. Res.* **2015**, *329*, 1–10. [CrossRef] [PubMed]
28. Kujawa, S.G.; Liberman, M.C. Synaptopathy in the noise-exposed and aging cochlea: Primary neural degeneration in acquired sensorineural hearing loss. *Hear. Res.* **2015**, *330*, 191–199. [CrossRef] [PubMed]
29. Furman, A.C.; Kujawa, S.G.; Liberman, M.C. Noise-induced cochlear neuropathy is selective for fibers with low spontaneous rates. *J. Neurophysiol.* **2013**, *110*, 577–586. [CrossRef] [PubMed]
30. Liberman, M.C. Noise-induced hearing loss: Permanent versus temporary threshold shifts and the effects of hair cell versus neuronal degeneration. *Adv. Exp. Med. Biol.* **2016**, *875*, 1–7.
31. Chen, G.-D.; Fechter, L.D. The relationship between noise-induced hearing loss and hair cell loss in rats. *Hear. Res.* **2003**, *177*, 81–90. [CrossRef]
32. Sha, S.-H.; Taylor, R.; Forge, A.; Schacht, J. Differential vulnerability of basal and apical hair cells is based on intrinsic susceptibility to free radicals. *Hear. Res.* **2001**, *155*, 1–8. [CrossRef]
33. Kurabi, A.; Keithley, E.M.; Housley, G.D.; Ryan, A.F.; Wong, A.C.Y. Cellular mechanisms of noise-induced hearing loss. *Hear. Res.* **2017**, *349*, 129–137. [CrossRef] [PubMed]
34. Lin, H.W.; Furman, A.C.; Kujawa, S.G.; Liberman, M.C. Primary neural degeneration in the guinea pig cochlea after reversible noise-induced threshold shift. *JARO* **2011**, *12*, 605–616. [CrossRef] [PubMed]
35. Liberman, L.D.; Liberman, M.C. Dynamics of cochlear synaptopathy after acoustic overexposure. *JARO* **2015**, *16*, 205–219. [CrossRef] [PubMed]
36. Suzuki, J.; Corfas, G.; Liberman, M.C. Round-window delivery of neurotrophin 3 regenerates cochlear synapses after acoustic overexposure. *Sci. Rep.* **2016**, *6*, 24907. [CrossRef] [PubMed]
37. Roman, D.L.; Blazer, L.L.; Monroy, C.A.; Neubig, R.R. Allosteric inhibition of the regulator of G protein signaling–Gα protein–protein interaction by CCG-4986. *Mol. Pharmacol.* **2010**, *78*, 360–365. [CrossRef]
38. Kimple, A.J.; Willard, F.S.; Giguère, P.M.; Johnston, C.A.; Mocanu, V.; Siderovski, D.P. The RGS protein inhibitor CCG-4986 is a covalent modifier of the RGS4 Gα-interaction face. *Biochim. Biophys. Acta (BBA)-Proteins Proteom.* **2007**, *1774*, 1213–1220. [CrossRef]
39. Ramkumar, V.; Whitworth, C.A.; Pingle, S.C.; Hughes, L.F.; Rybak, L.P. Noise induces A1 adenosine receptor expression in the chinchilla cochlea. *Hear. Res.* **2004**, *188*, 47–56. [CrossRef]
40. Ford, M.S.; Maggirwar, S.B.; Rybak, L.P.; Whitworth, C.; Ramkumar, V. Expression and function of adenosine receptors in the chinchilla cochlea. *Hear. Res.* **1997**, *105*, 130–140. [CrossRef]
41. Cunha, R.A. Neuroprotection by adenosine in the brain: From A1 receptor activation to A2A receptor blockade. *Purinergic Signal.* **2005**, *1*, 111–134. [CrossRef]
42. Sheth, S.; Brito, R.; Mukherjea, D.; Rybak, L.; Ramkumar, V. Adenosine receptors: Expression, function and regulation. *Int. J. Mol. Sci.* **2014**, *15*, 2024–2052. [CrossRef] [PubMed]
43. Viberg, A.; Canlon, B. The guide to plotting a cochleogram. *Hear. Res.* **2004**, *197*, 1–10. [CrossRef] [PubMed]
44. Vlajkovic, S.M.; Ambepitiya, K.; Barclay, M.; Boison, D.; Housley, G.D.; Thorne, P.R. Adenosine receptors regulate susceptibility to noise-induced neural injury in the mouse cochlea and hearing loss. *Hear. Res.* **2017**, *345*, 43–51. [CrossRef] [PubMed]

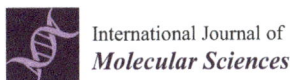 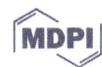

Article

Altered Gap Junction Network Topography in Mouse Models for Human Hereditary Deafness

Sara Eitelmann [1,2], Laura Petersilie [2], Christine R. Rose [2] and Jonathan Stephan [1,2,*]

[1] Animal Physiology Group, Department of Biology, University of Kaiserslautern, Erwin Schrödinger-Straße 13, D 67663 Kaiserslautern, Germany; sara.eitelmann@uni-duesseldorf.de
[2] Institute of Neurobiology, Heinrich Heine University Düsseldorf, Universitätsstraße 1, D 40225 Düsseldorf, Germany; laura.petersilie@hhu.de (L.P.); rose@uni-duesseldorf.de (C.R.R.)
* Correspondence: jonathan.stephan@uni-duesseldorf.de; Tel.: +49-211-81-13486

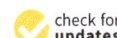

Received: 21 August 2020; Accepted: 2 October 2020; Published: 6 October 2020

Abstract: Anisotropic gap junctional coupling is a distinct feature of astrocytes in many brain regions. In the lateral superior olive (LSO), astrocytic networks are anisotropic and oriented orthogonally to the tonotopic axis. In $Ca_V1.3$ knock-out (KO) and otoferlin KO mice, where auditory brainstem nuclei are deprived from spontaneous cochlea-driven neuronal activity, neuronal circuitry is disturbed. So far it was unknown if this disturbance is also accompanied by an impaired topography of LSO astrocyte networks. To answer this question, we immunohistochemically analyzed the expression of astrocytic connexin (Cx) 43 and Cx30 in auditory brainstem nuclei. Furthermore, we loaded LSO astrocytes with the gap junction-permeable tracer neurobiotin and assessed the network shape and orientation. We found a strong elevation of Cx30 immunoreactivity in the LSO of $Ca_V1.3$ KO mice, while Cx43 levels were only slightly increased. In otoferlin KO mice, LSO showed a slight increase in Cx43 as well, whereas Cx30 levels were unchanged. The total number of tracer-coupled cells was unaltered and most networks were anisotropic in both KO strains. In contrast to the WTs, however, LSO networks were predominantly oriented parallel to the tonotopic axis and not orthogonal to it. Taken together, our data demonstrate that spontaneous cochlea-driven neuronal activity is not required per se for the formation of anisotropic LSO astrocyte networks. However, neuronal activity is required to establish the proper orientation of networks. Proper formation of LSO astrocyte networks thus necessitates neuronal input from the periphery, indicating a critical role of neuron-glia interaction during early postnatal development in the auditory brainstem.

Keywords: astrocytes; auditory brainstem; lateral superior olive; gap junctions; voltage-activated calcium channel 1.3; otoferlin; spontaneous activity; deafness

1. Introduction

In many brain regions, astrocytes and oligodendrocytes form large panglial gap junction (GJ)-mediated networks [1–4]. In the hippocampus, where only few oligodendrocytes are located [1,5], networks mainly consist of astrocytes [6]. GJ networks exhibit a heterogeneous topography throughout the CNS. In particular areas, astrocytes are unequally interconnected to each other leading to an anisotropic network topography. Such limitations are present, for example, in sensory systems, which exhibit a strong anatomo-functional organization. In the barrel cortex and the barreloid thalamus, tracer coupling is restricted to the barrels [7,8]. Moreover, anisotropic tracer spread is present in the lateral superior olive (LSO) and the inferior colliculus (IC) [1,2,9]—two nuclei of the auditory brainstem, in which tracer-coupled networks are oriented orthogonally to the tonotopic axis. Both LSO and IC are tonotopically organized [10–12] and principal neurons refer to this organization, as their dendritic trees exhibit a narrow morphology with an orientation orthogonal to the tonotopic axis [13–17]. The correlation of astrocyte network anisotropy with the topography of principal neurons suggests that they are causally linked to each other, though the mechanism is still unknown.

Before hearing onset, which takes place at around postnatal day 12 in mice, circuits undergo substantial refinement [10,18,19]. In the superior olivary complex (SOC) of some species, namely rats and gerbils, but not in mice, principal neurons in the medial nucleus of the trapezoid (MNTB) change their synaptic phenotype from GABAergic towards glycinergic [20–22]. Furthermore, the number of MNTB–LSO projections decreases within the first two postnatal weeks, and MNTB–LSO synapses become consolidated [22,23]. This developmental refinement requires spontaneous cochlea-driven neuronal activity [24–26]. Even interfering with cholinergic efferent signaling onto hair cells in the cochlea alters spontaneous cochlea-driven neuronal activity and causes disturbed tonotopic map formation and impairment of sound source localization [27,28]. Mutations in various genes, for example coding for the voltage-activated calcium channel (Ca_V) 1.3 or the calcium sensor otoferlin in inner hair cells of the cochlea, cause hereditary deafness [29–32]. For both deafness genes, mouse models are available: $Ca_V1.3$ knock-out (KO) mice [33] and otoferlin KO mice [34]. In these mice, the auditory brainstem lacks spontaneous cochlea-driven neuronal activity, which in the SOC results in malformed nuclei and impaired circuit formation, i.e., reduced refinement and strengthening of MNTB–LSO synapses as well as impaired reorganization of the dendrite topography of LSO principal neurons [26,35,36]. In the wild type (WT), LSO astrocyte networks are anisotropic and predominantly oriented orthogonally to the tonotopic axis, thus correlating with dendrite topography and tonotopy. It has been suggested that network anisotropy might be beneficial for directed redistribution of, e.g., ions to limit crosstalk between neighboring isofrequency bands [1]. Accordingly, any impairment of network anisotropy and preferential orientation would further undermine tonotopic information processing. However, it was unknown so far if astrocytes and astrocytic networks are affected in the two KOs models.

Our results show that LSO astrocytes assessed at postnatal days 10–12 maintain an electrophysiologically earlier developmental phenotype in $Ca_V1.3$ KO and otoferlin KO mice. The expression of connexin (Cx) 43 and Cx30 was increased, but the degree of GJ coupling was unaltered. However, network topography was strongly altered in $Ca_V1.3$ KO and otoferlin KO mice. Most networks were anisotropic, but in contrast to the WT, networks were now predominantly oriented parallel (and not orthogonal) to the tonotopic axis. Thus, our data show that spontaneous cochlea-driven neuronal activity is not only mandatory for proper formation of neuronal circuitry, but in addition is required for proper orientation of astrocyte networks in the LSO.

2. Results

2.1. Expression of Cx43 and Cx30 in the Auditory Brainstem

In $Ca_V1.3$ KO and otoferlin KO mice, neuronal circuitry and nuclei topography are altered in the auditory brainstem [26,35,36]. To assess putative changes in astrocytic coupling, we first analyzed the expression of Cx43 and Cx30 in the SOC containing the MNTB, superior paraolivary nucleus (SPN), and the LSO. As observed before, immunohistochemistry directed against Cx43 and Cx30 resulted in punctate labeling of auditory brainstem nuclei, whereas Cx levels outside of the nuclei, e.g. in the internuclear space, were low (Figure 1Aa–Cb; [1]). Compared to the WT, expression of Cx43 was increased in the SPN from both KO models ($Ca_V1.3$ KO: $p = 0.020$; otoferlin KO: $p = 0.010$) and in the LSO from otoferlin KO ($p = 0.006$; Figure 1D). Cx30 levels were elevated in the SPN ($p = 0.001$) and LSO ($p < 0.001$) from $Ca_V1.3$ KO, but not from the otoferlin KO (Figure 1E). Cx43 and Cx30 levels were not significantly altered in MNTB from either KO model as compared to the WT (Figure 1D–E).

It was previously shown that deprivation of spontaneous cochlea-driven neuronal activity alters nuclei topography [35]. Thus, we analyzed the size of nuclei and found a 50% smaller coronal nucleus area for the SPN and LSO in both KO models ($p < 0.001$ for all comparisons), however, the coronal MNTB area was not altered (Figure 1F). Notably, the LSO in the $Ca_V1.3$ KO lost its typical kidney-like shape (Figure 1B; [35]), whereas this topography was maintained in the otoferlin KO (Figure 1C). Thus, our initial results indicated that astrocytic GJ coupling might be altered due to altered Cx expression and nucleus size.

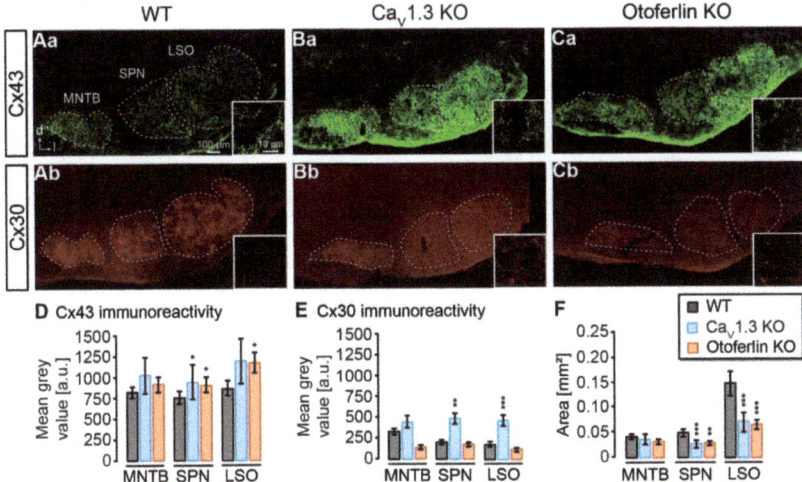

Figure 1. Expression of astrocyte-related connexins in the superior olivary complex (SOC). (**A–C**), widefield images showing immunoreactivity of Cx43 and Cx30 in the mouse SOC from the wild type (WT) (**Aa** (Cx43), **Ab** (Cx30)), CaV1.3 knock-out (KO) (**Ba** (Cx43), **Bb** (Cx30)) and otoferlin KO (**Ca** (Cx43), **Cb** (Cx30)). Regions used for mean grey value und area analysis are indicated with dashed lines. Insets: Close ups showing the punctate Cx labeling in the lateral superior olive (LSO) center. (**D**), mean grey values of Cx43 immunofluorescence. Cx43 levels were increased in the SPN from both KO models and in the LSO from otoferlin KO. (**E**), mean grey values of Cx30 immunofluorescence. Cx30 was elevated in the SPN and LSO of $Ca_V1.3$ KO. (**F**), area of nuclei in the SOC. SPN and LSO from both KO models exhibited a reduced area compared to the WT. Mean grey values were background subtracted. (**D–F**) show mean ± SD. Significance levels in panels (**D–F**) were Šidák corrected for two comparisons. The sample size is given in the text of Section 4.2. * $p < 0.025$, ** $p < 0.005$, *** $p < 0.0005$.

2.2. Electrophysiological Properties of LSO Astrocytes

To investigate the effect of reduced spontaneous neuronal activity on astrocytic GJ coupling in the auditory brainstem, we chose the LSO as a model region. In previous studies we could show that LSO astrocyte networks are predominantly anisotropic and oriented orthogonally to the tonotopic axis [1,9]. LSO astrocytes were a priori identified using sulforhodamine (SR) 101-labeling [37]. In the WT and both KO models, astrocytes were brightly labeled and were more numerous within the LSO as compared to the area around the nucleus. Analogous to the results from the immunohistochemistry experiment, the astrocyte distribution reflected the typical kidney-like shape of the LSO from the WT and otoferlin KO, and in the $Ca_V1.3$ KO astrocytes occupied an elliptic area (Figure 2Aa,Ba,Ca). As described above, the LSO size was reduced in both KO models. In the WT, astrocytes in the LSO center preferentially exhibited a dorsoventral orientation, which is roughly orthogonal to the tonotopic axis (Figure 2Aa; [1]). In contrast, astrocytes in the LSO center from both KO models appeared to be oriented in mediolateral direction, which approximately reflects the tonotopic axis (Figure 2Ba,Ca).

Neuronal circuitry in both KO models shows impaired development, but it was unknown, if the loss of spontaneous cochlea-driven neuronal activity interferes with astrocyte development. We patch-clamped individual LSO astrocytes and characterized their basic electrophysiological properties. Astrocytes from the WT exhibited a highly negative membrane potential (−82.9 ± 4.0 mV, $n = 63$) and a very low membrane resistance (3.7 ± 2.5 MΩ, $n = 63$), which is typical for LSO astrocytes [1,37]. LSO astrocytes from both KO models did not differ in their membrane potential (Ca$_V$1.3 KO: −83.2 ± 4.8 mV, n = 21, p = 0.814; otoferlin KO: −79.0 ± 8.1 mV, n = 17, p = 0.413) or membrane resistance (Ca$_V$1.3 KO: 3.5 ± 1.5 MΩ, n = 21, p = 0.833; otoferlin KO: 3.7 ± 1.7 MΩ, n = 17, p = 0.991).

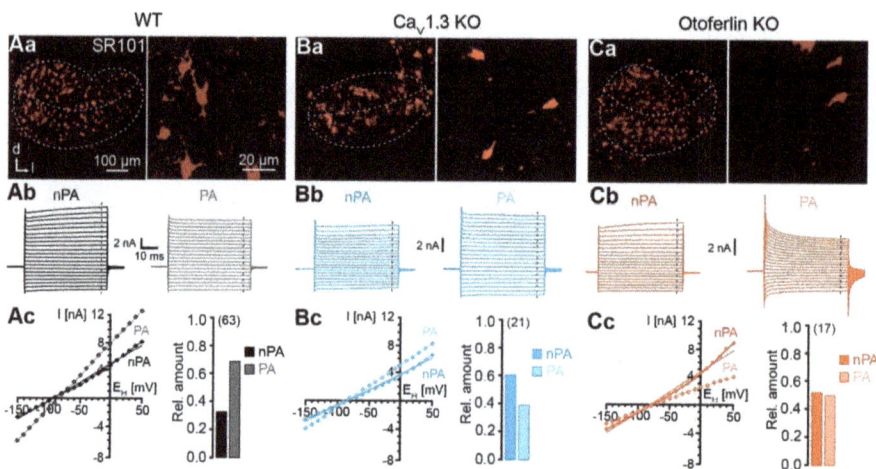

Figure 2. Identification and characterization of LSO astrocytes. (**A–C**), identification of astrocytes in the LSO. Confocal images of SR101-labeled astrocytes in the LSO (**left**). SR101-labeling was independent from genetic modification of mouse strains (**Aa,Ba,Ca**). The border of the LSO and the tonotopic axis are highlighted with dashed lines. In the WT and otoferlin KO mice, the LSO displayed the typical kidney-like shape (**Aa,Ca**). In Cav1.3 KO mice, the LSO was elliptic (**Ba**). Higher magnification of SR101-labeled astrocytes in the center of the LSO (**right**). Electrophysiological characterization of astrocytes (**Ab–Cc**). Astrocytes were recorded in voltage-clamp mode and step-wise hyper- and depolarized. Non-passive astrocytes (nPA) expressed time- and voltage-dependent outward currents (**left**). Passive astrocytes (PA) exhibited only ohmic currents (**right**) (**Ab,Bb,Cb**). Current-voltage (I/V) relationship was determined at the end of the voltage steps (dashed lines in **Ab,Bb,Cb**). Due to the presence of outward currents, nPAs and PAs exhibited non-linear and linear I/V relationships, respectively (**left**) (**Ac,Bc,Cc**). Relative amount of n/PAs (**right**). The number of analyzed cells is given in parentheses. The WT data (**Aa–Ac**) were part of [9]. Panels Aa left, Ab right, and parts of Ac left were reused from that publication.

We next hyper- and depolarized astrocytes from the WT and the two KO models to analyze the expression of inward and outward currents (Figure 2Ab,Bb,Cb). According to their elicited current traces, astrocytes could be classified as non-passive astrocytes (nPAs) and passive astrocytes (PAs). Astrocytes mainly showing voltage-activated outward currents resulting in a non-linear current-voltage (I/V) relationship were designated as nPAs. In turn, astrocytes that primarily expressed ohmic currents and hence displayed a preferentially linear I/V relationship, represented PAs. Both astrocytes subtypes are present in the WT and both KO models (Figure 2Ab,Cb). In the WT, most astrocytes exhibited a non-passive phenotype (nPA/PA: 32%/68%, n = 63; Figure 2Ac). Interestingly, the relative proportion shifted from PAs towards nPAs in both KO models. In Ca$_V$1.3 KO, there are more nPAs than PAs (62%/38%, n = 21, p < 0.001, X^2 test; Figure 2Bc). In the otoferlin KO, there is an almost equal amount of nPAs and PAs (nPA/PA: 53%/47%, n = 17, p < 0.001, X^2 test; Figure 2Cc). Thus, our data indicate that astrocytes in KO models do not undergo the normal postnatal transition from nPAs, expressing voltage-activated K$^+$ channels, towards PAs, predominantly expressing inwardly rectifying and leak K$^+$ channels, and thus partially maintain a phenotype characteristic of an earlier developmental stage [38,39].

2.3. Unaltered LSO Astrocyte Network Properties

Astrocyte coupling increases during postnatal development, which results in larger networks containing more cells [40,41]. As the percentage of astrocytes that maintained an electrophysiologically earlier developmental phenotype (nPAs) was increased in KO models, we next investigated, if coupling of LSO astrocytes was altered, too. During whole-cell recording the patch-clamped astrocytes were loaded with GJ-permeable tracer neurobiotin. Subsequent tracer visualization revealed labeling of coupled cells, whose brightness declined exponentially with increased distance to the patched cell (Figure 3Aa–Cc). Notably, the LSO borders did not restrict the tracer diffusion.

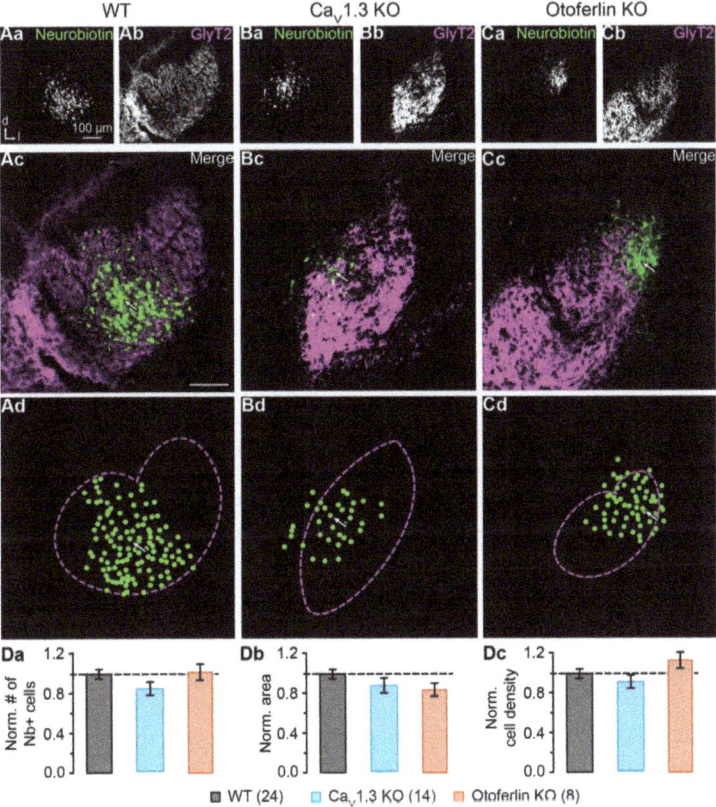

Figure 3. Reconstruction of LSO astrocyte networks. (**A–C**), tracer-coupled networks of the WT, Ca$_V$1.3 KO, and otoferlin KO mice. The tracer neurobiotin diffused from the patch-clamped astrocyte into coupled cells (**Aa–Ac,Ba–Bc,Ca–Cc**). Immunohistochemical labeling for glycine transporter (GlyT) 2 highlighted the LSO (**Ab,Bb,Cb**) and allowed the localization of the network within the nucleus (**Ac,Bb,Cc**). Cells with fluorescence intensity of at least 1.75-fold background intensity were transferred to a schematized representation and are displayed by green dots (**Ad,Bd,Cd**). The dotted magenta lines indicate the LSO border as derived from GlyT2 labeling (**Ab,Bb,Cb**). The arrows in (**Ac,Ad,Bc,Bd,Cc,Cd**) mark the patched cell. (**D**), network properties. Values were normalized to the WT data, indicated with the dashed line. There were no differences between the number of coupled cells (**Da**), network area (**Db**), or density of coupled cells (**Dc**). The WT data (**Aa–Ad**) were part of [9]. Panel (**Aa–Ac**) was reused from that publication. (**Da–Dc**) show mean ± SD. Number of slices is given in parentheses.

The semi-automated intensity-based cell detection [9] showed that networks did not differ significantly in basic properties between WT and KO models, i.e. cell number (WT: 64 ± 15, $n = 24$; Ca$_V$1.3 KO: 54 ± 12, $n = 14$, $p = 0.468$; otoferlin KO: 65 ± 14, $n = 8$, $p = 0.129$; Figure 3Da), area (WT: 0.043 ± 0.009 mm^2, $n = 24$; Ca$_V$1.3 KO: 0.039 ± 0.007 mm^2, $n = 14$, $p = 0.513$; otoferlin KO: 0.036 ± 0.007 mm^2, $n = 8$, $p = 0.644$; Figure 3Db), and cell density (WT: 1484 ± 331 cells/mm^2, $n = 24$; Ca$_V$1.3 KO: 1398 ± 331 cells/mm^2, $n = 14$, $p = 0.493$; otoferlin KO: 1816 ± 384 cells/mm^2, $n = 8$, $p = 0.137$; Figure 3Dc). Thus, in contrast to the electrophysiological phenotype, the network size in both KO models was unchanged and did thereby not reflect the properties of an earlier developmental stage.

2.4. Disturbed LSO Astrocyte Network Topography

LSO astrocyte networks are predominantly orthogonal to the tonotopic axis [1,9]. We next analyzed, if this preferential orientation is maintained in KO models. Network anisotropy was analyzed using our vector-based approach with subsequent meta-analysis [9]. Therefore, we applied a sinusoidal fit to the data to calculate the shape (R_{max}) and orientation (α) relative to the dorsoventral axis (Figure 4Aa,Ba,Ca). In case of anisotropic tracer-coupled networks comprising two axes of symmetry, rotating the coordinate system resulted in a ratio that oscillates two times per full turn (Figure 4Aa,Ba). In contrast, spherical networks with more than two axes of symmetry oscillated with a considerably higher frequency (Figure 4Ca).

As expected (cf. [1]), the WT LSO astrocyte networks were predominantly anisotropic and oriented orthogonally to the tonotopic axis (71%, 17/24; Figure 4Ab,Db). Only 13% (3/24) of the WT tracer-coupled networks were spherical and 17% (4/24) were anisotropic with a preferential orientation parallel to the tonotopic axis (Figure 4Ab,Db). Similar to this, most LSO astrocyte networks in Ca$_V$1.3 KO and otoferlin KO mice were anisotropic (Figure 4Bb,Cb). However, tracer-coupled networks in both KO models showed a different predominant orientation. Half of the networks in Ca$_V$1.3 KO (7/14) and otoferlin KO mice (4/8) were oriented parallel to the tonotopic axis (Figure 4Bb,Cb,Db). Less were spherical (Ca$_V$1.3: 29%, 4/14; Figure 4Bb,Db; Otof: 25%, 2/8; Figure 4Cb,Db) or oriented orthogonally to the tonotopic axis (Ca$_V$1.3 KO: 21%, 3/14; Figure 4Bb,Db; otoferlin KO: 25%, 2/8; Figure 4Cb,Db). Thus, the predominant direction of tracer spread and, accordingly, the preferred orientation of LSO astrocytes networks turned in both KO models by 90°, as compared to the WT. As a consequence, there might be increased gap junction-related cross-talk along the tonotopic axis (Figure 5).

Taken together, our results show that deprivation of spontaneous cochlea-driven neuronal activity does not per se distort astrocyte coupling in the LSO. However, LSO astrocyte network orientation is largely altered.

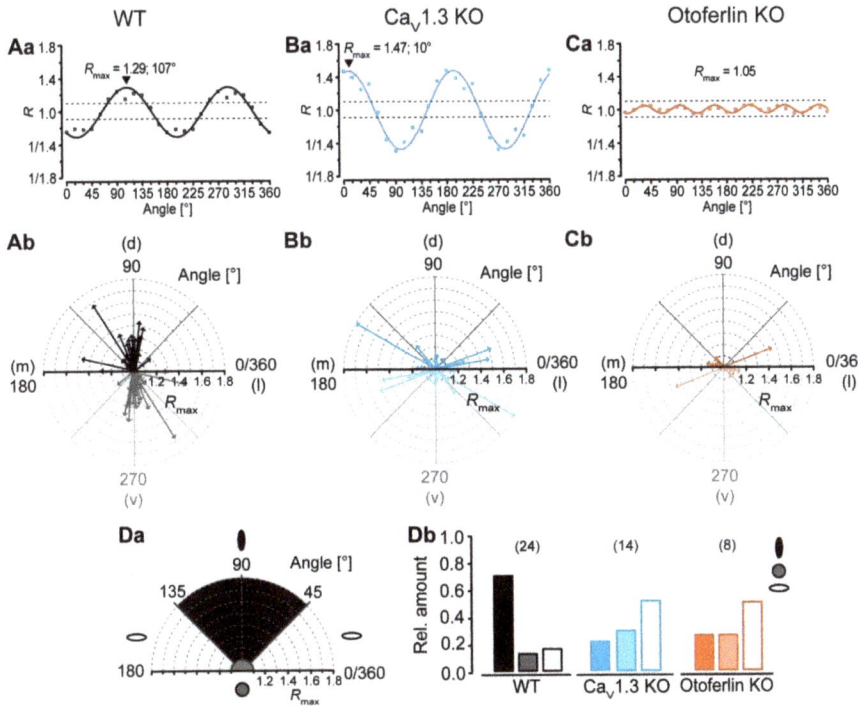

Figure 4. LSO astrocyte networks show a disturbed topography in Ca$_V$1.3 KO and otoferlin KO mice. (**A–C**), analysis of network topography. The coordinate system was step wise rotated and the ratio of tracer extent was calculated using the vector means approach. The anisotropy and orientation of networks in the center of the LSO were determined using a sinusoidal function (**Aa–Ca**). Shown, are representative sinusoidal fits of the anisotropic networks that were oriented orthogonally (WT; **Aa**) and parallel to the tonotopic axis (Ca$_V$1.3 KO; **Ba**) as well as a fit of an isotropic network with no preferential orientation (otoferlin KO; **Ca**). (**Aa–Ca**) refer to networks shown in Figure 3Aa–Cd. Radar diagrams displaying the anisotropy (R_{max} > 1.1: anisotropic; R_{max} ≤ 1.1: isotropic) and orientation α of tracer-coupled networks (**Ab–Cb**). The mediolateral (m-l) axis resembles the tonotopic axis, the dorsoventral (d-v) axis resembles the orientation of isofrequency bands, which are oriented orthogonal to the tonotopic axis. In WT mice, most tracer-coupled networks showed a preferential orientation orthogonal to the tonotopic axis (d–v; 45 ≤ α < 135°) (**Ab**). In contrast, the majority of anisotropic astrocyte networks in Ca$_V$1.3 KOs and otoferlin KOs were aligned parallel to the tonotopic axis (m-l; α < 45° and α ≥ 135°) (**Bb–Cb**). (**D**), classification of networks. Astrocyte networks were affiliated to three classes by their shape R_{max} and orientation α (class 1, black ellipse: anisotropic and oriented orthogonally to tonotopic axis; class 2, grey circle: isotropic; class 3: anisotropic and oriented parallel to the tonotopic axis; **Da**). In WT mice, most LSO astrocyte networks were categorized into class 1. In contrast, tracer-coupled networks in KOs were predominantly affiliated to class 3 (**Db**). The WT data (**Aa–Ab**) were already part of the following study: [9]. Panel Ab was reused from that publication.

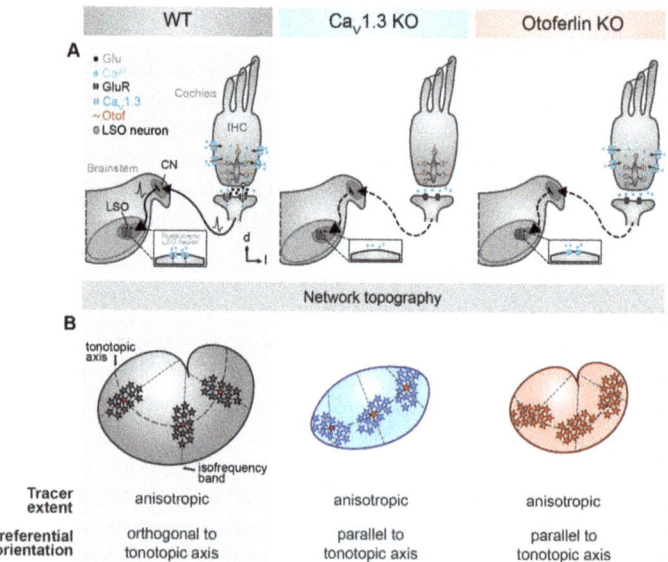

Figure 5. Summary of LSO astrocyte network topography in mouse models for human hereditary deafness. (**A**) schematic drawings depicting the subcellular modifications of the different mouse models. Compared to the WT (**left**), absence of Ca$_V$1.3 (**middle**) and otoferlin (**right**) from cochlear inner hair cells prevents Ca^{2+} entry into the inner hair cell and Ca^{2+} detection, respectively. Subsequently, exocytotic glutamate release is inhibited. Thereby, spontaneous activity of inner hair cells does not result in vesicle fusion, synaptic transmission, and subsequent activation of the auditory pathway. (**B**) main result of network analysis. LSO astrocyte networks are preferentially anisotropic and oriented orthogonally to the tonotopic axis (**left**). By contrast, networks in Ca$_V$1.3 KO (**middle**) and otoferlin KO mice (**right**) are predominantly oriented parallel to the tonotopic axis. Furthermore, the area of the LSO is reduced in both KO models. Moreover, the kidney-like shape of the LSO is lost in the Ca$_V$1.3 KO.

3. Discussion

In the present study, we have investigated the influence of absent spontaneous cochlea-driven neuronal activity on gap junctional tracer coupling in LSO astrocytes. To do so, we used two mouse models of hereditary deafness—a Ca$_V$1.3 KO and an otoferlin KO. As we have previously demonstrated a strong anatomo-functional correlation between neuronal circuitry and glial GJ network topography, we hypothesized that the altered neuronal circuitry in these two mouse models is also reflected in altered astrocytic networks. Our data show that the expression of astrocytic Cx is partially increased in the LSO, but the extent of tracer coupling is not altered. Most GJ networks are still anisotropic, but are oriented along the tonotopic axis in the KOs, thus correlating with the disturbed neuronal circuitry.

3.1. Connexin Expression in KO Models

GJ coupling depends on Cx expression levels. In the barrel cortex, high Cx expression within barrels correlates with strong GJ coupling, whereas lower Cx levels in the septa between the barrels result in weaker coupling [7,42]. Furthermore, Cx expression is upregulated during development [1,2,43,44], which increases GJ coupling [40,41]. Accordingly, loss of spontaneous cochlea-driven neuronal activity leading to impaired developmental maturation of neuronal circuitry [25,26,35,36] might have kept Cx expression in the LSO at an earlier developmental state as well. Here, we even found moderately increased Cx levels in the LSO, while the nucleus area was reduced in Ca$_V$1.3 KO and otoferlin KO mice (Figure 1; [35]). However, neither the increase in Cx levels nor the reduced nucleus size affected the size of tracer-coupled networks (Figure 3).

3.2. Activity-Dependent Alteration of Astrocyte Network Topography

LSO astrocytes in the two KO models exhibited similar basic membrane properties as reported earlier for the WT, namely a very negative membrane potential and a low membrane resistance [1,37]. Thus, expression of Kir and K_2P channels, which set both membrane potential and membrane resistance [45], is independent from spontaneous cochlea-driven neuronal activity. However, LSO astrocytes in both KO models exhibited more often a non-linear I/V relationship (Figure 2), which is indicative of partially impaired development, as they stayed in an earlier developmental state (cf. [38,39]). There was no significant alteration of network size, which is a bit surprising as Cx levels were moderately increased. Moreover, most tracer-coupled networks were anisotropic in both KO models (Figure 4). However, the disturbed refinement of neuronal circuitry is paralleled by an altered network orientation. Whereas networks in the WT were predominantly oriented orthogonally to the tonotopic axis [1,9], networks in KO models were predominantly oriented parallel to the tonotopic axis (Figure 4). Thus, spontaneous cochlea-driven neuronal activity per se is not required for the formation of anisotropic LSO astrocyte networks. However, it drives astrocytes and networks to be predominantly oriented orthogonally to the tonotopic axis.

3.3. Mechanism Underlying the Altered Network Topography

There must be at least two mechanisms in the LSO directing, on the one hand, network anisotropy and on the other hand, network orientation. In the two KO models used, loss of spontaneous cochlea-driven neuronal activity only interferes with network orientation, but not with network anisotropy per se (Figure 4). Anisotropic tracer coupling is present in different brain regions and can have different origins. In the barrel cortex and barreloid thalamus, anisotropy of glial GJ networks arises from restricted coupling across the barrels [7,8]. So far, such restrictions were not found in the LSO, since GJ networks cross nuclear borders [1]. In contrast, network anisotropy in the hippocampus and in the LSO originates from anisotropic topography of astrocyte processes [1,9,46,47]. The astrocyte polarization in the hippocampus depends on a non-channel function of Cx30 [46]. However, polarization of astrocytes and subsequent orientation of GJ networks in the LSO must be independent from Cx30 as it is virtually absent at the early postnatal stage (P10–12) investigated in this study [1]. Moreover, it is rather unlikely that the slightly elevated Cx30 expression in the $Ca_V1.3$ KO interferes with GJ network orientation, as there is no elevation of Cx30 expression in the otoferlin KO (Figure 1) and both KO models show the same alteration of GJ network orientation (Figure 4).

Astrocyte morphology correlates with topography of GJ networks in the auditory brainstem [1,2]. The changed orientation of astrocyte processes in the LSO in both KO models is likely to be responsible for the alteration of preferred GJ network orientation (Figures 2 and 4). However, the following question needs to be answered: What is the link between the lack of spontaneous cochlea-driven neuronal activity and alteration of astrocyte and GJ network topography?

3.4. Signaling between Astrocytes and Neurons

Spontaneous cochlea-driven neuronal activity is not only important for postnatal refinement of neuronal circuitry and dendrite topography [26,35,36], but is also required for the formation of GJ networks that are oriented predominantly orthogonally to the tonotopic axis. However, the interplay between astrocytes and neurons during this early postnatal phase is not clear as we do not know who signalizes whom to mature. There are basically two opposing possibilities: (1) Astrocyte topography and subsequent GJ network orientation precede and induce neuronal refinement, or (2) neuronal circuitry directs astrocytes and subsequently GJ networks to arrange properly. Another aspect is the question—until which point do the astrocyte and network maturation processes require cochlea-driven neuronal activity? This question can be addressed in future studies using, for example, the Pou4f3[DTR] mouse line, in which inner hair cells can be ablated by injection of diphtheria toxin [48].

In the avian auditory brainstem astrocyte-secreted factors are required to modulate dendrite topography and synapse distribution [49,50]. Therefore, the absence of spontaneous cochlea-driven neuronal activity likely does not induce neuronal refinement directly, but requires astrocyte–neuron signaling. However, GJ networks are affected themselves. This suggests that there must be in addition a communication between neurons and astrocytes, whose absence renders GJ network orientation in the KO models. This idea is further supported by the fact that the knocked-out targets, namely $Ca_V1.3$ and otoferlin, are localized in neurons and inner hair cells, respectively, but not in astrocytes [51,52]. In contrast, the still maintained preferred anisotropic topography of GJ networks indicates that this is an intrinsic property of LSO astrocytes and is independent from spontaneous cochlea-driven neuronal activity.

3.5. Conclusion

Taken together, our results demonstrate that spontaneous cochlea-driven neuronal activity is not exclusively mandatory for the proper formation of neuronal circuitry, but in addition, is crucial for the proper formation of GJ networks. Hence, GJ network topography reflects disturbed neuronal topography in the investigated mouse models. The signaling path between astrocytes and neurons has to be further analyzed.

4. Materials and Methods

Experiments were performed on WT C57BL/6 mice, $Ca_V1.3$ KO mice [33] and otoferlin KO mice [34] of both genders at postnatal days 10–12 in accordance with the German law for conducting animal experiments. Animals were bred at a 12 h day/night cycle and received food and water ad libitum. Breeding was approved by the regional council of Rhineland-Palatinate (23 177-07/G 15-2-076; 24 August 2016). In accordance with the German animal welfare act (TSchG), no additional approval for post mortem removal of brain tissue was necessary. All chemicals were purchased from Sigma-Aldrich (St. Louis, MO, USA) or AppliChem (Darmstadt, Germany), if not stated otherwise.

4.1. Genotyping

At 3–5 days after birth and directly after preparation of brain tissue, a tail biopsy was taken. First, biopsies were digested in 200 µL 25 mM NaOH and 0.2 mM ethylenediaminetetraacetic acid (EDTA) for 1 h at 95° Celcius (C) at 300 rpm in a twitter (Thriller, Peqlab, VWR, Darmstadt, Germany) to isolate the DNA. Afterwards, 200 µL 40 mM tris(hydroxymethyl)aminomethane (Tris)—HCl, pH 5, was added to neutralize the solution and products were centrifuged for 9–10 min at 15–20 °C at 13,000 rpm (Biofuge fresco, Heraeus, Thermo Fisher Scientific, Waltham, MA, USA). For the following polymerase chain reaction (PCR), 200 µL of the supernatant was decanted, since this contained the DNA. The PCR solution contained the master mix (Table 1) as well as the decanted supernatant. PCR protocols were performed as listed in Table 1. For otoferlin PCR, a restriction enzyme was used to determine genotypes. Therefore, a second digestion was performed with a solution containing 3 µL autoclaved H_2O, 1 µL 10× NEB 3 enzyme buffer and 1 µL BGI II-enzyme (Biolabs, Frankfurt am Main, Germany) times the samples plus 5 µL of the PCR product.

Next, visualization of the DNA bands in the gel was achieved by adding 4 µL sample buffer (40 mM Tris, 20 mM acetic acid, 1 mM EDTA with 40% glycerol and Xylene cyanol). Then, 5 µL DNA ladder (Hyperladder Bio-33040, Bioline, Meridian Biosciences, Memphis, TN, USA) was loaded into the first lane of each 1.5% agarose gel (1.5% agarose and 0.001% EtBr diluted in tris-acetate-EDTA buffer). The other lanes were filled with 14 µL of each probe and were run for 30–35 min at 90–95 V. To develop the gel and visualize the bands, gels were put into a chamber (Biometra Tl1, LTF Labortechnik, Wasserburg, Germany).

Table 1. Master mixes for PCR solutions and protocols used for genotyping of WT and KO mice.

Geno-Type	H$_2$O	5× PCR Buffer	Forward Primer	Reverse Primer	Taq Poly-Merase	PCR Protocol	Amplicon Size (bp)
WT	7.7 µL	4.0 µL	2.0 µL, 5 pmol/µL, 5'-GCA AAC TAT GCA AGA GGC ACC AGA-3'	2.0 µL, 5 pmol/µL, 5'-TAC TTC CAT TCC ACT ATA CTA ATG CAG GCT-3'	0.3 µL	2 min 92 °C; 20 s 52 °C; 30 s 72 °C; 30 cycles (20 s 92 °C; 20 s 52 °C; 30 s 72 °C); 7 min 72 °C; 15 °C cool down	300
CaV1.3 KO	7.9 µL	4.0 µL	2.0 µL, 5 pmol/µL, 5'-TTC CAT TTG TCA CGT CCT GCA CCA-3'	2.0 µL, 5 pmol/µL, 5'-TAC TTC CAT TCC ACT ATA CTA ATG CAG GCT-3'	0.1 µL	2 min 92 °C; 20 s 52 °C; 30 s 72 °C; 43 cycles (25 s 92 °C; 20 s 52 °C; 30 s 72 °C); 7 min 72 °C; 15 °C cool down	450
Otoferlin KO	7.9 µL	4.0 µL	0.5 µL, 10 pmol/µL, 5'-TAC TGC CCA CAT GAG CTT TG-3'	0.5 µL, 10 pmol/µL, 5'-CAG AGG AAT CCA GCT GAA GG-3'	0.1 µL	2 min 95 °C; 30 s 95 °C; 34 cycles (20 s 57 °C; 30 s 72 °C); 5 min 72 °C; 15 °C cool down	186/163 (WT), 349 (KO)

4.2. Immunohistochemistry

Animal perfusion and tissue preparations were performed as described earlier [1]. The tissue was subsequently processed for Cx43 and Cx30 antibody labeling. Tissues were transferred to phosphate buffered saline (PBS) and cut into 25–30 µm thick slices using a microtome (HM650V, Microtome, Microm International GmbH, Thermo Fisher Scientific, Waltham, MA, USA). Slices were mounted on glass slides (SuperFrost Plus, VWR, Darmstadt, Germany) for on-slide labeling. Unspecific binding sites were blocked with 0.25% triton X-100 and 2% normal goat serum (NGS; Gibco, Thermo Fisher Scientific, Waltham, MA, USA) for 1 h at room temperature (RT). Primary antibodies (rabbit anti-connexin 43, C6219, Sigma-Aldrich, St. Louis, MO, USA; rabbit anti-connexin 30, 700258, Invitrogen, Thermo Fisher Scientific, Waltham, MA, USA) were diluted 1:500 in 0.25% triton X-100 and 2% NGS and applied over night at +4 °C. Since both Cx antibodies were raised in the same host species, stainings were performed on separate sets of fixed slices. After washing with 0.25% triton X-100 and 2% NGS, tissue slices were incubated with secondary antibody (Alexa Fluor (AF) 488 goat anti-rabbit, A-11034, Invitrogen, Thermo Fisher Scientific, Waltham, MA, USA) diluted 1:100 in 2% NGS for 70 min at RT. After washing with PBS, slices were provided with coverslips in 10% DABCO (Fluka, Sigma-Aldrich, St. Louis, MO, USA) in MOWIOL (Calbiochem, Merck, Darmstadt, Germany).

Overview images were documented using a motorized upright widefield microscope (Nikon Eclipse 90i: Plan Fluor 10×/0.30, Nikon Instruments, Tokio, Japan) equipped with a DS-Q1Mc camera (Nikon Instruments, Tokio, Japan) and a FITC filter set (EX: 465–495 nm; DM: 505 nm; BA: 515–555 nm). All settings were kept constant when comparing immunolabeled areas and stainings. High-resolution images showing the center of auditory brainstem nuclei were taken on a motorized confocal laser scanning microscope (Nikon Eclipse C1 mounted at an E600FN: Plan Apo VC 60x/1.40 Oil, Nikon Instruments, Tokio, Japan). Fluorophores were detected with an Argon laser (excitation: 488 nm; emission collected at >515 nm; Melles Griot, Bensheim, Germany) in combination with EZ-C1 3.91 Silver Version software (Nikon Instruments, Tokio, Japan). A minimum of 3 slices were analyzed per nucleus and genotype: WT (Cx43/30): n = 3–5/3–8; Ca$_V$1.3 KO: n = 19–23/11–12; otoferlin KO: n = 5/6–8. The number of slices used for the analysis of nucleus area is the cumulated number of slices used for Cx43 and Cx30 for each nucleus and genotype. Selection and documentation of slices was done blind. For background correction of signal intensities, negative controls were performed and resulting mean background levels for each nucleus were subtracted.

4.3. Preparation of Acute Tissue Slices

Acute coronal brainstem slices were prepared as described earlier [37]. In brief, brains were quickly dissected after decapitation and transferred into ice-cold cutting solution containing (in mM): 26 $NaHCO_3$, 1.25 NaH_2PO_4, 2.5 KCl, 1 $MgCl_2$, 2 $CaCl_2$, 260 D-glucose, 2 Na-pyruvate, and 3 myo-inositol, pH 7.4, bubbled with carbogen (95% O_2, 5% CO_2). Thereafter, slices were transferred to artificial cerebrospinal fluid (ACSF) containing (in mM): 125 NaCl, 25 $NaHCO_3$, 1.25 NaH_2PO_4, 2.5 KCl, 1 $MgCl_2$, 2 $CaCl_2$, 10 D-glucose, 2 Na-pyruvate, 3 myo-inositol, and 0.44 ascorbic acid, pH 7.4, bubbled with carbogen. 270-µm-thick slices were cut using a vibratome (VT1200 S, Leica, Wetzlar, Germany). For a priori identification of astrocytes, slices were incubated for 30 min at 37 °C in 0.5–1 µM SR101 dissolved in ACSF and washed for another 30 min at 37 °C in SR101-free ACSF. Afterwards, slices were kept at RT until experiments were performed.

4.4. Electrophysiology and Tracer Loading

Whole-cell patch-clamp experiments were performed at RT with an upright microscope equipped with infrared differential interference contrast (Eclipse FN1, Nikon Instruments, 60× water immersion objective, N.A. 1.0, Tokio, Japan) and an infrared video camera (XC-ST70CE, Hamamatsu, Shizuoka, Japan) using a patch-clamp EPC10 amplifier and "PatchMaster" software (HEKA Elektronik, Lambrecht, Germany). The pipette solution contained (in mM): 140 K-gluconate, 5 EGTA (glycol-bis(2-aminoethylether)-N,N',N',N'-tetraacetic acid), 10 HEPES (*N*-(2-hydroxyethyl)piperazine-N'-2-ethanesulfonic acid), 1 $MgCl_2$, 2 Na_2ATP, and 0.3 Na_2GTP, pH 7.3. The pipette solution additionally contained a cocktail of the GJ-impermeable dye AF568 (100 µM, Invitrogen, Thermo Fisher Scientific, Waltham, MA, USA) and the GJ-permeable tracer neurobiotin (1%, Vector Laboratories, Inc., Peterborough, UK) to mark the patched cell and label the coupling network, respectively [1,2]. Patch pipettes were pulled from borosilicate glass capillaries (GB150(F)-8P, Science Products, Hofheim am Taunus, Germany) using a horizontal puller (P-87, Sutter Instruments, Novato, CA, USA) and had a resistance of 2–8 MΩ.

Astrocytes were patched in the central part of the LSO, where the mediolateral and dorsoventral axes are roughly tangential and orthogonal to the tonotopic axis, respectively. Astrocytes were recorded in voltage-clamp mode and held at −85 mV, which is close to their resting membrane potential [1,37]. The (fast) pipette capacitance was compensated. In standard whole-cell configuration the total input resistance (R_{In}) consists of membrane resistance (R_M) and series resistance (R_S) that are arranged in series [53]. They were calculated from currents recorded during hyperpolarizing voltage steps (ΔU = 5 mV). R_{In} is given by (Equation (1)):

$$R_{In} = \frac{U_2 - U_1}{I_2 - I_1} \quad (1)$$

with U_1 is −85 mV, U_2 is −90 mV. I_1 and I_2 are the recorded steady-state currents at U_1 and U_2, respectively. R_S was calculated by (Equation (2)):

$$R_S = \frac{U_2 - U_1}{I_{peak} - I_1} \quad (2)$$

with U_1, U_2, and I_2 are the same parameters as given in Equation (1) and I_{peak} is the maximal current at the initial phase when clamping from U_1 to U_2. Finally, R_M was calculated by (Equation (3); [54]):

$$R_M = R_{In} - R_S \quad (3)$$

Measurements were rejected if the R_S exceeded 15 MΩ to ensure sufficient electrical and diffusional access to the patched cell [55]. The liquid junction potential was not corrected. Astrocytes were characterized by applying a standard step protocol ranging from −150 mV to +50 mV with 10 mV increments and step duration of 50 ms to determine their *I/V* relationship. The resulting current traces were sampled at 50 kHz and online filtered at 2.9 kHz. Data were analyzed using "IGOR Pro" software (WaveMetrics, Lake Oswego, OR, USA).

4.5. Visualization of Coupled Cells

GJ networks and nucleus boundaries were visualized as described earlier [1,9]. Fixed slices were processed at RT. First, slices were washed three times in PBS (containing NaCl, $Na_2HPO_4*2H_2O$, $NaH_2PO_4*H_2O$; pH 7.4). Membrane permeabilization was achieved by incubation in 0.25% triton X-100 for 30 min. Thereafter, slices were washed again in PBS. Neurobiotin was identified by incubating slices for 3 h with avidin AF488 (50 µg/mL, Invitrogen, Thermo Fisher Scientific, Waltham, MA, USA) and slices were washed again. Since tracer coupling differs within and dorsal to the LSO [1], glycine transporter (GlyT) 2-staining was used to identify the relative position of the patched cell and the network within the LSO. Avidin-labeled slices were again permeabilized for 30 min in 0.25% triton X-100. Unspecific binding sites were blocked for 1 h in a solution containing 2% bovine serum albumin (BSA), 11.1% NGS (PAA laboratories, Cölbe, Germany), and 0.3% triton X-100. The slices were then incubated overnight (about 20 h) at +4 °C with primary antibody (rabbit anti-GlyT2, AB1773, Millipore, Burlington, MA, USA) diluted 1:2000 in 1% BSA, 1% NGS, and 0.3% triton X-100. The next steps were performed at RT. After washing in PBS, slices were incubated for 90 min with the secondary antibody (goat anti-rabbit AF647, A-21450, Invitrogen, Thermo Fisher Scientific, Waltham, MA, USA) diluted 1:300 in 1% BSA, 1% NGS, and 0.3% triton X-100. Finally, slices were washed in PBS and mounted in 2.5% Dabco on glass slides.

SR101-labeling, network tracing and immunohistochemical stainings were documented at a confocal microscope (Zeiss LSM700: EC Plan-Fluor 10x/0.3; Plan-Apochromat 63x/1.4 Oil) in combination with ZEN software (Zeiss, Oberkochen, Germany), respectively. Fluorophores were detected as follows (excitation wavelength/filtered emission wavelength): AF488 (488 nm/505–530 nm), AF568 (543 nm/>560 nm), AF647 (639 nm/>640 nm), and SR101 (561 nm/580–620 nm). To improve the quality of confocal micrographs and reduce background fluorescence, a Kalman filter was used (averaging of four identical image sections). Images were processed using "FIJI" software [56].

4.6. Analysis of Network Topography

To avoid unconscious experimenter-based corruption of data, coupled cells were identified using an intensity-based detection method [9]. Only cells surpassing a threshold of 1.75 times background intensity were incorporated in the analysis (Figure 3Ad,Bb,Cd). Subsequent vector-based calculation of network topography was used for an automated analysis [9]. Here, the network was divided into four 90° sectors and the sum vector for each sector was calculated. The length of these vectors was normalized to the number of cells in each sector. R is the quotient of the normalized y value and the normalized x value (Equation (4)):

$$R = \frac{\frac{|\vec{y_{1A}}|}{n_{1A}} + \frac{|\vec{y_{1B}}|}{n_{1B}}}{\frac{|\vec{x_{2A}}|}{n_{2A}} + \frac{|\vec{x_{2B}}|}{n_{2B}}} \quad (4)$$

where $|\vec{y_{1A}}|, |\vec{y_{1B}}|, |\vec{x_{2A}}|, |\vec{x_{2B}}|$ are the absolute values of the sum vectors of the sectors 1A, 1B, 2A, and 2B, respectively, and n_{1A}, n_{1B}, n_{2A} and n_{2B} are the number of cells in respective sectors. Then, the coordinate system was rotated and the ratio was recalculated in 15° steps. A sinusoidal function (Figure 4Aa,Ba,Ca; Equation (5)) was fitted to the data:

$$R = A_0 + A \sin(\omega \alpha + (\varphi + \frac{3}{4}\pi)) \quad (5)$$

where A_0 is the offset, ω is the circular frequency, α is the angle and φ is the phase shift. The highest Ratio ($R_{max} = A_0 + A$) of the fit reveals the angle of maximal anisotropy of a single network. Therefore, networks were classified into three groups depending on R_{max} and their preferential orientation α (Figure 4Da): (1) $R_{max} > 1.1$ and $45° < \alpha \leq 135°$, anisotropic and orthogonal to the tonotopic axis, (2) $R_{max} \leq 1.1$, round and (3) $R_{max} > 1.1$ and $0° \leq \alpha < 45°$ or $135° < \alpha \leq 180°$, anisotropic and parallel to the tonotopic axis.

4.7. Statistics

Results are provided as mean ± SD. Data were statistically analyzed using WinSTAT (R. Fitch Software, Bad Krozingen, Germany) and tested for normal distribution with the Kolmogorov–Smirnov test. In case of normal distribution, results were assessed by two-tailed, unpaired Student's *t*-tests. Otherwise, results were assessed by a Mann–Whitney *U*-test. Differences in distribution of classes were analyzed between the WT and the two mouse models using a X^2 test. *p* represents the error probability, * $p < 0.05$, ** $p < 0.01$, *** $p < 0.001$. *n* represents the number of recorded cells or analyzed networks (/slices). In case of multiple comparisons data were statistically analyzed by the tests described above under post hoc Šidák correction of critical values [57]: two comparisons: Figure 1D–F and Figure 3D: * $p < 0.025$, ** $p < 0.005$, *** $p < 0.0005$.

4.8. Additional Information

The WT data, as well as Figure 2Aa left, Ab right, and parts of Ac, Figure 3Aa–Ac, and Figure 4Ab were taken from [9] in accordance to the terms and conditions of the Creative Commons Attribution (CC BY) license (http://creativecommons.org/licenses/by/4.0/).

Author Contributions: Conceptualization, J.S.; methodology, S.E., L.P., and J.S.; validation, J.S.; formal analysis, S.E.; investigation, S.E. and L.P.; resources, J.S. and C.R.R.; data curation, S.E. and L.P.; writing—original draft preparation, S.E. and J.S.; writing—review and editing, S.E., C.R.R., and J.S.; visualization, S.E.; supervision, J.S.; project administration, J.S.; funding acquisition, C.R.R. and J.S. All authors have read and agreed to the published version of the manuscript.

Funding: This study was supported by institutional funding (TU Kaiserslautern) and the GERMAN RESEARCH FOUNDATION (DFG Priority Program 1608 "Ultrafast and temporally precise information processing: Normal and dysfunctional hearing": STE 2352/2-1; Priority Program 1757 "Functional Specializations of Neuroglia as Critical Determinants of Brain Activity": RO 2327/8-2).

Acknowledgments: We thank Eckhard Friauf for critical comments on the manuscript. Additionally, we thank Ralph Reiss for genotyping, and Tina Kehrwald and Simone Durry for preparing transgenic mice and immunohistochemical processing of the tissue, respectively.

Conflicts of Interest: The authors declare no conflict of interest.

Abbreviations

ACSF	Artificial cerebrospinal fluid
AF	Alexa fluor
BSA	Bovine serum albumin
Ca_V	Voltage-activated calcium channel
Cx	Connexin
EDTA	Ethylenediaminetetraacetic acid
EGTA	Glycol-bis(2 aminoethylether)-N,N′,N′,N′-tetraacetic acid
GJ	Gap junction
GlyT	Glycine transporter
HEPES	N (2 hydroxyethyl)piperazine-N′ 2 ethanesulfonic acid
IC	Inferior colliculus
KO	Knock-out
LSO	Lateral superior olive
MNTB	Medial nucleus of the trapezoid body
NGS	Normal goat serum

nPA   Non-passive astrocyte
PA   Passive astrocyte
PBS   Phosphate buffered solution
PCR   Polymerase chain reaction
R Ratio
RT   Room temperature
SOC   Superior olivary complex
SPN   Superior paraolivery nucleus
SR101 Sulforhodamine 101
Tris   Tris(hydroxymethyl)aminomethane
WT   Wild type

References

1. Augustin, V.; Bold, C.; Wadle, S.L.; Langer, J.; Jabs, R.; Philippot, C.; Weingarten, D.J.; Rose, C.R.; Steinhauser, C.; Stephan, J. Functional anisotropic panglial networks in the lateral superior olive. *Glia* **2016**, *64*, 1892–1911. [CrossRef] [PubMed]
2. Wadle, S.L.; Augustin, V.; Langer, J.; Jabs, R.; Philippot, C.; Weingarten, D.J.; Rose, C.R.; Steinhauser, C.; Stephan, J. Anisotropic Panglial Coupling Reflects Tonotopic Organization in the Inferior Colliculus. *Front. Cell. Neurosci.* **2018**, *12*, 431. [CrossRef] [PubMed]
3. Maglione, M.; Tress, O.; Haas, B.; Karram, K.; Trotter, J.; Willecke, K.; Kettenmann, H. Oligodendrocytes in mouse corpus callosum are coupled via gap junction channels formed by connexin47 and connexin32. *Glia* **2010**, *58*, 1104–1117. [CrossRef] [PubMed]
4. Moshrefi-Ravasdjani, B.; Hammel, E.L.; Kafitz, K.W.; Rose, C.R. Astrocyte Sodium Signalling and Panglial Spread of Sodium Signals in Brain White Matter. *Neurochem. Res.* **2017**, *42*, 2505–2518. [CrossRef] [PubMed]
5. Griemsmann, S.; Hoft, S.P.; Bedner, P.; Zhang, J.; von Staden, E.; Beinhauer, A.; Degen, J.; Dublin, P.; Cope, D.W.; Richter, N.; et al. Characterization of Panglial Gap Junction Networks in the Thalamus, Neocortex, and Hippocampus Reveals a Unique Population of Glial Cells. *Cereb. Cortex* **2015**, *25*, 3420–3433. [CrossRef] [PubMed]
6. Wallraff, A.; Kohling, R.; Heinemann, U.; Theis, M.; Willecke, K.; Steinhauser, C. The impact of astrocytic gap junctional coupling on potassium buffering in the hippocampus. *J. Neurosci.* **2006**, *26*, 5438–5447. [CrossRef]
7. Houades, V.; Koulakoff, A.; Ezan, P.; Seif, I.; Giaume, C. Gap junction-mediated astrocytic networks in the mouse barrel cortex. *J. Neurosci.* **2008**, *28*, 5207–5217. [CrossRef]
8. Claus, L.; Philippot, C.; Griemsmann, S.; Timmermann, A.; Jabs, R.; Henneberger, C.; Kettenmann, H.; Steinhauser, C. Barreloid Borders and Neuronal Activity Shape Panglial Gap Junction-Coupled Networks in the Mouse Thalamus. *Cereb. Cortex* **2018**, *28*, 213–222. [CrossRef]
9. Eitelmann, S.; Hirtz, J.J.; Stephan, J. A Vector-Based Method to Analyze the Topography of Glial Networks. *Int. J. Mol. Sci.* **2019**, *20*, 2821. [CrossRef]
10. Kandler, K.; Clause, A.; Noh, J. Tonotopic reorganization of developing auditory brainstem circuits. *Nat. Neurosci.* **2009**, *12*, 711–717. [CrossRef]
11. Huang, C.M.; Fex, J. Tonotopic organization in the inferior colliculus of the rat demonstrated with the 2-deoxyglucose method. *Exp. Brain Res.* **1986**, *61*, 506–512. [CrossRef]
12. Merzenich, M.M.; Reid, M.D. Representation of the cochlea within the inferior colliculus of the cat. *Brain Res.* **1974**, *77*, 397–415. [CrossRef]
13. Rietzel, H.J.; Friauf, E. Neuron types in the rat lateral superior olive and developmental changes in the complexity of their dendritic arbors. *J. Comp. Neurol.* **1998**, *390*, 20–40. [CrossRef]
14. Malmierca, M.S.; Blackstad, T.W.; Osen, K.K. Computer-assisted 3-D reconstructions of Golgi-impregnated neurons in the cortical regions of the inferior colliculus of rat. *Hear. Res.* **2011**, *274*, 13–26. [CrossRef]
15. Sanes, D.H.; Song, J.; Tyson, J. Refinement of dendritic arbors along the tonotopic axis of the gerbil lateral superior olive. *Brain Res. Dev. Brain Res.* **1992**, *67*, 47–55. [CrossRef]
16. Bal, R.; Green, G.G.; Rees, A.; Sanders, D.J. Firing patterns of inferior colliculus neurons-histology and mechanism to change firing patterns in rat brain slices. *Neurosci. Lett.* **2002**, *317*, 42–46. [CrossRef]

17. Ghirardini, E.; Wadle, S.L.; Augustin, V.; Becker, J.; Brill, S.; Hammerich, J.; Seifert, G.; Stephan, J. Expression of functional inhibitory neurotransmitter transporters GlyT1, GAT-1, and GAT-3 by astrocytes of inferior colliculus and hippocampus. *Mol. Brain* **2018**, *11*, 4. [CrossRef]
18. Kandler, K.; Gillespie, D.C. Developmental refinement of inhibitory sound-localization circuits. *Trends Neurosci.* **2005**, *28*, 290–296. [CrossRef]
19. Friauf, E.; Krächan, E.G.; Müller, N.I.C. Lateral superior olive. In *The Oxford Handbook of the Auditory Brainstem*; Kandler, K., Ed.; Oxford University Press: New York, NY, USA, 2019; pp. 328–394. [CrossRef]
20. Kotak, V.C.; Korada, S.; Schwartz, I.R.; Sanes, D.H. A developmental shift from GABAergic to glycinergic transmission in the central auditory system. *J. Neurosci.* **1998**, *18*, 4646–4655. [CrossRef]
21. Nabekura, J.; Katsurabayashi, S.; Kakazu, Y.; Shibata, S.; Matsubara, A.; Jinno, S.; Mizoguchi, Y.; Sasaki, A.; Ishibashi, H. Developmental switch from GABA to glycine release in single central synaptic terminals. *Nat. Neurosci.* **2004**, *7*, 17–23. [CrossRef]
22. Fischer, A.U.; Muller, N.I.C.; Deller, T.; Del Turco, D.; Fisch, J.O.; Griesemer, D.; Kattler, K.; Maraslioglu, A.; Roemer, V.; Xu-Friedman, M.A.; et al. GABA is a modulator, rather than a classical transmitter, in the medial nucleus of the trapezoid body-lateral superior olive sound localization circuit. *J. Physiol.* **2019**, *597*, 2269–2295. [CrossRef] [PubMed]
23. Kim, G.; Kandler, K. Elimination and strengthening of glycinergic/GABAergic connections during tonotopic map formation. *Nat. Neurosci.* **2003**, *6*, 282–290. [CrossRef] [PubMed]
24. Tritsch, N.X.; Yi, E.; Gale, J.E.; Glowatzki, E.; Bergles, D.E. The origin of spontaneous activity in the developing auditory system. *Nature* **2007**, *450*, 50–55. [CrossRef] [PubMed]
25. Sanes, D.H.; Takacs, C. Activity-dependent refinement of inhibitory connections. *Eur. J. Neurosci.* **1993**, *5*, 570–574. [CrossRef]
26. Muller, N.I.C.; Sonntag, M.; Maraslioglu, A.; Hirtz, J.J.; Friauf, E. Topographic map refinement and synaptic strengthening of a sound localization circuit require spontaneous peripheral activity. *J. Physiol.* **2019**, *597*, 5469–5493. [CrossRef]
27. Clause, A.; Kim, G.; Sonntag, M.; Weisz, C.J.; Vetter, D.E.; Rubsamen, R.; Kandler, K. The precise temporal pattern of prehearing spontaneous activity is necessary for tonotopic map refinement. *Neuron* **2014**, *82*, 822–835. [CrossRef]
28. Clause, A.; Lauer, A.M.; Kandler, K. Mice Lacking the Alpha9 Subunit of the Nicotinic Acetylcholine Receptor Exhibit Deficits in Frequency Difference Limens and Sound Localization. *Front. Cell. Neurosci.* **2017**, *11*, 167. [CrossRef]
29. Choi, B.Y.; Ahmed, Z.M.; Riazuddin, S.; Bhinder, M.A.; Shahzad, M.; Husnain, T.; Riazuddin, S.; Griffith, A.J.; Friedman, T.B. Identities and frequencies of mutations of the otoferlin gene (OTOF) causing DFNB9 deafness in Pakistan. *Clin. Genet.* **2009**, *75*, 237–243. [CrossRef]
30. Duman, D.; Sirmaci, A.; Cengiz, F.B.; Ozdag, H.; Tekin, M. Screening of 38 genes identifies mutations in 62% of families with nonsyndromic deafness in Turkey. *Genet. Test. Mol. Biomark.* **2011**, *15*, 29–33. [CrossRef]
31. Baig, S.M.; Koschak, A.; Lieb, A.; Gebhart, M.; Dafinger, C.; Nurnberg, G.; Ali, A.; Ahmad, I.; Sinnegger-Brauns, M.J.; Brandt, N.; et al. Loss of Ca(v)1.3 (CACNA1D) function in a human channelopathy with bradycardia and congenital deafness. *Nat. Neurosci.* **2011**, *14*, 77–84. [CrossRef]
32. Iwasa, Y.; Nishio, S.Y.; Yoshimura, H.; Kanda, Y.; Kumakawa, K.; Abe, S.; Naito, Y.; Nagai, K.; Usami, S. OTOF mutation screening in Japanese severe to profound recessive hearing loss patients. *BMC Med. Genet.* **2013**, *14*, 95. [CrossRef] [PubMed]
33. Platzer, J.; Engel, J.; Schrott-Fischer, A.; Stephan, K.; Bova, S.; Chen, H.; Zheng, H.; Striessnig, J. Congenital deafness and sinoatrial node dysfunction in mice lacking class D L-type Ca^{2+} channels. *Cell* **2000**, *102*, 89–97. [CrossRef]
34. Longo-Guess, C.; Gagnon, L.H.; Bergstrom, D.E.; Johnson, K.R. A missense mutation in the conserved C2B domain of otoferlin causes deafness in a new mouse model of DFNB9. *Hear. Res.* **2007**, *234*, 21–28. [CrossRef] [PubMed]
35. Hirtz, J.J.; Boesen, M.; Braun, N.; Deitmer, J.W.; Kramer, F.; Lohr, C.; Muller, B.; Nothwang, H.G.; Striessnig, J.; Lohrke, S.; et al. Cav1.3 calcium channels are required for normal development of the auditory brainstem. *J. Neurosci.* **2011**, *31*, 8280–8294. [CrossRef]

36. Hirtz, J.J.; Braun, N.; Griesemer, D.; Hannes, C.; Janz, K.; Lohrke, S.; Muller, B.; Friauf, E. Synaptic refinement of an inhibitory topographic map in the auditory brainstem requires functional Cav1.3 calcium channels. *J. Neurosci.* **2012**, *32*, 14602–14616. [CrossRef]
37. Stephan, J.; Friauf, E. Functional analysis of the inhibitory neurotransmitter transporters GlyT1, GAT-1, and GAT-3 in astrocytes of the lateral superior olive. *Glia* **2014**, *62*, 1992–2003. [CrossRef]
38. Kafitz, K.W.; Meier, S.D.; Stephan, J.; Rose, C.R. Developmental profile and properties of sulforhodamine 101–Labeled glial cells in acute brain slices of rat hippocampus. *J. Neurosci. Methods* **2008**, *169*, 84–92. [CrossRef] [PubMed]
39. Zhou, M.; Schools, G.P.; Kimelberg, H.K. Development of GLAST(+) astrocytes and NG2(+) glia in rat hippocampus CA1: Mature astrocytes are electrophysiologically passive. *J. Neurophysiol.* **2006**, *95*, 134–143. [CrossRef]
40. Langer, J.; Stephan, J.; Theis, M.; Rose, C.R. Gap junctions mediate intercellular spread of sodium between hippocampal astrocytes in situ. *Glia* **2012**, *60*, 239–252. [CrossRef]
41. Schools, G.P.; Zhou, M.; Kimelberg, H.K. Development of gap junctions in hippocampal astrocytes: Evidence that whole cell electrophysiological phenotype is an intrinsic property of the individual cell. *J. Neurophysiol.* **2006**, *96*, 1383–1392. [CrossRef]
42. Kiyoshi, C.M.; Du, Y.; Zhong, S.; Wang, W.; Taylor, A.T.; Xiong, B.; Ma, B.; Terman, D.; Zhou, M. Syncytial isopotentiality: A system-wide electrical feature of astrocytic networks in the brain. *Glia* **2018**, *66*, 2756–2769. [CrossRef] [PubMed]
43. Kunzelmann, P.; Schroder, W.; Traub, O.; Steinhauser, C.; Dermietzel, R.; Willecke, K. Late onset and increasing expression of the gap junction protein connexin30 in adult murine brain and long-term cultured astrocytes. *Glia* **1999**, *25*, 111–119. [CrossRef]
44. Nagy, J.I.; Patel, D.; Ochalski, P.A.; Stelmack, G.L. Connexin30 in rodent, cat and human brain: Selective expression in gray matter astrocytes, co-localization with connexin43 at gap junctions and late developmental appearance. *Neuroscience* **1999**, *88*, 447–468. [CrossRef]
45. Felix, L.; Stephan, J.; Rose, C.R. Astrocytes of the early postnatal brain. *Eur. J. Neurosci.* **2020**. [CrossRef]
46. Ghezali, G.; Calvo, C.F.; Pillet, L.E.; Llense, F.; Ezan, P.; Pannasch, U.; Bemelmans, A.P.; Etienne Manneville, S.; Rouach, N. Connexin 30 controls astroglial polarization during postnatal brain development. *Development* **2018**, *145*, dev155275. [CrossRef] [PubMed]
47. Anders, S.; Minge, D.; Griemsmann, S.; Herde, M.K.; Steinhauser, C.; Henneberger, C. Spatial properties of astrocyte gap junction coupling in the rat hippocampus. *Philos. Trans. R Soc. Lond. B Biol. Sci.* **2014**, *369*, 20130600. [CrossRef] [PubMed]
48. Golub, J.S.; Tong, L.; Ngyuen, T.B.; Hume, C.R.; Palmiter, R.D.; Rubel, E.W.; Stone, J.S. Hair cell replacement in adult mouse utricles after targeted ablation of hair cells with diphtheria toxin. *J. Neurosci.* **2012**, *32*, 15093–15105. [CrossRef]
49. Korn, M.J.; Koppel, S.J.; Cramer, K.S. Astrocyte-secreted factors modulate a gradient of primary dendritic arbors in nucleus laminaris of the avian auditory brainstem. *PLoS ONE* **2011**, *6*, e27383. [CrossRef]
50. Korn, M.J.; Koppel, S.J.; Li, L.H.; Mehta, D.; Mehta, S.B.; Seidl, A.H.; Cramer, K.S. Astrocyte-secreted factors modulate the developmental distribution of inhibitory synapses in nucleus laminaris of the avian auditory brainstem. *J. Comp. Neurol.* **2012**, *520*, 1262–1277. [CrossRef]
51. Xu, J.H.; Long, L.; Tang, Y.C.; Hu, H.T.; Tang, F.R. Ca(v)1.2, Ca(v)1.3, and Ca(v)2.1 in the mouse hippocampus during and after pilocarpine-induced status epilepticus. *Hippocampus* **2007**, *17*, 235–251. [CrossRef]
52. Schug, N.; Braig, C.; Zimmermann, U.; Engel, J.; Winter, H.; Ruth, P.; Blin, N.; Pfister, M.; Kalbacher, H.; Knipper, M. Differential expression of otoferlin in brain, vestibular system, immature and mature cochlea of the rat. *Eur. J. Neurosci.* **2006**, *24*, 3372–3380. [CrossRef] [PubMed]
53. Hamill, O.P.; Marty, A.; Neher, E.; Sakmann, B.; Sigworth, F.J. Improved patch-clamp techniques for high-resolution current recording from cells and cell-free membrane patches. *Pflugers. Arch.* **1981**, *391*, 85–100. [CrossRef] [PubMed]
54. Stephan, J.; Haack, N.; Kafitz, K.W.; Durry, S.; Koch, D.; Hochstrate, P.; Seifert, G.; Steinhauser, C.; Rose, C.R. Kir4.1 channels mediate a depolarization of hippocampal astrocytes under hyperammonemic conditions in situ. *Glia* **2012**, *60*, 965–978. [CrossRef] [PubMed]
55. Pusch, M.; Neher, E. Rates of diffusional exchange between small cells and a measuring patch pipette. *Pflugers. Arch.* **1988**, *411*, 204–211. [CrossRef] [PubMed]

56. Schindelin, J.; Arganda-Carreras, I.; Frise, E.; Kaynig, V.; Longair, M.; Pietzsch, T.; Preibisch, S.; Rueden, C.; Saalfeld, S.; Schmid, B.; et al. Fiji: An open-source platform for biological-image analysis. *Nat. Methods* **2012**, *9*, 676–682. [CrossRef]
57. Abdi, H. The Bonferroni and Šidák corrections for multiple comparisons. In *Encyclopedia of Measurement and Statistics*; Salkind, N., Ed.; Sage Publications: Thousand Oaks, CA, USA, 2007; pp. 103–107.

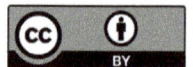

© 2020 by the authors. Licensee MDPI, Basel, Switzerland. This article is an open access article distributed under the terms and conditions of the Creative Commons Attribution (CC BY) license (http://creativecommons.org/licenses/by/4.0/).

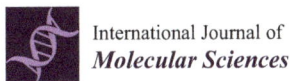 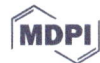

Article

Expression and Localization of BDNF/TrkB System in the Zebrafish Inner Ear

Antonino Germanà, Maria Cristina Guerrera *, Rosaria Laurà, Maria Levanti, Marialuisa Aragona, Kamel Mhalhel, Germana Germanà, Giuseppe Montalbano and Francesco Abbate

Zebrafish Neuromorphology Lab, Department of Veterinary Sciences, University of Messina, 98168 Messina, Italy; agermana@unime.it (A.G.); laurar@unime.it (R.L.); mblevanti@unime.it (M.L.); mlaragona@unime.it (M.A.); kmhalhel@unime.it (K.M.); pgermana@unime.it (G.G.); gmontalbano@unime.it (G.M.); abbatef@unime.it (F.A.)
* Correspondence: mguerrera@unime.it; Tel.: +39-090-6766542

Received: 25 June 2020; Accepted: 10 August 2020; Published: 12 August 2020

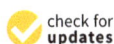

Abstract: Brain-derived neurotrophic factor (BDNF), a member of the neurotrophin family, is involved in multiple and fundamental functions of the central and peripheral nervous systems including sensory organs. Despite recent advances in knowledge on the functional significance of BDNF and TrkB in the regulation of the acoustic system of mammals, the localization of BDNF/TrkB system in the inner ear of zebrafish during development, is not well known. Therefore, the goal of the present study is to analyze the age-dependent changes using RT-PCR, Western Blot and single and double immunofluorescence of the BDNF and its specific receptor in the zebrafish inner ear. The results showed the mRNA expression and the cell localization of BDNF and TrkB in the hair cells of the crista ampullaris and in the neuroepithelium of the utricle, saccule and macula lagena, analyzed at different ages. Our results demonstrate that the BDNF/TrkB system is present in the sensory cells of the inner ear, during whole life. Therefore, this system might play a key role in the development and maintenance of the hair cells in adults, suggesting that the zebrafish inner ear represents an interesting model to study the involvement of the neurotrophins in the biology of sensory cells

Keywords: brain-derived neurotrophic factor; TrkB; inner ear; development; zebrafish

1. Introduction

According to the World Health Organization, around 466 million people (5% of the populations) worldwide have disabling hearing loss. The onset of the hearing disorders originate from genetic problems to pharmacological treatments, through infectious diseases and exposure to strong noise. Particularly, the non-sensorineural hearing loss represents the most common hearing disorder, caused by a serious morphofunctional alterations of cochlear hair cells. Brain-derived neurotrophic factor (BDNF) belongs to the neurotrophin family and is involved in the development, maintenance and neuronal plasticity of the different neuronal subpopulations of the central and peripheral nervous systems [1]. BDNF acts on cell surfaces through a specific receptor called TrkB. Brain-derived neurotrophic factor (BDNF) and neurotrophin 3 (NT-3) with their specific receptors (TrkB and TrkC) play a key role in the regulation of the acoustic system of mammals [2]. Recently, the expression and localization of neurotrophins and their receptors have been found in the inner ear and lateral line system of different teleosts [3–5]. It was demonstrated that the BDNF and TrkB sequences are well preserved during evolution [6] and therefore these two proteins have been identified and analyzed thoroughly in the fish nervous system with a specific focus on the zebrafish sensory organs. BDNF and its specific receptor TrkB were localized in different areas of both adult and developing zebrafish brain [7–11], in the photoreceptor layer of the retina, from larval to adult stage, under both physiological and experimental conditions with an identical pattern of distribution and cell localization [12], in the hair cells of the lateral line system during development [13] and in the chemosensory cells of the taste buds [14]. In teleosts, the auditory system is formed by the inner ear and lateral line system. The inner ear, more specifically, consists of the labyrinth formed by three semicircular canals, connected to a sacciform structure, the utricle, which connects, in the lower part, to a second sacciform structure, the saccule. Adjacent to the saccule is the lagena. At the base of each canal, the bony region is enlarged and has a dilated sac at one end, called the osseous ampullae. Each ampulla contains a patch of sensory epithelium with an evident round shape, called crista ampullaris. Utricle, saccule and lagena are provided with a thickening of sensory cells called macula, whose kinocilia and stereocilia are connected to dense limestone structures, the otoliths [15]. It is well-known that the utricle is usually considered to be a vestibular organ; the sacculus is involved in sound reception and the lagena assists with sacculus functions playing an important role in orientation and hearing too [16]. The zebrafish is now recognized as an important experimental animal for studying developmental biology and genetics as well as for modeling human disorders including sensorineural hearing loss mainly resulting from damage to the sensory hair cells of the inner ear [17–19]. The hair cells of the zebrafish inner ear present structural and molecular homology with the sensory cells of the mammalian inner ear including that of humans. Moreover, numerous genes as ATOH1, POU4F3, GFI1 and other genes, are expressed in the sensory cells of zebrafish, mainly during embryonic development, also expressed in mammals [20]. It is well known that zebrafish is able to regenerate, within a few days, the hair cells damaged or lost by acoustic trauma, chemical exposure or genetics [21–25]. Therefore, based on the peculiar ability of zebrafish to regenerate new hair cells, this study was undertaken to analyze the cellular localization of BDNF and its specific receptor TrkB location in the inner ear of the zebrafish.

2. Results

2.1. Anatomical Study of Zebrafish Inner Ear

The inner ear in zebrafish is located in a bone capsule in the cranial cavity, posterolaterally to the optic tectum, just behind the eyes (Figure 1a,b). It is divided into an upper part including three semicircular canals related to the utricle and the lower part made up of the saccule and lagena, also called otolith organs. The semicircular canals are spatially oriented in three mutually perpendicular planes following the main axis and orthogonally among them. The anterior and posterior canals are placed vertically and the lateral canal horizontally. The opposite parts of the anterior and posterior canals considering the ampullary end, converge in a common part called crus communis (Figure 1).

At the end of each semicircular canals a dilated sac is present, called ampulla ossea, containing a cluster of sensory cells called crista ampullaris and a thick gelatinous cap called cupula (Figure 2a). The crista ampullaris shows a cuboidal epithelium. In the apical part a sensory epithelium with hair, supporting and basal cells is present (Figure 2b).

Each otolith organ, containing an oval thickening called maculae of supporting cells, interdigitates among hair sensory cells (Figure 3).

Dense calcareous structures are present in close proximity to sensory epithelium, the utricular otolith (lapillus), saccular otolith (arrow) and lagenar otolith (asterisk) located in a small cavity in the temporal bone (Figure 1d–f). In the larval stage, at 8 days post fertilization (dpf), the pars inferior shows little resemblance to the final adult form but is merely a slight ventromedial pouch containing the posterior macula (Figure 4).

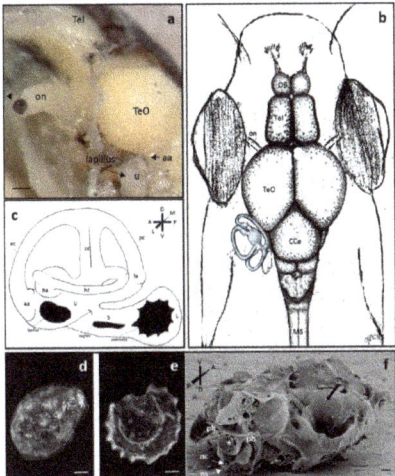

Figure 1. (**a**) Stereomicrograph: Cranial cavity dissection in adult zebrafish, lateral view: the bone skull has been removed in order to highlight the brain and the topographical relationships with the inner ear; some bony labyrinth was dissected away to improve visualization of membranous labyrinth: Tel—Telencephalon; TeO—Optic tectum; on—optic nerve with optic papilla (arrowhead) u—utricle, lapillus in the utricle, aa—anterior ampulla; (**b**) schematic drawing of the dorsal view zebrafish head without the skull: the topographical relationship of the inner ear with respect to TeO and eyes is represented. OB—olfactory bulb, Tel—Telencephalon, TeO—Optic tectum, CCe—cerebellar corpus, MS—spinal cord. (**c**) schematic drawing of the membranous labyrinth in adult zebrafish: lateral view; Orientation: D-dorsal, V-ventral, A—anterior, P—posterior, L—lateral, M—medial; aa—anterior ampulla; ac—anterior canal; cc—crus commune; ha—horizontal ampulla; hc—horizontal canal; la—lateral ampulla; pc—posterior canal; S—saccule; U—utricle; L—lagena. The otoliths (lapillus, sagitta, asteriscus) have been depicted in the respective otolithic organs, utricle, saccule and lagena. (**d**–**f**) Scanning electron microscopy: lapillus (**d**), asteriscus (**e**), base of the neurocranium, ventro-dorsal view: cervical vertebra in posterior view (asterisk) (**f**). The black arrow shows a landmark of the inner ear area placed inside the bone capsule; ph—parapophysis, nc—neural canal, ns—neural spine. Scale bar: (**a**) 1 mm, (**d**–**f**) 100 µm.

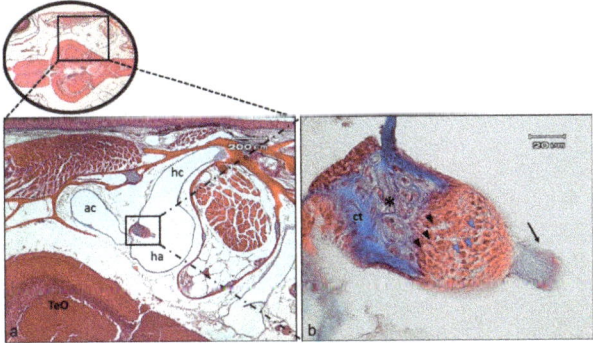

Figure 2. (**a**) Light micrographs (Masson Trichrome with Anylin blue staining) of adult zebrafish head; dorso-ventral view, horizontal section: semicircular horizontal canal (hc) of the inner ear, with its ampulla (ha) containing the crista ampullaris, placed near Optic tectum (TeO), are visible; ac—semicircular anterior canal; (**b**) High magnification of ampullary crest in the horizontal canal: the connective tissue (ct) supports nerve fibers (asterisk). The black arrowheads indicate the supporting cells, blue arrowheads indicate the hair cells, the arrow points to the cupula.

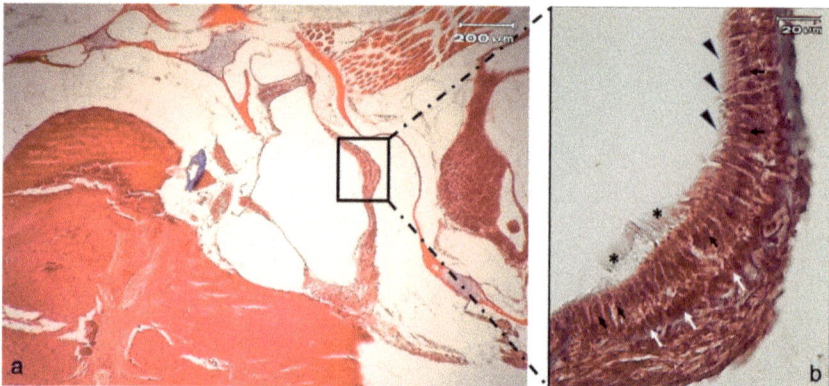

Figure 3. (**a**) Light micrographs (Masson Trichrome with Anylin blue staining) of adult zebrafish head; dorso-ventral view, horizontal section: macula of utricle (rectangle); (**b**) High magnification of utricular macula. The portion of the utricle that forms the macula shows a sort of pouch. The sensory hair cells (black arrows) with numerous stereocilia (arrowheads) and less numerous but longer kinocilia (asterisk) are visible. The white arrows indicate the supporting cells.

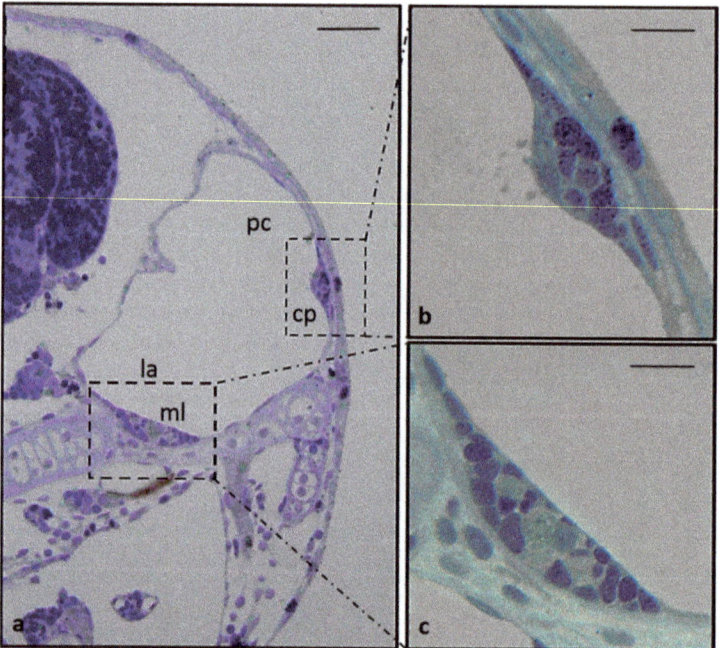

Figure 4. (**a**) Transverse section of the larval stage head (8 dpf), semithin section, toluidine blue staining. Structure of an 8 days old inner ear: crista ampullaris (square) and macula (rectangle). (**b**) High magnification of sensory epithelial cells of lateral cristae: (**c**) High magnification saccular macula. ml—macula lagena; la—lagena; pc—posterior canal, cp—crista posterior. Scale bars: (**a**) 30µm, (**b**,**c**) 9 µm.

Although its dimensions have increased, the 15, 30 and 50 dpf ear is characterized by the semicircular canals and utricle, and the anatomical spatial organization and the histological features of the neuroepithelium are very similar to the adult zebrafish (data not shown).

2.2. Expression and Occurrence of Bdnf and TrkB in Zebrafish Inner Ear

The expression of *Bdnf* and *ntrk2b* mRNA was assayed in the homogenates of zebrafish inner ear using reverse transcriptase PCR. Our observations demonstrated that *Bdnf* and *ntrk2b* are expressed at 8, 15, 30, 50 dpf and adult stage. *B-actin* controls for each condition were also conducted (Figure 5).

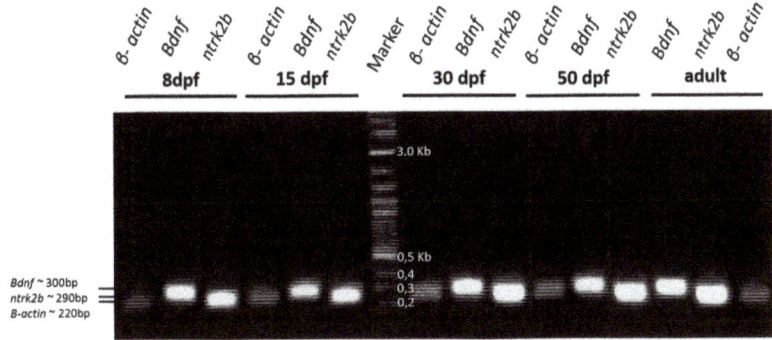

Figure 5. RT-PCR, *Bdnf* and *ntrk2b* mRNA expression in the inner ear from larval to adult stage. *B-actin* controls for each condition are also shown. Lines 1, 2 and 3: detection of *β-actin*, *Bdnf* and *ntrk2b* at 8 dpf. Lines 4, 5 and 6: detection of *β-actin*, *Bdnf* and *ntrk2b* at 15 dpf. Line 7 Marker. Lines 8, 9 and 10: detection of *β-actin*, *Bdnf* and *ntrk2b* at 30 dpf. Lines 11, 12 and 13: detection of *β-actin*, *Bdnf* and *ntrk2b* at 50 dpf. Lines 14, 15 and 16: *Bdnf*, *ntrk2b* and *β-actin* in the adult stage. The size of the amplified fragment is indicated.

The negative (not shown) and positive controls were performed to validate the obtained results. Moreover, in order to test the specificity of the antibodies utilized, we performed western blot analysis at the same age. Two specific protein bands with a molecular weight of 14 and 145 kDa, corresponding to the mammalian isoform of BDNF and TrkB respectively, were observed. β-Actin protein was used as an endogenous control to allow the normalization of BDNF and TrkB proteins (Figure 6).

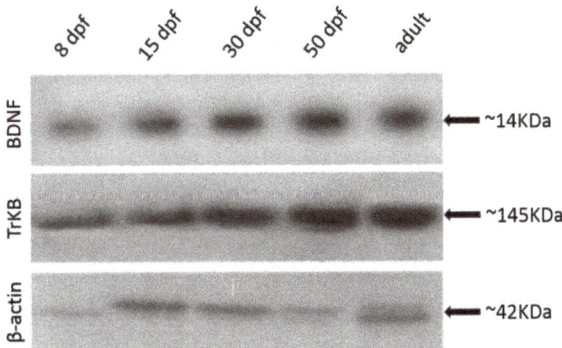

Figure 6. Western blot: detection of BDNF at 8 dpf (line 1), 15 dpf (line 2), 30 dpf (line 3), 50 dpf (line 4), adult stage (line 5). Detection of TrkB at 8 dpf (line 1), 15 dpf (line 2), 30 dpf (line 3), 50 dpf (line 4), adult stage (line 5). β-Actin protein was used as an endogenous control: 8 dpf (line 1), 15 dpf (line 2), 30 dpf (line 3), 50 dpf (line 4), adult stage (line 5).

2.3. Immunofluorescence

An immunohistochemical analysis was carried out in serial sections using single and double immunofluorescence. Cellular localization was performed in zebrafish larvae using double immunofluorescence with a monoclonal antibody against pro-BDNF and a polyclonal antibody against TrkB. Moreover, in order to identify the positive cells, we used a morpho-topographical approach based on the observation of the cellular histological features. The results, using confocal laser microscopy, demonstrated that pro-BDNF and TrkB were found only in the hair cells of the macule and cristae lateralis with an identical pattern of expression (Figure 7a–f). To make clear what is signal and what is background, both negative and positive controls are provided (Supplementary Materials).

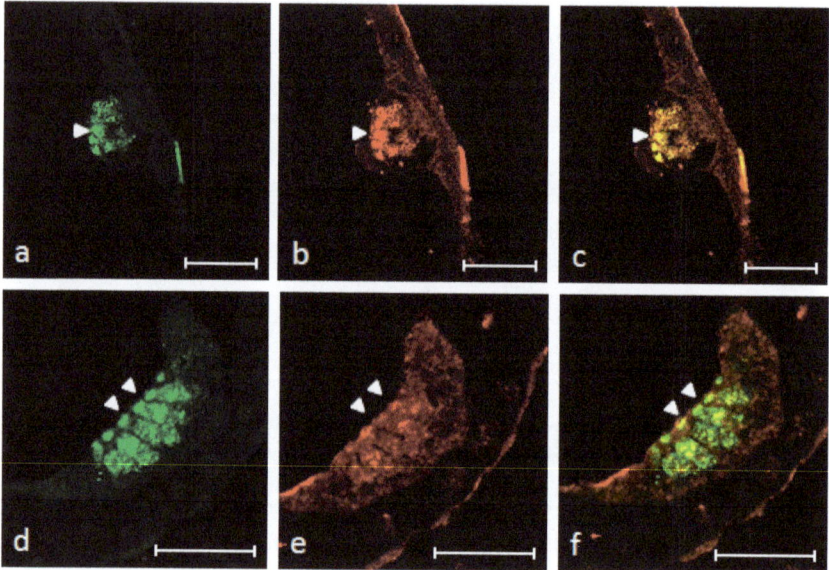

Figure 7. Inner ear of zebrafish larva 8 dpf: immunohistochemical detection of proBDNF (**a**), trkB (**b**) and colocalization of both antibodies (**c**) in utricular macula; Immunohistochemical detection of proBDNF (**d**), trkB (**e**) and colocalization of both antibodies (**f**) in lateral crista. Immunoreactivity was found in the sensory epithelial cells of utricular macula and lateral crista. Scale bars = 20 µm.

Regarding the adult zebrafish, an intense and strong immunostaining for BDNF, and its specific receptor TrkB, was observed in the maculae of the utricle, saccule and lagena and more specifically in the hair bundle of the sensory cells (Figure 8a,b).

Moreover, the immunohistochemical detection performed in serial sections, also using S100 protein as specific marker for hair cells in order to identify the cells displaying BDNF and TrkB, demonstrated a similar pattern of distribution (Figure 9). Both BDNF and TrkB were localized in the cytoplasm of cylindrical cells placed in the apical part of the sensory patches of the different macules. These cells were identified as sensory hair cells because of their morphology and localization as well as their S100 protein immunoreactivity (Figure 9). In fact, S100 proteins are a large subfamily of EF-hand Ca2+-binding proteins localized in the cytoplasm and/or nucleus of a wide range of cells, participating in the regulation of intracellular Ca2+ homeostasis as trigger or activator proteins. S-100 immunoreactivity, in previous studies, has been localized within the sensory epithelium of the saccular macula, hair cells and myelinated saccular nerve fibers [14,25–30].

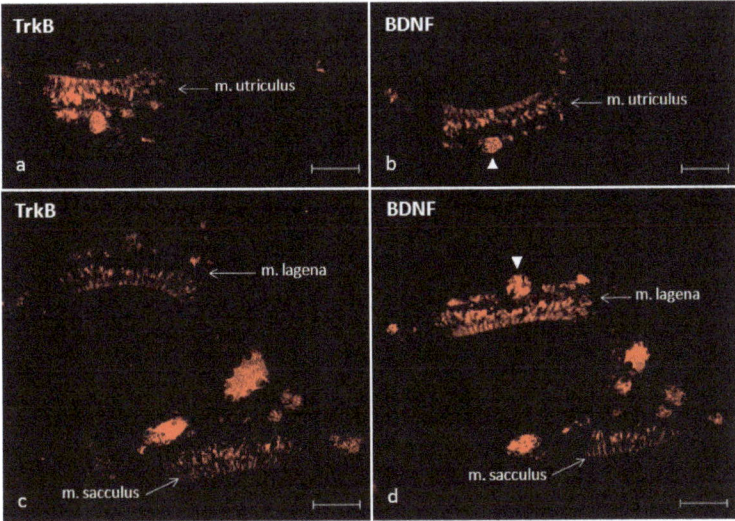

Figure 8. Inner ear of adult zebrafish. Immunohistochemical localization of TrkB (**a**) and BDNF (**b**) in the macula of the utricle. Immunohistochemical localization of TrkB (**c**) and BDNF (**d**) in the macula of the lagena and saccule. Arrowheads in (**b**,**d**) indicate nerves. Scale bars = 50 μm.

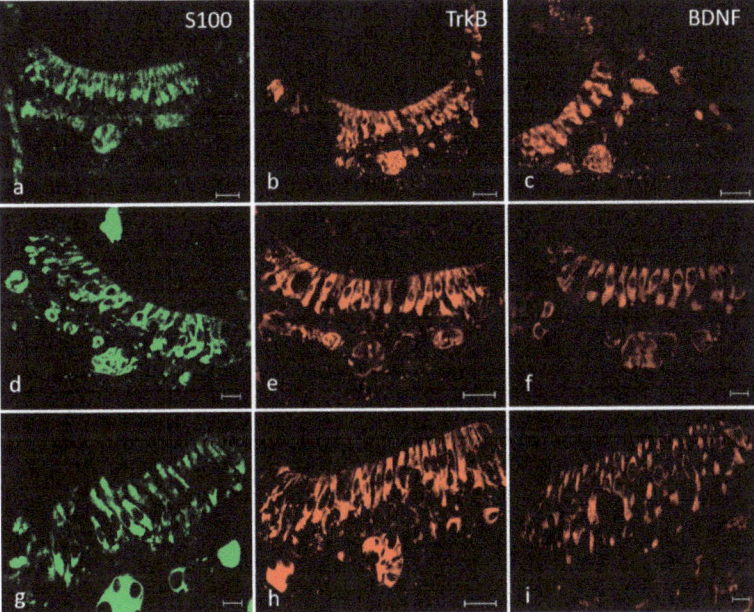

Figure 9. Inner ear of adult zebrafish. Immunohistochemical detection of S100 protein* in the macula of the utricle (**a**), saccule (**d**) and lagena (**g**), of TrkB in the macula of the utricle (**b**), saccule (**e**) and lagena (**h**). Immunohistochemical detection of BDNF in the macula of the utricle (**c**), saccule (**f**) and lagena (**i**). The utricular and saccular maculae consist of a cylindrical epithelium formed by sensory hair, supporting, mantle and basal cells. Cytoplasmic immunoreactivity for these antibodies was found in the sensory epithelial cells of the utriculus, sacculus and lagena. Scale bars = 10 μm (**a**,**c**,**d**,**f**,**g**,**i**). Scale bar s = 20 μm (**b**,**e**,**h**). The authors specify that the green channel was chosen to differentiate the immunofluorescence for protein S100.

In addition, BDNF, TrkB and S100 proteins were detected in the cristae ampullaris of the semicircular canals. Specific staining was found in a subpopulation of hair cells localized in the central and peripheral part of the sensory cells cluster respectively (Figure 10).

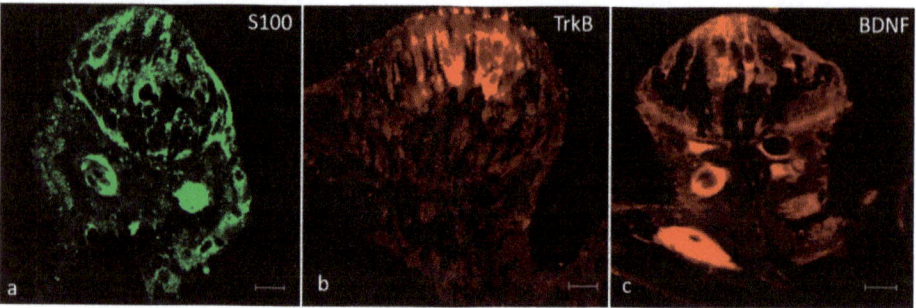

Figure 10. Inner ear of adult zebrafish. The cristae ampullaris in the apical portion contain sensory hair, supporting and basal cells. The sensory hair cells of the cristae ampullaris displayed cytoplasmic immunoreactivity for S100 protein. (**a**), TrkB (**b**) and BDNF (**c**). Scale bars= 10 µm. The authors specify that the green channel was chosen to differentiate the immunofluorescence for protein S100.

3. Discussion

This study demonstrates the expression and cell localization of the BDNF, and its specific receptor TrkB in the inner ear of zebrafish from larval to adult stages. Moreover, the S100 protein was also found in the sensory cells of the zebrafish inner ear. This finding is in complete agreement with previous results, demonstrating the presence and specificity of the S100 protein used as a specific marker for the identification of hair cells in the inner ear and lateral line system of zebrafish at different stages of development [14,26–30]. The expression and the presence of the BDNF and TrkB at mRNA and protein levels and a specific immunoreactivity for the BNDF and TrkB in the sensory cells of the inner ear were found [31]. The specificity of the antibodies used in this study has been also previously demonstrated by our research group using cross pre-absorption analysis and the western blot technique on homogenates of the whole head of the zebrafish [12,13,32]. It is well known that neurotrophins are involved in the development and maintenance of the auditory system. Particularly, BDNF is expressed in sensory epithelium of the utricle and saccule of mammals, birds and amphibians [33–35]. The data, present in literature, regarding the presence and distribution of BDNF and TrkB in the inner ear of zebrafish, is scarce and there are only a few reports related to the expression of neurotrophins and their specific receptors in the sensory organs of different teleosts [3–5]. Specifically, BDNF and TrkB in zebrafish are expressed and localized in the mechanosensory cells of the lateral line system from embryo to adult stage [13]. BDNF and TrkB in the sensory patches of both macula and crista ampullaris were found. These findings are in part consistent with previous studies performed in mammals where the BDNF is restricted only to the hair cells of maculae and to the crista ampullaris [2]. Neurotrophins and their receptors including BDNF and TrkB have been well preserved during vertebrate evolution [36]. TrkB also known as neurotrophic tyrosine kinase receptor (ntrk) has two isoforms in zebrafish, ntrk2a and ntrk2b. In this study we investigate the expression of ntrk2b because it is the most expressed isoform in mechanosensory systems, if compared to ntrk2a [13,37]. In the last decades, several animal models, including zebrafish, have been used in biomedicine in order to model sensorineural hearing loss and study the morpho-functional alteration and ototoxic lesions due to pharmacological treatments mainly carried out with aminoglycoside antibiotics in the sensory cells of the inner ear [38,39]. It is well known that the spontaneous regeneration of hair cells is not possible in mammals whereas fish maintain the capacity to regenerate damaged hair cells within a few days [25,40,41]. Moreover, we demonstrated that the anatomical structures and the histological aspects of the inner ear neuroepithelium in fish resemble those observed in mammals [42]. In vertebrates, the neurotrophins play an important role during the development and maintenance of the auditory system in adult stage. Recent findings have showed that sensorineural hearing loss leads to an evident reduction of the cochlear hair cells with a decrease of the spiral ganglion neurons probably due to less availability of neurotrophic factors. However, the exogenous treatment with BDNF and NT-3 partially restores the loss of cochlear hair cells [43,44] and also implements neurite outgrowth [45]. The findings that the BDNF/TrkB system is present in the sensory patches of the inner ear during the whole life cycle, the morpho-functional and molecular analogy, the similarity of the localization pathway as well as the role of the BNDF/TrkB system in the biology of the auditory system, both in zebrafish and mammals, indicates a possible important role of this complex in the development, maintenance and mainly in the regenerative process of the hair cells in zebrafish. Finally, based on the obtained results, we can assume that the zebrafish inner ear represents a perfect model to study the growth factors in the biology of sensory cells with special attention to the regenerative events within the sensory patches of the inner ear. Studies are in progress in our laboratory targeted at creating mutant zebrafish for BDNF and TrkB to deeply analyze the functional activity of BDNF in the mechanical-sensory organs of zebrafish

4. Materials and Methods

4.1. Zebrafish Breeding and Tissue Treatments

In this study, we used eighty (80) zebrafish from larval to adult stage. Particularly, we utilized samples at 8 days post-fertilization (dpf), 15 dpf, 30 dpf, 50 dpf and adulthood. The fish were obtained from CISS (Center of Experimental Ichthyiopathology of Sicily, University of Messina, Italy) and kept on a 14 h day, 10 h night cycle at a constant temperature of 28.5 °C and were fed twice a day. All embryos were collected after natural spawning and staged according to Kimmel et al. [46]. The fishes, at the above-mentioned stage, were sacrificed with a lethal dose of tricaine methane sulfonate (MS222; 1000–10,000 mg L-1. The heads of 5 zebrafish for each group were quickly removed, fixed in 4% paraformaldehyde in phosphate buffered saline (PBS) 0.1 m (pH = 7.4) for 12–18 h, dehydrated trough graded ethanol series, clarified in xylene, for paraffin wax embedding. Included tissues were then cut in to 7 μm thick serial sections and collected on gelatin-coated microscope slides and then routinely processed for histological and immunohistochemical analysis. Furthermore, three adult and two larval zebrafish heads (8 dpf) were fixed in 2.5% glutaraldehyde in 0.1 M Phosphate buffer, and processed, partly for scanning electron and stereo microscopy analysis and partly embedded in epoxy resin for histological study using semi-thin section (0.99 μm) stained with toluidine blue [47]. In the remaining animals (50) the inner ear was dissected and used to isolate mRNA (25) and proteins (25); there were 5 zebrafish heads for each group. The heads have been deprived of the brain, the gills, the snout including the olfactory system and the eyes and then collected in a pool per age group.

4.2. RT-PCR

For the isolation of RNA and Reverse Transcription PCR, total RNAs were extracted using Trizol reagent (Sigma; St. Louis, MO, USA). The integrity of RNA was checked using agarose gel electrophoresis. RNA extracted was reverse-transcribed in a final volume of 20 μL using 20 U of Superscript RNA-ase H2 Reverse Transcriptase (Gibco BRL, Gaithersburg, MD, USA) in the manufacturer's buffer containing 2 μg RNA, 5 μM oligo (dT), 12–18 mM dNTPs 40 U RNA-ase inhibitor (Amersham Pharmacia Biotech, Little Chalfont, Buckinghamshire, UK), 0.1 μg/μL BSA and 10 mM DTT. The reaction took place at 42 °C for 90 min. The sequences of the oligonucleotide primers were based upon the published sequences for, *Brachidanio rerio* bdnf (GenBank accession number NM_131595) *Brachidanio rerio* ntrk2b (GenBank accession number NM_001197161.2) and *Brachidanio rerio* β-actin (GenBank accession number NM_131031) and were: bdnf forward: 5′AACTCCAAAGGATCCGCTCA3′, reverse: 5′GCAGCTCTCATGCAACTGA3′, for ntrk2b forward: 5′ACGAGG-ACCACATGAAGTTC3′, reverse: 5′GCAGAACGTCTCTTTCACTG3′ and for β-actin forward: 5′ CACAGATCATGTTCGAGACC3′, reverse 5′GGTCAGGATCTTCATCAGGT3′. The conditions of amplification were as follows: 2 U Taq

DNA Polymerase (Promega, Madison, WI), 1 µM primers, 10 ng zebrafish brain cDNA, 0.2 mM each dNTP in 15 µLTaq DNA Polymerase buffer. The reaction was performed in a thermal cycler (Hyband Th. Cycler) with the following program: 1 min at 94 °C initial denaturation, then 10 cycles of 94 °C for 1 min, 65 °C for 30 s and 72 °C for 45 s, followed by 20 cycles of 94 °C for 1 min, 61 °C for 30 s, 72 °C for 45 s and a 5 min final extension at 72 °C. The PCR products were visualized by ethidium bromide staining under UV light following electrophoresis on a 2% agarose gel.

4.3. Western Blot

Frozen material was processed for Western blot. Experiments were performed in triplicate as follows: they were rinsed in cold saline, then pooled and homogenized (1:2, *w/v*) with a Potter homogenizer in Tris–HCl buffered saline (Tris-HCl 0.1 M, pH = 7.5) containing 1 µM leupeptin, 10 µM pepstatin and 2 mM phenylmethylsulfonyl fluoride. The homogenates were then centrifuged at 25,000× *g* for 15 min at 4 °C, and the resulting pellet dissolved in 10 mM Tris–HCl, pH = 6.8, 2% SDS, 100 mM DTT, and 10% glycerol at 4 °C. The pellets were thawed and analyzed by electrophoresis in 10% (for Trks) or 15% (for NTs) polyacrylamide SDS gels. After electrophoresis, proteins were transferred to a nitrocellulose membrane and unspecific binding was blocked by incubation for 3 h in phosphate-buffered saline containing 5% dry milk, and 0.1% Tween 20. The membranes were then incubated at 4 °C for 2 h with primary antibodies against BDNF and TrkB proteins. We used rabbit polyclonal antibodies against an amino-terminal sequence of mouse BDNF (sequence H2N-HSDPARRGEL-COOH; dilution 1:500; Chemicon International Inc., Temecula, CA, USA; catalog #AB1534SP) and TrkB (dilution 1:500, directed against the residues 794–808 of the intracytoplasmatic domain of human TrkB; Santa Cruz Biotechnology, Santa Cruz, CA, USA; catalog #sc-12). These antibodies have been characterized elsewhere for use in zebrafish and are suitable for use in Western blot and immunohistochemistry [5,13]. β-Actin protein was used as an endogenous control to allow the normalization of BDNF and TrKB proteins. We used mouse monoclonal beta Actin antibody (GT5512), validated in WB and also tested in Zebrafish (dilution 1:500, Gene Tex, Cat No. GTX629630) After incubation the membranes were washed with TBS pH = 7.6 containing 20% Tween 20, and incubated at room temperature for 1 h with goat anti-rabbit IgG secondary antibodies diluted 1:100. Membranes were washed again and incubated with the plasmin-alpha-2-antiplasmin (PAP) complex diluted 1: 100 for 1 h at room temperature and the reaction was visualized using Amersham™ ECL™ Western Blotting Detection Reagents (Amersham Pharmaceuticals). Marker proteins were visualized by staining with Brilliant Blue.

4.4. Localization of BDNF, TrkB and S100 Protein Using Single and Double Immunofluorescence Staining

To analyze the expression of different proteins in the sensory patches of inner ear, sections were deparaffinized and rehydrated, washed in Phosphate-Buffered Saline (PBS) 0.1 M pH = 7.4 and incubated for 30 min in a PBS solution of fetal bovine serum to avoid non-specific binding, followed by incubation with the primary antibodies. Incubation was carried out overnight at 4 °C in a humid chamber. We used mouse monoclonal antibody pro-BDNF, also designated preproprotein BDNF antibody (Santa Cruz Bio- Biotechnology, CA, USA catalog no. sc-65513) and rabbit polyclonal antibodies against a sequence of amino-terminal mouse BDNF (dilution 1:500; Chemicon International Inc., Temecula, CA, USA; catalog no. AB1534SP), TrkB (dilution 1:500, directed against the residue 794–808 of the intracytoplasmatic domain of human TrkB; Santa Cruz Biotechnology, catalog no. sc-12) and S100 protein directed against bovine S100 protein (Dako, Glostrup, Denmark; code no. Z0311; diluted 1:1000) and it detects both S100A and S100B proteins (manufacturer's notice) [27,28,48]. After rinsing in PBS, the sections were incubated for 1 h and incubated overnight at 4 °C with Alexa Fluor 488 (Invitrogen, diluted 1:200) and/or with Alexa Fluor 568 (Invitrogen, diluted 1:20) in PBS. Both steps were performed at room temperature in a dark humid chamber. Finally washed, dehydrated and mounted with Fluoromount Aqueous Mounting Medium (Sigma Aldrich, St. Louis, MO, USA). The immunofluorescence was detected using a Zeiss LSMDUO confocal laser scanning microscope with META module (Carl Zeiss Micro Imaging GmbH, Germany) and the images captured were processed using Zen 2011 (LSM 700 Zeiss software). Double fluorescence. Each image was rapidly acquired in order to minimize photodegradation. Digital images were cropped, and the figure montage prepared using Adobe Photoshop 7.0 (Adobe Systems, San Jose, CA, USA). To provide negative controls, representative sections were incubated with specifically preabsorbed antisera as described above. Under these conditions, no positive immunostaining was observed (data not shown).

4.5. Scanning Electron Microscopy

Defleshing (Stripping)

Two heads of adult zebrafish utilized for the anatomical study before being fixed, were put in a tank containing tap water for one month in order to accelerate the tissues maceration process [49,50]. During this period the water was changed every two days. Then the samples were fixed in 2.5% glutaraldehyde in Sörensen phosphate buffer 0.1 M. After several rinsing in the same buffer, they were dehydrated in a graded alcohols series, critical-point dried in a Balzers CPD 030, sputter coated with 3 nm gold in a Balzers BAL-TEC SCD 050 and examined under a Zeiss EVO LS 10.2.2 [51,52].

Supplementary Materials: The following are available online at http://www.mdpi.com/1422-0067/21/16/5787/s1.

Author Contributions: A.G. designed the experiments, wrote the manuscript and coordinated the study; M.A. and K.M. performed the experiments; M.C.G. carried out the experiments, draft and edited the manuscript; R.L., M.L., G.M. and G.G. critically revised the manuscript; F.A. supervised the experiments and co-coordinated the study. All authors have read and agreed to the published version of the manuscript.

Funding: This study was supported by a grant from Sicily Region (FISH PATHNET–Potenziamento dei Centri di Ittiopatologia Siciliani) and University of Messina (reserch and mobility project).

Conflicts of Interest: The authors declare no conflict of interest.

References

1. Huang, E.J.; Reichardt, L.F. Neurotrophins: Roles in neuronal development and function. *Annu. Rev. Neurosci.* **2001**, *24*, 677–736. [CrossRef] [PubMed]
2. Fritzsch, B.; Tessarollo, L.; Coppola, E.; Reichardt, L.F. Neurotrophins in the ear: Their roles in sensory neuron survival and fiber guidance. *Prog. Brain Res.* **2004**, *146*, 265–278. [PubMed]
3. Hannestad, J.; Marino, F.; Germanà, A.; Catania, S.; Abbate, F.; Ciriaco, E.; Vega, J. Trk neurotrophin receptor-like proteins in the teleost Dicentrarchus labrax. *Cell Tissue Res.* **2000**, *300*, 1–9. [CrossRef] [PubMed]
4. Germanà, A.; Catania, S.; Cavallaro, M.; González-Martínez, T.; Ciriaco, E.; Hannestad, J.; Vega, J. Immunohistochemical localization of BDNF-, TrkB- and TrkA-like proteins in the teleost lateral line system. *J. Anat.* **2002**, *200*, 477–485. [CrossRef] [PubMed]
5. Catania, S.; Germana, A.; Cabo, R.; Ochoa-Erena, F.; Guerrera, M.; Hannestad, J.; Represa, J.; Vega, J. Neurotrophin and Trk neurotrophin receptors in the inner ear of Salmo salar and Salmo trutta. *J. Anat.* **2007**, *210*, 78–88. [CrossRef] [PubMed]
6. Hallböök, F. Evolution of the vertebrate neurotrophin and Trk receptor gene families. *Curr. Opin. Neurobiol.* **1999**, *9*, 616–621. [CrossRef]
7. Lucini, C.; D'Angelo, L.; Cacialli, P.; Palladino, A.; de Girolamo, P. BDNF, Brain, and Regeneration: Insights from Zebrafish. *Int. J. Mol. Sci.* **2018**, *19*, 3155. [CrossRef]
8. Montalbano, G.; Mania, M.; Guerrera, M.C.; Abbate, F.; Laurà, R.; Navarra, M.; Vega, J.A.; Ciriaco, E.; Germanà, A. Morphological differences in adipose tissue and changes in BDNF/Trkb expression in brain and gut of a diet induced obese zebrafish model. *Ann. Anat.* **2016**, *204*, 36–44. [CrossRef]
9. Cacialli, P.; Gueguen, M.-M.; Coumailleau, P.; D'Angelo, L.; Kah, O.; Lucini, C.; Pellegrini, E. BDNF expression in larval and adult zebrafish brain: Distribution and cell identification. *PLoS ONE* **2016**, *11*, e0158057. [CrossRef]
10. De Felice, E.; Porreca, I.; Alleva, E.; De Girolamo, P.; Ambrosino, C.; Ciriaco, E.; Germanà, A.; Sordino, P. Localization of BDNF expression in the developing brain of zebrafish. *J. Anat.* **2014**, *224*, 564–574. [CrossRef]

11. Abbate, F.; Guerrera, M.C.; Montalbano, G.; Levanti, M.B.; Germanà, G.P.; Navarra, M.; Laurà, R.; Vega, J.; Ciriaco, E.; Germanà, A. Expression and anatomical distribution of TrkB in the encephalon of the adult zebrafish (Danio rerio). *Neurosci. Lett.* **2014**, *563*, 66–69. [CrossRef] [PubMed]
12. Sánchez-Ramos, C.; Bonnin-Arias, C.; Guerrera, M.C.; Calavia, M.; Chamorro, E.; Montalbano, G.; López-Velasco, S.; López-Muñiz, A.; Germanà, A.; Vega, J.A. Light regulates the expression of the BDNF/TrkB system in the adult zebrafish retina. *Microsc. Res. Tech.* **2013**, *76*, 42–49. [CrossRef] [PubMed]
13. Germanà, A.; Laurà, R.; Montalbano, G.; Guerrera, M.C.; Amato, V.; Zichichi, R.; Campo, S.; Ciriaco, E.; Vega, J. Expression of brain-derived neurotrophic factor and TrkB in the lateral line system of zebrafish during development. *Cell. Mol. Neurobiol.* **2010**, *30*, 787–793. [CrossRef] [PubMed]
14. Germana, A.; Abbate, F.; González-Martínez, T.; del Valle, M.; de Carlos, F.; Germanà, G.; Vega, J. S100 protein is a useful and specific marker for hair cells of the lateral line system in postembryonic zebrafish. *Neurosci. Lett.* **2004**, *365*, 186–189. [CrossRef] [PubMed]
15. Bang, P.I.; Sewell, W.F.; Malicki, J.J. Morphology and cell type heterogeneities of the inner ear epithelia in adult and juvenile zebrafish (Danio rerio). *J. Comp. Neurol.* **2001**, *438*, 173–190. [CrossRef]
16. Monroe, J.D.; Rajadinakaran, G.; Smith, M.E. Sensory hair cell death and regeneration in fishes. *Front. Cell. Neurosci.* **2015**, *9*, 131. [CrossRef]
17. Harris, J.A.; Cheng, A.G.; Cunningham, L.L.; MacDonald, G.; Raible, D.W.; Rubel, E.W. Neomycin-induced hair cell death and rapid regeneration in the lateral line of zebrafish (Danio rerio). *J. Assoc. Res. Otolaryngol.* **2003**, *4*, 219–234. [CrossRef]
18. Owens, K.N.; Santos, F.; Roberts, B.; Linbo, T.; Coffin, A.B.; Knisely, A.J.; Simon, J.A.; Rubel, E.W.; Raible, D.W. Identification of genetic and chemical modulators of zebrafish mechanosensory hair cell death. *PLoS Genet.* **2008**, *4*, e1000020. [CrossRef]
19. Nicolson, T. The genetics of hair-cell function in zebrafish. *J. Neurogenet.* **2017**, *31*, 102–112. [CrossRef]
20. Blanco-Sánchez, B.; Clément, A.; Phillips, J.; Westerfield, M. Zebrafish models of human eye and inner ear diseases. In *Method Cell Biology*; Academic Press: Cambridge, MA, USA, 2017; Volume 138, pp. 415–467.
21. Rubel, E.W.; Furrer, S.A.; Stone, J.S. A brief history of hair cell regeneration research and speculations on the future. *Hear. Res.* **2013**, *297*, 42–51. [CrossRef]
22. Montalbano, G.; Abbate, F.; Levanti, M.B.; Germanà, G.P.; Laurà, R.; Ciriaco, E.; Vega, J.A.; Germanà, A. Topographical and drug specific sensitivity of hair cells of the zebrafish larvae to aminoglycoside-induced toxicity. *Ann. Anat.* **2014**, *196*, 236–240. [CrossRef] [PubMed]
23. Montalbano, G.; Capillo, G.; Laurà, R.; Abbate, F.; Levanti, M.; Guerrera, M.C.; Ciriaco, E.; Germanà, A. Neuromast hair cells retain the capacity of regeneration during heavy metal exposure. *Ann. Anat.* **2018**, *218*, 183–189. [CrossRef] [PubMed]
24. He, Y.; Bao, B.; Li, H. Using zebrafish as a model to study the role of epigenetics in hearing loss. *Expert Opin. Drug Discov.* **2017**, *12*, 967–975. [CrossRef]
25. Chen, Y.; Zhang, S.; Chai, R.; Li, H. Hair Cell Regeneration. *Adv. Exp. Med. Biol.* **2019**, *1130*, 1–16. [CrossRef] [PubMed]
26. Montalbano, G.; Mania, M.; Guerrera, M.C.; Laurà, R.; Abbate, F.; Levanti, M.; Maugeri, A.; Germanà, A.; Navarra, M. Effects of a Flavonoid-Rich Extract from Citrus sinensis Juice on a Diet-Induced Obese Zebrafish. *Int. J. Mol. Sci.* **2019**, *20*, 5116. [CrossRef]
27. Germanà, A.; Marino, F.; Guerrera, M.C.; Campo, S.; De Girolamo, P.; Montalbano, G.; Germanà, G.P.; Ochoa-Erena, F.J.; Ciriaco, E.; Vega, J. Expression and distribution of S100 protein in the nervous system of the adult zebrafish (Danio rerio). *Microsc. Res. Tech.* **2008**, *71*, 248–255. [CrossRef]
28. Germanà, A.; Paruta, S.; Germanà, G.P.; Ochoa-Erena, F.J.; Montalbano, G.; Cobo, J.; Vega, J.A. Differential distribution of S100 protein and calretinin in mechanosensory and chemosensory cells of adult zebrafish (Danio rerio). *Brain Res.* **2007**, *1162*, 48–55. [CrossRef]
29. Germana', A.; Montalbano, G.; Laura, R.; Ciriaco, E.; Del Valle, M.; Vega, J.A. S100 protein-like immunoreactivity in the crypt olfactory neurons of the adult zebrafish. *Neurosci. Lett.* **2004**, *371*, 196–198. [CrossRef]
30. Abbate, F.; Catania, S.; Germana, A.; González, T.; Diaz-Esnal, B.; Germana, G.; Vega, J. S-100 protein is a selective marker for sensory hair cells of the lateral line system in teleosts. *Neurosci. Lett.* **2002**, *329*, 133–136. [CrossRef]

31. Guerrera, M.C.; Montalbano, G.; Germana, A.; Maricchiolo, G.; Ciriaco, E.; Abbate, F. Morphology of the tongue dorsal surface in white sea bream (Diplodus sargus sargus). *Acta Zool.* **2015**, *96*, 236–241. [CrossRef]
32. Germanà, A.; Sánchez-Ramos, C.; Guerrera, M.C.; Calavia, M.; Navarro, M.; Zichichi, R.; García-Suárez, O.; Pérez-Piñera, P.; Vega, J.A. Expression and cell localization of brain-derived neurotrophic factor and TrkB during zebrafish retinal development. *J. Anat.* **2010**, *217*, 214–222. [CrossRef] [PubMed]
33. Montcouquiol, M.; Valat, J.; Travo, C.; Sans, A. A role for BDNF in early postnatal rat vestibular epithelia maturation: Implication of supporting cells. *Eur. J. Neurosci.* **1998**, *10*, 598–606. [CrossRef]
34. Pirvola, U.; Hallböök, F.; Xing-Qun, L.; Virkkala, J.; Saarma, M.; Ylikoski, J. Expression of neurotrophins and Trk receptors in the developing, adult, and regenerating avian cochlea. *J. Neurobiol.* **1997**, *33*, 1019–1033. [CrossRef]
35. Don, D.M.; Newman, A.N.; Micevych, P.E.; Popper, P. Expression of brain-derived neurotrophic factor and its receptor *mRNA* in the vestibuloauditory system of the bullfrog. *Hear. Res.* **1997**, *114*, 10–20. [CrossRef]
36. Heinrich, G.; Lum, T. Fish neurotrophins and Trk receptors. *Int. J. Dev. Neurosci.* **2000**, *18*, 1–27. [CrossRef]
37. Nittoli, V.; Sepe, R.M.; Coppola, U.; D'Agostino, Y.; De Felice, E.; Palladino, A.; Vassalli, Q.A.; Locascio, A.; Ristoratore, F.; Spagnuolo, A.; et al. A comprehensive analysis of neurotrophins and neurotrophin tyrosine kinase receptors expression during development of zebrafish. In *J. Comp. Neurol.*; 2018; Volume 526, pp. 1057–1072. [CrossRef]
38. Coffin, A.B.; Ramcharitar, J. Chemical ototoxicity of the fish inner ear and lateral line. In *Fish Hearing and Bioacoustics*; Springer: Cham, Switzerland, 2016; pp. 419–437.
39. Stawicki, T.M.; Esterberg, R.; Hailey, D.W.; Raible, D.W.; Rubel, E.W. Using the zebrafish lateral line to uncover novel mechanisms of action and prevention in drug-induced hair cell death. *Front. Cell. Neurosci.* **2015**, *9*, 46. [CrossRef]
40. Thomas, E.D.; Raible, D.W. Distinct progenitor populations mediate regeneration in the zebrafish lateral line. *eLife* **2019**, *8*, e43736. [CrossRef]
41. Zhang, Q.; Li, S.; Wong, H.-T.C.; He, X.J.; Beirl, A.; Petralia, R.S.; Wang, Y.-X.; Kindt, K.S. Synaptically silent sensory hair cells in zebrafish are recruited after damage. *Nat. Commun.* **2018**, *9*, 1–16. [CrossRef]
42. Thomas, J.; Gangappa, S.; Kanangat, S.; Rouse, B. On the essential involvement of neutrophils in the immunopathologic disease: Herpetic stromal keratitis. *J. Immunol.* **1997**, *158*, 1383–1391.
43. Nicolson, T. The genetics of hearing and balance in zebrafish. *Annu. Rev. Genet.* **2005**, *39*, 9–22. [CrossRef]
44. Shepherd, R.K.; Coco, A.; Epp, S.B.; Crook, J.M. Chronic depolarization enhances the trophic effects of brain-derived neurotrophic factor in rescuing auditory neurons following a sensorineural hearing loss. *J. Comp. Neurol.* **2005**, *486*, 145–158. [CrossRef] [PubMed]
45. Budenz, C.L.; Pfingst, B.E.; Raphael, Y. The use of neurotrophin therapy in the inner ear to augment cochlear implantation outcomes. *Anat. Rec.* **2012**, *295*, 1896–1908. [CrossRef]
46. Schmidt, N.; Schulze, J.; Warwas, D.P.; Ehlert, N.; Lenarz, T.; Warnecke, A.; Behrens, P. Long-term delivery of brain-derived neurotrophic factor (BDNF) from nanoporous silica nanoparticles improves the survival of spiral ganglion neurons in vitro. *PLoS ONE* **2018**, *13*, 3. [CrossRef] [PubMed]
47. Kimmel, C.B.; Ballard, W.W.; Kimmel, S.R.; Ullmann, B.; Schilling, T.F. Stages of embryonic development of the zebrafish. *Dev. Dyn.* **1995**, *203*, 253–310. [CrossRef] [PubMed]
48. Laurà, R.; Abbate, F.; Germanà, G.; Montalbano, G.; Germanà, A.; Levanti, M. Fine structure of the canal neuromasts of the lateral line system in the adult zebrafish. *Anat. Histol. Embryol.* **2018**, *47*, 322–329. [CrossRef]
49. Amato, V.; Vina, E.; Calavia, M.; Guerrera, M.C.; Laurà, R.; Navarro, M.; De Carlos, F.; Cobo, J.; Germanà, A.; Vega, J. TRPV4 in the sensory organs of adult zebrafish. *Microsc. Res. Tech.* **2012**, *75*, 89–96. [CrossRef] [PubMed]
50. Gier, R. Preparation of great horned owl skeleton. *Trans. Kans. Acad. Sci. (1903-)* **1951**, *54*, 344–345. [CrossRef]
51. Mairs, S.; Swift, B.; Rutty, G.N. Detergent: An alternative approach to traditional bone cleaning methods for forensic practice. *Am. J. Forensic Med. Pathol.* **2004**, *25*, 276–284. [CrossRef]
52. Modina, S.; Abbate, F.; Germana, G.P.; Lauria, A.; Luciano, A.M. β-Catenin localization and timing of early development of bovine embryos obtained from oocytes matured in the presence of follicle stimulating hormone. *Anim. Reprod. Sci.* **2007**, *100*, 264–279. [CrossRef]

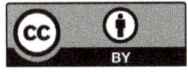

© 2020 by the authors. Licensee MDPI, Basel, Switzerland. This article is an open access article distributed under the terms and conditions of the Creative Commons Attribution (CC BY) license (http://creativecommons.org/licenses/by/4.0/).

in
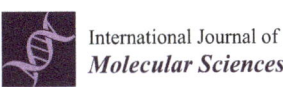

Review

Activation of KCNQ4 as a Therapeutic Strategy to Treat Hearing Loss

John Hoon Rim [1], Jae Young Choi [2], Jinsei Jung [2,*] and Heon Yung Gee [1,*]

1. Department of Pharmacology, Graduate School of Medical Science, Brain Korea 21 Project, Yonsei University College of Medicine, Seoul 03722, Korea; JOHNHOON1@yuhs.ac
2. Department of Otorhinolaryngology, Graduate School of Medical Science, Brain Korea 21 Project, Yonsei University College of Medicine, Seoul 03722, Korea; JYCHOI@yuhs.ac
* Correspondence: JSJUNG@yuhs.ac (J.J.); hygee@yuhs.ac (H.Y.G.)

Abstract: Potassium voltage-gated channel subfamily q member 4 (KCNQ4) is a voltage-gated potassium channel that plays essential roles in maintaining ion homeostasis and regulating hair cell membrane potential. Reduction of the activity of the KCNQ4 channel owing to genetic mutations is responsible for nonsyndromic hearing loss, a typically late-onset, initially high-frequency loss progressing over time. In addition, variants of KCNQ4 have also been associated with noise-induced hearing loss and age-related hearing loss. Therefore, the discovery of small compounds activating or potentiating KCNQ4 is an important strategy for the curative treatment of hearing loss. In this review, we updated the current concept of the physiological role of KCNQ4 in the inner ear and the pathologic mechanism underlying the role of KCNQ4 variants with regard to hearing loss. Finally, we focused on currently developed KCNQ4 activators and their pros and cons, paving the way for the future development of specific KCNQ4 activators as a remedy for hearing loss.

Keywords: potassium voltage-gated channel subfamily q member 4; potassium; hearing loss; nonsyndromic hearing loss; KCNQ4 activator

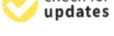

Citation: Rim, J.H.; Choi, J.Y.; Jung, J.; Gee, H.Y. Activation of KCNQ4 as a Therapeutic Strategy to Treat Hearing Loss. *Int. J. Mol. Sci.* **2021**, *22*, 2510. https://doi.org/10.3390/ijms22052510

Academic Editor: Srdjan M Vlajkovic

Received: 20 January 2021
Accepted: 22 February 2021
Published: 2 March 2021

Publisher's Note: MDPI stays neutral with regard to jurisdictional claims in published maps and institutional affiliations.

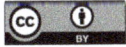

Copyright: © 2021 by the authors. Licensee MDPI, Basel, Switzerland. This article is an open access article distributed under the terms and conditions of the Creative Commons Attribution (CC BY) license (https://creativecommons.org/licenses/by/4.0/).

1. Introduction

Hearing impairment, the most common sensory deficit in humans, affects 466 million people (over 6% of the world's population) according to the World Health Organization (WHO) (https://www.who.int/news-room/fact-sheets/detail/deafness-and-hearing-loss) (accessed on 20 January 2021) [1,2]. Approximately 1 in 500–1000 individuals suffer from congenital hearing loss, of which approximately 50% are known to be caused by genetic mutations [3,4]. The prevalence of hearing loss has been reported to double with every 10-y increase in age, with almost two-thirds of individuals over the age of 70 y having a hearing impairment associated with sounds ≥ 25 dB [2]. The main causes of adult-onset hearing loss are noise exposure, aging, genetic mutations, exposure to therapeutic drugs that have ototoxic side-effects, viruses, or ototoxic drugs or chemicals, resulting in damage to the auditory hair cells and neurons [1,2]. As the number of aging adults is increasing globally, hearing loss poses a high economic burden, with an estimated cost of $750 billion annually [5]. Despite this, all available treatment options for hearing loss to date are limited to hearing devices, such as hearing aids and cochlear implants. Medical treatments are both lacking and required.

As with almost all other sensory transduction systems, hearing involves the modulation of potassium (K^+) channels at an early stage of the process of turning mechanical sound into electrical signals. Potassium voltage-gated channel subfamily q member 4 (KCNQ4) is known to play an essential role in the auditory function of the inner ear, contributing to potassium recycling and homeostasis maintenance. Reduction of the activity of the KCNQ4 channel has been associated with a genetic form of hearing loss, noise-induced hearing loss, and age-related hearing loss [6–8]; therefore, small compounds that activate KCNQ4, the so-called "channel openers", have been developed as a strategy for the treatment of these hearing impairments [9]. In this review, we focused on the developmental status of KCNQ4 activators and compared their advantages and shortcomings in terms of their potential to be used for the specific activation of KCNQ4.

2. KCNQ Potassium Channels

The KCNQ family of voltage-gated potassium channels (Kv7) includes five members (Kv7.1–Kv7.5) that have important roles in the brain, heart, kidney, and inner ear [10]. In particular, KCNQ channels consist of a K^+ channel pore-forming subunit (α-subunit) with six transmembrane domains (S1–S6) and a single pore-loop (P-loop), and two intracellular termini (Figure 1). Functional KCNQ channels are assembled in homo- or heterotetramer pore-forming subunits. The proteins have been shown to share between 30 and 65% amino acid identity, with particularly high homology in the transmembrane regions (Figure 1) [11,12]. The S4 transmembrane domain containing a regular distribution of positively charged amino acids acts as the voltage sensor, while the P-loop contains the K^+ pore TxxTxGYG signature sequence (Figure 1). The length of the N-terminus, which is in the order of 100 amino acids, is similar between the five subtypes, whereas the length of the C-terminus varies greatly between the subtypes. All five proteins display a highly homologous region on their intracellular C-terminus termed "A-domain" (Figure 1) [11]. The high homology in critical residues, such as the voltage sensor domain and P-loot, has hindered the development of subtype-specific activators, including KCNQ4-specific activators.

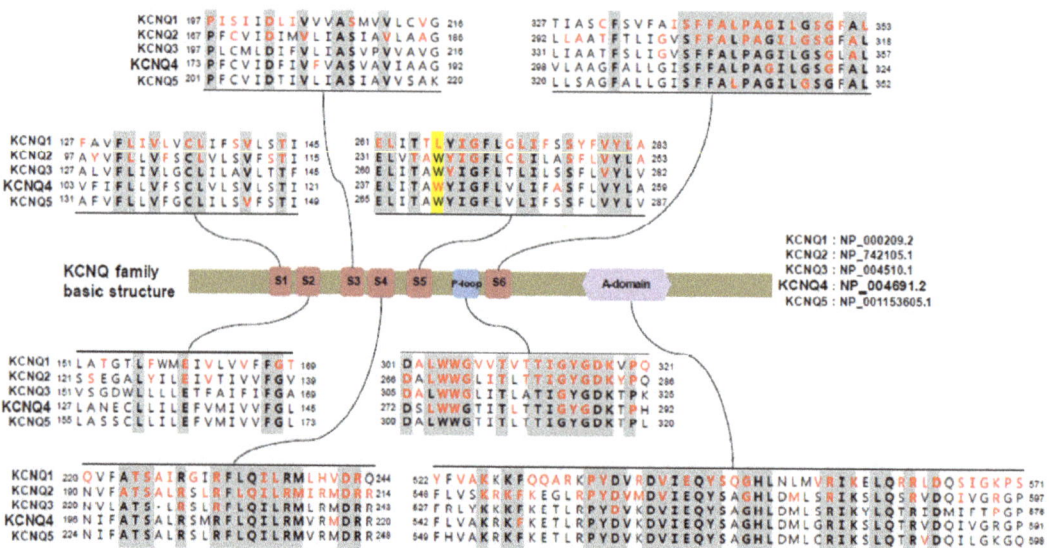

Figure 1. Comparative sequence analysis among voltage-gated channel subfamily q (KCNQ) family genes and mutational spectrum in protein sequences. Conserved sequences are presented in bold characters. Amino acids affected by pathogenic mutations reported in associated Mendelian diseases were collected from the HGMD and ClinVar databases and are presented in red characters. KCNQ2–4 share the tryptophan residue (Trp242 in KCNQ4, highlighted in yellow), which is critical for the activity of several KCNQ activators, including retigabine; however, KCNQ1 has a leucine at this position, and not a tryptophan.

All five Kv7 members map to a human disease locus. Mutations in KCNQ genes have been shown to cause inherited syndromic diseases. More specifically, mutations of *KCNQ1* are known to cause heart diseases, including long QT syndrome (MIM 192500), and Jervell and Lange-Nielsen syndrome (MIM 220400) in autosomal dominant and recessive manners, respectively [13–15]. Mutations of *KCNQ2* have been found to cause autosomal dominant benign familial neonatal seizures (MIM 121200) [16,17]. Mutations of *KCNQ3* have also been shown to cause autosomal dominant benign neonatal seizures (MIM 121201) [18], while mutations of *KCNQ4* result in autosomal dominant nonsyndromic hearing loss (DFNA2, MIM 600101) [6]. Finally, mutations of *KCNQ5* have been reported to cause autosomal dominant intellectual disability (MIM 617601) [19].

Among the 30 genes associated with autosomal dominant hearing loss, KCNQ4 is one of the most commonly mutated genes [20,21]. *KCNQ4* mutations explained 6.62% (19/287) in Japanese families with autosomal dominant nonsyndromic hearing loss and c.211delC was identified as a founder mutation in Japanese individuals, explaining 68.4% (13/19) among families with *KCNQ4* mutations [20]. In addition, in our Korean adult-onset hearing loss patient cohort (i.e., Yonsei University Hearing Loss or YUHL cohort) without noise exposure history, *KCNQ4* presented the highest prevalence for mutations (9/213 patients, unpublished). In particular, DFNA2 resulting from mutations in *KCNQ4* is characterized by progressive sensorineural hearing loss at all frequencies [6,22]. The progressive nature of DFNA2 is advantageous for treatment because it provides a wide therapeutic window if the causative mutations could be detected early. Since the first clinical report of a mutation of *KCNQ4* responsible for deafness in 1999 [6], over 40 pathogenic mutations have been identified in individuals with DFNA2 (www.deafnessvariationdatabase.org or www.hgmd.cf.ac.uk/ac/index.php, accessed on 31 December 2020) [21]. The mutation hotspots in *KCNQ4* associated with DFNA2 have been shown to be clustered around the pore region [21]. Variants in the pore region of KCNQ4 are known to be unresponsive to KCNQ activators, such as retigabine or zinc pyrithione [21,23,24]. In addition, it was found that among pore region variants, variants that result in almost null potassium activity did not respond to KCNQ activators, whereas variants with residual voltage-activated K^+ currents could be activated by KCNQ activators [21]. In addition, variants occurring in the N- and C-terminal cytoplasmic termini had higher chances to be rescued by KCNQ4 activators [21,25]. However, the relationship between each mutation and drug responsiveness remains unclear.

3. Potassium Recycling and KCNQ4 in the Inner Ear

The inner ear of mammals contains two sensory organs, the cochlea and the vestibule, which are responsible for hearing and balance, respectively. The cochlea consists of three fluid-filled compartments with different ion compositions: (1) scala vestibuli; (2) scala media; and (3) scala tympani. The scala vestibule and scala tympani are filled with perilymph, whereas the scala media is filled with the endolymph, which has a high K^+ concentration and a positive potential [26]. The mammalian cochlear contains two types of sensory cells with a bundle of actin-based stereocilia on their apical surface: (1) outer hair cells (OHCs), which amplify sound stimuli; and (2) inner hair cells (IHCs), which transmit sound stimuli to the central nervous system [27]. The sensory cells of cochlea are bathed in endolymph and a difference in K^+ concentration is maintained between the endolymph and the sensory cells in the scala media. As K^+ is the major charge carrier for the sensory transduction, its proper recycling is of great importance for the process of hearing. Briefly, K^+ ions are secreted into the endolymph by the stria vascularis, enter the sensory OHCs through apical mechanosensitive K^+ channels, probably including transmembrane channel like 1 (TMC1) and TMC2 [28], thereby triggering neurotransmission, and are released from these cells into the perilymph via basolateral K^+ channels, including KCNQ4. Then, they migrate through supporting cells and fibrocytes toward the stria vascularis using a network of gap junctions [26]. Accordingly, K^+ recycling genes were shown to be indispensable for the process of hearing, as evidenced by the fact that multiple mutations in these genes (*GJB1* (Cx32), *GJB2* (Cx26), *GJB3* (Cx31), *GJB4* (Cx30.3), *GJB6* (Cx30), *KCNE1*, *KCNQ1*, and *KCNQ4*) lead to both syndromic and nonsyndromic forms of hearing loss [6,14,15]. Moreover, mice deficient for SLC12A2, a $Na^+/2Cl^-/K^+$ cotransporter, and KCNJ10 were reported to develop hearing loss due to collapsed endolymphatic spaces and the inability to generate an endocochlear potential, respectively [29,30].

In order for the cochlear to respond to the dynamic range and speed of sound, fast electromechanical amplification of sound and fast repolarization of the receptor potential by OHCs is required [31]. The K$^+$ current that is known to dominate in OHCs is termed $I_{K,n}$ [32]. Mechanoelectrical transducer channels have been shown to be opened by deflections of the hair cell bundles at cochlear regions of specific frequencies, causing an influx of K$^+$, which would in turn lead to the depolarization of the membrane and contraction of OHCs by the motor protein prestin [33]. The fast amplification process depends on the capacitance of OHCs at resting membrane potential, which is determined by the conductance of OHCs maintained through the KCNQ4-mediated efflux current $I_{K,n}$ [34]. The expression and current of KCNQ4 were reported to be detected prior to hearing onset along the entire basolateral membrane of OHCs in mice [34,35]; however, after the onset of hearing (postnatal day 12–14), its expression was redistributed and restricted to the basal pole [36]. This expression pattern was demonstrated to correlate with its function in extruding K$^+$ ions [32,37,38]. Moreover, KCNQ4 is known to be also expressed in IHCs, spiral ganglion neurons, and several nuclei along the auditory pathway, for example, cochlear nuclei and inferior colliculus [37,39,40]. However, it remains controversial whether it is expressed in IHCs or spiral ganglions, and whether there is a tonotopy in the expression in IHCs [41,42]. Accordingly, $Kcnq4^{-/-}$ mice were reported to exhibit progressive hearing loss, with OHCs slowly decreasing at a young age with increasing cell loss leading up to complete degeneration at the oldest ages [42,43]. Degeneration of IHCs, particularly at the basal turn was also observed, but only in the adult stage [30]. The loss of this important K$^+$ channel in OHCs is known to result in a chronic depolarization, possibly increasing Ca^{2+} influx through voltage-gated Ca^{2+} channels and causing their subsequent degeneration due to chronic cellular stress [44].

When expressed alone in CHO cells, KCNQ4 displays a half-activation voltage of −19 mV and a slope constant of 10 mV. The activation onset has been found to be exponential, except at very positive voltages, displaying little or no inactivation [45]. In oocytes, the half-activation voltage has been demonstrated to be −10 mV, the slope constant 18 mV, and the activation slow, with a time constant of 600 msec at +40 mV [6].

4. Association of KCNQ4 and Noise-Induced Hearing Loss

Noise-induced hearing loss is estimated to affect 12% or more of the global population and has become a leading occupational health risk in developed countries [46]. The World Health Organization estimated that 1.1 billion young people worldwide are at risk of developing hearing loss due to noise exposure [47].

Genetic factors are also known to contribute to noise-induced hearing loss [48]. Therefore, the association of K$^+$ recycling gene variants with susceptibility to noise has been examined. Van Laer et al. investigated the association of 35 single nucleotide polymorphisms (SNPs) in 10 genes including *GJB1*, *GJB2*, *GJB3*, *GJB4*, *GJB6*, *KCNJ10*, *KCNQ4*, *KCNQ1*, *KCNE1*, *KCNQ3*, and *SLC12A2* on 104 noise-susceptible and 114 noise-resistant individuals selected from a population of 1261 Swedish noise-exposed workers [7]. They found that three SNPs in *KCNE1*, one SNP in *KCNQ1*, and one SNP in *KCNQ4* were significantly associated with noise-induced hearing loss [7]. Another association study was performed in 119 noise-susceptible and 119 noise-resistant individuals selected from a population of 3860 Polish noise-exposed workers [49]. Pawelczyk et al. examined 99 SNPs in 10 K$^+$ recycling genes and found a significant association of SNPs in 7 out of 10 genes (*KCNE1*, *KCNQ4*, *GJB1*, *GJB2*, *GJB4*, *KCNJ10*, and *KCNQ1*) [49]. Two SNPs, the rs2070358 G allele in *KCNE1* and rs34287852 G allele (c.1365T>G, p.H455Q) in *KCNQ4*, were reported to be significant in both populations, with the rs2070358 G allele increasing the susceptibility to noise-induced hearing loss [7,49]. Interestingly, the rs34287852 G allele in *KCNQ4* exhibited the opposite effect in these two populations, as it was found to decrease the risk of developing noise-induced hearing loss in the Swedish population, but increased the susceptibility of noise-induced hearing loss in the Polish population [7,49]. This discrepancy could be theoretically explained by differences in allele frequency or linkage disequilibrium patterns in both populations, slightly different selection procedures applied in both studies, the influence of various environmental factors, or, finally, by a false positive association with noise-induced hearing loss of the rs34287852 G allele of *KCNQ4* [50]. The allele frequency of rs34287852 is 0.1763 in total; however, ethnic differences exist. It has been shown to be more common in Europeans with an allele frequency of over 0.15, whereas it is less than 0.07 in eastern Asians and Africans. This SNP is known to result in a missense change (p.H455Q). Jung et al. showed that the activity of the K^+ channel of this variant was not different from that of wild-type KCNQ4 and increased to a level similar to wild-type KCNQ4 following administration of retigabine [21]. Last, Guo et al. examined three SNPs (rs709688, rs2769256 and rs4660468) for an association with noise-induced hearing loss on 571 cases and 639 normal controls selected from about 2700 noise-exposed Chinese workers [51]. They found that one synonymous SNP, the rs4660468 T allele, was significant, conferring a higher risk of noise-induced hearing loss [51].

Acoustic noise exposure has been suggested to decrease the functionality of KCNQ4 on the surface membrane, thereby playing a pivotal role in noise-induced hearing loss. Loss of KCNQ4 on the membranes of OHCs in cochlear regions of high frequency was reported to precede the loss of OHCs in mouse models [44,52]. Likewise, KCNQ4 was also reported to be lost from the surface membrane of OHCs in cochlear regions of low frequency following exposure to low frequency noise [53]. Therefore, KCNQ4 was assumed to protect OHCs from Ca^{2+} overload triggered by noise exposure [42,53].

5. KCNQ4 Activators

As we discussed, the common molecular basis of DFNA2 and noise-induced hearing loss is the reduction of the activity of KCNQ4 in OHCs, resulting from either mutations or noise exposure; therefore, restoration of the activity of KCNQ4 is a logical strategy for the treatment and prevention of these conditions. To this end, a number of synthetic compounds that potentiate KCNQ channels have been developed to treat diseases resulting from neuronal hyperexcitability, such as epilepsy and neuropathic pain [54]. Some of these chemicals have been examined for their ability to activate KCNQ4. In addition, efforts have been made to develop compounds specific to KCNQ4 over other KCNQ channels.

5.1. Retigabine

Retigabine, also known as ezogabine, is a first-in-class drug for the treatment of epilepsy, approved by the US Food and Drug Administration [55–58]. Retigabine has been the most characterized activator of KCNQ channels and has been shown to potentiate KCNQ2, KCNQ3, KCNQ4, and KCNQ5, without activating KCNQ1, thereby avoiding potential cardiac effects [56,59–61]. Due to its broad effect on various subtypes of KCNQ channels, retigabine is also utilized as an antidepressant [62], an antihypertensive [63], an analgesic [64], an anxiolytic [65], and even as an antimanic [66]. However, its administration has been associated with side-effects, such as retinal pigmentation, urinary retention, and skin discoloration [58,67]. Although it is known to serve as an activator, it has also been shown to inhibit KCNQ channels at positive potentials [68]. In addition, retigabine is known to act on other channels, including g-aminobutyric acid receptor channels [69].

Retigabine has an effective concentration for half-maximum response (EC_{50}) of 1.4 µM at −30 mV [70] and 3.7 µM at 0 mV [23] for KCNQ4 in vitro, with 10 µM of retigabine increasing the native $I_{k,n}$ currents by 1.4-fold at −60 mV to 2.2-fold at −110 mV [23]. Moreover, retigabine has been shown to shift voltages of activation to hyperpolarized potentials [23]. Li et al. determined the structures of KCNQ4 and its complex with retigabine using cryoelectron microscopy [71]. Four retigabine molecules were demonstrated to bind to one KCNQ4 tetramer, with each retigabine residing in a single hydrophobic fenestration site in the middle of the membrane. Retigabine contains three major functional groups: the fluorophenyl group, the middle phenyl ring, and the carbamate group (Figure 2). The Trp242, Phe246, Leu249, Leu305, Leu306, Ser309, Phe310, Phe311, Pro314, and Leu318 residues of KCNQ4 have been shown to be involved in the binding of retigabine (Figure 2) [71]. Using systematic mutagenesis studies, it was identified that the tryptophan residue (Trp242 in KCNQ4) in S5 was crucial for the activity of retigabine and was further shown that it is conserved from KCNQ2 to KCNQ5 [61,72], but replaced by Leu266 in KCNQ1 (Figure 1) [71]. Both the side chain of Ser309 and the carbonyl oxygen of Leu305 can form hydrogen bonds with the amino group from the carbamate group of retigabine [71]. In addition, both the side chain of Ser309 and the carbonyl oxygen of Phe311 can form hydrogen bonds with the amino group from the middle phenyl ring of retigabine [71]. The side chain of Trp242 and the aromatic ring of Phe110 have been reported to interact with the carbonyl oxygen from the carbamate group and the fluorine atom of retigabine, respectively [71]. In particular, KCNQ4 was shown to be modulated by phosphatidylinositol 4,5-bisphosphate (PIP_2) which is known to activate KCNQ channels by coupling voltage-sensing domains and the central pore domain [73,74]; a single molecule of PIP_2 inserts its head group into a cavity within each voltage-sensing domain [71].

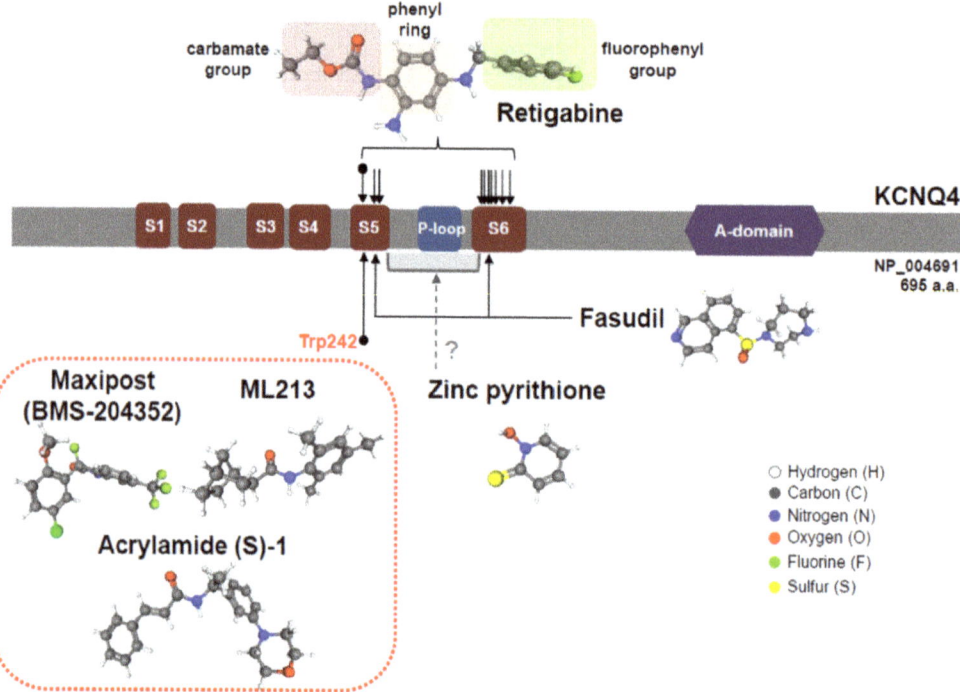

Figure 2. Pharmacological action sites of KCNQ4 activators along functional domains. Critical amino acid residues for the action of KCNQ4 activators are mostly located in the S5 and S6 regions, including the crucial site Trp242. Retigabine, maxipost, acrylamide (S)-1, and ML213 require this tryptophan residue for their activity.

Even though retigabine has been extensively studied and shown to prevent salicylate-induced ototoxicity in rats [75], its use against hearing loss has been limited due to the potential side-effects resulting from its broad action on KCNQ channels.

5.2. Retigabine Derivatives

Wang et al. reported several compounds that were made by modifying retigabine and showed better selectivity for KCNQ4 and KCNQ5 [76]. For instance, a N-1/3 substitution resulted in improved specificity for KCNQ4 and KCNQ5 compared with naïve retigabine [76]. Especially, 10 g of one of those derivatives showed the best potency for KCNQ4 and KCNQ5 with EC_{50} values of 0.78 and 1.68 µM, respectively, and had a minimal effect on homomeric KCNQ2 [76]. More specifically, 10 µM of 10 g of this compound was reported to increase the currents of KCNQ4 and KCNQ5 by 6.4- and 4.6-fold, respectively [76]. Further modification of this compound may lead to a drug with better specificity for KCNQ4 over KCNQ5. This study also demonstrated that alteration of chemical subunits from currently available KCNQ channel activators might serve as a promising platform for the discovery of novel compounds targeting KCNQ4 with higher specificity [77].

NS15370, which was developed as a chemical retigabine analog with higher potency [78], was shown to induce a shift in the voltage-dependence of activation, enhancing KCNQ4-mediated currents at potentials negative to 0 mV, but suppressing them at more positive membrane potentials [79].

5.3. Zinc Pyrithione

Zinc pyrithione (ZnPy), which is widely used for dandruff and psoriasis [80], has been shown to activate KCNQ channels, except KCNQ3 and KCNQ5 [81]. Accordingly, 10 µM ZnPy increased KCNQ4-mediated currents by 76.1-fold at −30 mV and 23.5-fold at +50 mV [81] and potentiated the native $I_{k,n}$ currents when combined with retigabine [23]. It should be mentioned that ZnPy is unique in that it increases the open probability of KCNQ2 and KCNQ4 in addition to inducing a hyperpolarizing shift in the voltage dependence of activation and increasing the current amplitude [81]. However, the activity of ZnPy does not depend on the tryptophan residue in S5, which is different from retigabine, but on the interaction with the pore region (Figure 2) [82]. Furthermore, both Zn^{2+} and pyrithione were demonstrated to be essential for activity, with the potency depending on the proper stoichiometry of 1:2 zinc-to-pyrithione [81].

5.4. Maxipost

Maxipost, formerly known as BMS-204352, was identified as a potent opener of calcium-activated maxi-K channels (BK channels) used for the control of convulsion and stroke [83]. Maxipost is known to be a potent activator of KCNQ channels with an EC_{50} of 2.4 µM for KCNQ4 at −30 mV [65,70], exhibiting protective effects against peripheral salicylate ototoxicity [75], and reported to abolish behavioral evidence of tinnitus [84]. Maxipost has been found to shift the voltages of activation to hyperpolarized potentials, which are dependent on the tryptophan residue in S5 (Figure 2) [65,70,85], but failed to potentiate native $I_{k,n}$; therefore, its application for hearing loss has been limited [23].

5.5. Acrylamide (S)-1

Acrylamide (S)-1 was synthesized as an orally bioavailable KCNQ2 activator for the control of migraines [86]. Despite its development for KCNQ4, acrylamide S-(1) was shown to be preferentially specific for KCNQ4 and KCNQ5 [85]. The EC_{50} for KCNQ4 determined for acrylamide S-(1) in *Xenopus* oocytes was 10.4 µM at 0 mV, with 100 µM acrylamide (S)-1 leading to a 20-fold enhancement of current amplitude [85]. The effect of acrylamide (S)-1 on KCNQ4 was reported to be potentiated across all voltage levels [85], whereas its effect on KCNQ2 and KCNQ3 was shown to be voltage-dependent [87]. Another study revealed that the hyperpolarizing shift induced by acrylamide (S)-1 depended on the conserved tryptophan residue in S5 (Figure 2) [79], which is also required for retigabine and maxipost, suggesting that these three compounds might exert their effects on KCNQ4 in a similar manner.

5.6. Other KCNQ4 Activators

There have been additional compounds reported to activate KCNQ4. AaTXKβ$_{(2-64)}$, a toxin isolated from the North African scorpion, was shown to specifically activate KCNQ3 and KCNQ4, without affecting KCNQ1 and KCNQ2 [88]. This peptide had an EC_{50} of 58 µg/mL at 0 mV, inducing a hyperpolarizing shift, and increasing KCNQ4 currents by 2-fold at 0 mV [88]. Fasudil, a rho-associated kinase inhibitor and a vasodilator, was found to potentiate KCNQ4 and KCNQ4/5 with EC_{50} values of 12.9 and 15.7 µM, at −30 mV, respectively, without affecting KCN2 and KCNQ2/3 [89]. Fasudil shifted the voltage-dependent activation curve in a more negative direction, for which the Val248 in S5 and Ile308 in the S6 segment of KCNQ4 were required [89]. ML213, identified by a high throughput fluorescent screen of the NIH Molecular Libraries Small Molecule Repository and structure–activity relationship, was initially characterized as specific for KCNQ2 and KCNQ4, with a 80-fold selectivity over other KCNQ channels [90]. The EC_{50} of ML213 for KCNQ4 was shown to be 1.8 µM at −10 mV, with ML213 inducing a hyperpolarizing shift, which was reported to be dependent on the crucial tryptophan residue in S5 and a 2-fold increase in currents following administration of 10 µM of the drug (Figure 2) [79]. In the cases of AaTXKβ$_{(2-64)}$, fasudil, and ML213, it is necessary to examine whether these drugs could induce the native $I_{k,n}$ currents of OHCs.

Through the Cortellis Drugs Discovery Intelligence™ service by Clarivate, we found that several pharmaceutical companies and universities are currently developing KCNQ4 activators. Most of them are being explored for their potential to treat neurological disorders, including epilepsy, pain, migraines, and many more conditions, and are currently in the phase of biological or preclinical testing. Acousia Therapeutics, which is a biotech company aiming for the development of small-molecule drugs for sensory neuronal hearing loss, has eight compounds targeting KCNQ4 in its pipeline.

6. Conclusions and Future Directions

Understanding of the function, structure, physiology, pharmacology, and genetics of KCNQ4 has indicated that KCNQ4 holds great promise for the discovery and development of drugs useful in genetic, age-related, and noise-induced hearing loss. Due to the growing prevalence and socioeconomic burden of hearing loss, the demand for drugs aimed in controlling these conditions have been increasing.

Application of available KCNQ4 activators has been currently restricted due to the lack of subtype specificity, especially for KCNQ2–KCNQ5, as well as due to their insufficient in vivo efficacy. As a member of voltage-gated K^+ channels, KCNQ4 shares structural and amino acid similarities with other KCNQ channels, which hinders the development of KCNQ4-specific drugs. As other KCNQ channels are involved in the physiology of diverse tissues and may also be associated with diseases, lack of specificity would lead to unwanted side-effects. As such, the selectivity for KCNQ4 could be achieved by the further refinement of existing compounds, as shown previously [76]. Based on the delineation of the crucial residues of the specific binding of retigabine with KCNQ4 and the molecular details of its activation [71], the discovery and optimization of related chemicals would be accelerated. Knowledge of the structure of KCNQ4 should also enable the design of compounds that induce conformational changes with an outcome similar to that normally caused by membrane depolarization. Moreover, simultaneous application of two activators with distinct modes of action may result in synergistic effects and reduced side-effects. In addition, considering the anatomical characteristic of the inner ear, as an isolated organ, using local administration as the effective delivery route might serve as both the main point of concern in the pharmacological development process, as well as an opportunity for reducing side-effects. Limited volume of therapeutic materials for administration in the inner ear without overloading the cochlea might require high efficacy and concentrations in order to reach the maximal impacts on hearing rescue.

Although some compounds could activate KCNQ4 in vitro, none of them were potent in inducing the native $I_{k,n}$ currents in OHCs [23]. The molecular basis for this discrepancy is not yet clear and OHC-specific modifiers were suggested [23]; however, more thorough studies regarding this aspect are required because many compounds have not been properly evaluated in this regard. The efficacy of KCNQ4 activators needs to be examined not only in OHCs in explants, but also in Kcnq4 mouse models. Besides, KCNQ4 activators would not be effective in Kcnq4$^{-/-}$ mice as there is no KCNQ4 to be activated. Similarly, they would not be effective in knock-in mice harboring the p.G286S (c.856G>A) pore region mutation, which results in unresponsiveness to KCNQ activators [21,42]. Therefore, it is necessary to generate additional Kcnq4 mice that would harbor pore region mutations with residual activity of K$^+$ channels or variants in the two cytoplasmic termini of KCNQ4 to investigate the in vivo efficacy of channel openers. In addition, the effectiveness of KCNQ4 activators needs to be examined in mouse models of noise-hearing loss.

More importantly, KCNQ4 activators should be validated in clinical trials, as there is no ongoing clinical trial targeting hearing loss by KCNQ4 activators currently. Target population, such as individuals with genetic hearing loss or noise-induced hearing, should be carefully selected. Both the therapeutic window and convenient application methods are important issues to be discussed in clinical trials. Drug repurposing and optimization for applicable specific *KCNQ4* mutation might also be an option for clinical application of KCNQ4 activators in deafness treatment with advantages of reducing the cost and shortening the time when compared to de novo drug discovery. In addition, the half-life duration and bioavailability of drugs targeting the activation of KCNQ4 would also be required to satisfy clinical degrees.

Author Contributions: Conceptualization, J.J. and H.Y.G.; investigation, J.H.R. and H.Y.G.; data curation, J.H.R. and H.Y.G.; writing—original draft preparation, J.H.R., J.J., and H.Y.G.; writing—review and editing, J.Y.C., J.J., and H.Y.G.; visualization, J.J. and H.Y.G.; supervision, J.Y.C., J.J., and H.Y.G.; funding acquisition, J.Y.C., J.J., and H.Y.G. All authors have read and agreed to the published version of the manuscript.

Funding: This research was supported by the Bio and Medical Technology Development Program of the National Research Foundation (NRF) funded by the Ministry of Science and ICT (NRF-2019M3E5D5066690 and 2018R1A5A2025079).

Acknowledgments: We thank the members of the Institute of Yonsei Ear Sciences (iYES) for their constructive comments and the Clarivate for the Cortellis Drugs Discovery Intelligence™.

Conflicts of Interest: The authors declare no conflict of interest.

Abbreviations

DFNA2	deafness nonsyndromic autosomal dominant 2
IHC	Inner hair cell
KCNQ	Potassium voltage-gated channel subfamily q
OHC	Outer hair cell

References

1. Petit, C.; El-Amraoui, A.; Avan, P. Audition: Hearing and Deafness. In *Neuroscience in the 21st Century*, 2nd ed.; Springer: New York, NY, USA, 2016.
2. Cunningham, L.L.; Tucci, D.L. Hearing Loss in Adults. *N. Engl. J. Med.* **2017**, *377*, 2465–2473. [CrossRef]
3. Petit, C.; Levilliers, J.; Hardelin, J.P. Molecular genetics of hearing loss. *Annu. Rev. Genet.* **2001**, *35*, 589–646. [CrossRef]
4. Raviv, D.; Dror, A.A.; Avraham, K.B. Hearing loss: A common disorder caused by many rare alleles. *Ann. N. Y. Acad. Sci.* **2010**, *1214*, 168–179. [CrossRef] [PubMed]
5. Chadha, S.; Cieza, A. World Health Organization and Its Initiative for Ear and Hearing Care. *Otolaryngol. Clin. N. Am.* **2018**, *51*, 535–542. [CrossRef] [PubMed]
6. Kubisch, C.; Schroeder, B.C.; Friedrich, T.; Lutjohann, B.; El-Amraoui, A.; Marlin, S.; Petit, C.; Jentsch, T.J. KCNQ4, a novel potassium channel expressed in sensory outer hair cells, is mutated in dominant deafness. *Cell* **1999**, *96*, 437–446. [CrossRef]
7. van Laer, L.; Carlsson, P.I.; Ottschytsch, N.; Bondeson, M.L.; Konings, A.; Vandevelde, A.; Dieltjens, N.; Fransen, E.; Snyders, D.; Borg, E.; et al. The contribution of genes involved in potassium-recycling in the inner ear to noise-induced hearing loss. *Hum. Mutat.* **2006**, *27*, 786–795. [CrossRef] [PubMed]
8. Peixoto Pinheiro, B.; Vona, B.; Löwenheim, H.; Rüttiger, L.; Knipper, M.; Adel, Y. Age-related hearing loss pertaining to potassium ion channels in the cochlea and auditory pathway. *Pflüg. Arch. Eur. J. Physiol.* **2020**. [CrossRef]
9. Wulff, H.; Castle, N.A.; Pardo, L.A. Voltage-gated potassium channels as therapeutic targets. *Nat. Rev. Drug Discov.* **2009**, *8*, 982–1001. [CrossRef]
10. Maljevic, S.; Wuttke, T.V.; Seebohm, G.; Lerche, H. KV7 channelopathies. *Pflüg. Arch. Eur. J. Physiol.* **2010**, *460*, 277–288. [CrossRef]

11. Schroeder, B.C.; Hechenberger, M.; Weinreich, F.; Kubisch, C.; Jentsch, T.J. KCNQ5, a novel potassium channel broadly expressed in brain, mediates M-type currents. *J. Biol. Chem.* **2000**, *275*, 24089–24095. [CrossRef]
12. Lerche, C.; Scherer, C.R.; Seebohm, G.; Derst, C.; Wei, A.D.; Busch, A.E.; Steinmeyer, K. Molecular cloning and functional expression of KCNQ5, a potassium channel subunit that may contribute to neuronal M-current diversity. *J. Biol. Chem.* **2000**, *275*, 22395–22400. [CrossRef]
13. Wang, Q.; Curran, M.E.; Splawski, I.; Burn, T.C.; Millholland, J.M.; VanRaay, T.J.; Shen, J.; Timothy, K.W.; Vincent, G.M.; de Jager, T.; et al. Positional cloning of a novel potassium channel gene: KVLQT1 mutations cause cardiac arrhythmias. *Nat. Genet.* **1996**, *12*, 17–23. [CrossRef] [PubMed]
14. Splawski, I.; Timothy, K.W.; Vincent, G.M.; Atkinson, D.L.; Keating, M.T. Molecular basis of the long-QT syndrome associated with deafness. *N. Engl. J. Med.* **1997**, *336*, 1562–1567. [CrossRef] [PubMed]
15. Neyroud, N.; Tesson, F.; Denjoy, I.; Leibovici, M.; Donger, C.; Barhanin, J.; Fauré, S.; Gary, F.; Coumel, P.; Petit, C.; et al. A novel mutation in the potassium channel gene KVLQT1 causes the Jervell and Lange-Nielsen cardioauditory syndrome. *Nat. Genet.* **1997**, *15*, 186–189. [CrossRef]
16. Singh, N.A.; Charlier, C.; Stauffer, D.; DuPont, B.R.; Leach, R.J.; Melis, R.; Ronen, G.M.; Bjerre, I.; Quattlebaum, T.; Murphy, J.V.; et al. A novel potassium channel gene, KCNQ2, is mutated in an inherited epilepsy of newborns. *Nat. Genet.* **1998**, *18*, 25–29. [CrossRef]
17. Biervert, C.; Schroeder, B.C.; Kubisch, C.; Berkovic, S.F.; Propping, P.; Jentsch, T.J.; Steinlein, O.K. A potassium channel mutation in neonatal human epilepsy. *Science* **1998**, *279*, 403–406. [CrossRef] [PubMed]
18. Charlier, C.; Singh, N.A.; Ryan, S.G.; Lewis, T.B.; Reus, B.E.; Leach, R.J.; Leppert, M. A pore mutation in a novel KQT-like potassium channel gene in an idiopathic epilepsy family. *Nat. Genet.* **1998**, *18*, 53–55. [CrossRef]
19. Lehman, A.; Thouta, S.; Mancini, G.M.S.; Naidu, S.; van Slegtenhorst, M.; McWalter, K.; Person, R.; Mwenifumbo, J.; Salvarinova, R.; Guella, I.; et al. Loss-of-Function and Gain-of-Function Mutations in KCNQ5 Cause Intellectual Disability or Epileptic Encephalopathy. *Am. J. Hum. Genet.* **2017**, *101*, 65–74. [CrossRef]
20. Naito, T.; Nishio, S.-Y.; Iwasa, Y.-I.; Yano, T.; Kumakawa, K.; Abe, S.; Ishikawa, K.; Kojima, H.; Namba, A.; Oshikawa, C.; et al. Comprehensive Genetic Screening of KCNQ4 in a Large Autosomal Dominant Nonsyndromic Hearing Loss Cohort: Genotype-Phenotype Correlations and a Founder Mutation. *PLoS ONE* **2013**, *8*, e63231.
21. Jung, J.; Lin, H.; Koh, Y.I.; Ryu, K.; Lee, J.S.; Rim, J.H.; Choi, H.J.; Lee, H.J.; Kim, H.Y.; Yu, S.; et al. Rare KCNQ4 variants found in public databases underlie impaired channel activity that may contribute to hearing impairment. *Exp. Mol. Med.* **2019**, *51*, 99. [CrossRef]
22. Gao, Y.; Yechikov, S.; Vazquez, A.E.; Chen, D.; Nie, L. Impaired surface expression and conductance of the KCNQ4 channel lead to sensorineural hearing loss. *J. Cell. Mol. Med.* **2013**, *17*, 889–900. [CrossRef] [PubMed]
23. Leitner, M.G.; Feuer, A.; Ebers, O.; Schreiber, D.N.; Halaszovich, C.R.; Oliver, D. Restoration of ion channel function in deafness-causing KCNQ4 mutants by synthetic channel openers. *Br. J. Pharmacol.* **2012**, *165*, 2244–2259. [CrossRef] [PubMed]
24. Jung, J.; Choi, H.B.; Koh, Y.I.; Rim, J.H.; Choi, H.J.; Kim, S.H.; Lee, J.; Kim, A.; Lee, J.S.; et al. Whole-exome sequencing identifies two novel mutations in KCNQ4 in individuals with nonsyndromic hearing loss. *Sci. Rep.* **2018**, *8*, 16659. [CrossRef]
25. Shin, D.H.; Jung, J.; Koh, Y.I.; Rim, J.H.; Lee, J.S.; Choi, H.J.; Joo, S.Y.; Yu, S.; Cha, D.H.; Lee, S.Y.; et al. A recurrent mutation in KCNQ4 in Korean families with nonsyndromic hearing loss and rescue of the channel activity by KCNQ activators. *Hum. Mutat.* **2019**, *40*, 335–346. [CrossRef]
26. Wangemann, P. K$^+$ cycling and the endocochlear potential. *Hear. Res.* **2002**, *165*, 1–9. [CrossRef]
27. Delmaghani, S.; El-Amraoui, A. Inner Ear Gene Therapies Take Off: Current Promises and Future Challenges. *J. Clin. Med.* **2020**, *9*, 2309. [CrossRef]
28. Pan, B.; Akyuz, N.; Liu, X.-P.; Asai, Y.; Nist-Lund, C.; Kurima, K.; Derfler, B.H.; György, B.; Limapichat, W.; Walujkar, S.; et al. TMC1 Forms the Pore of Mechanosensory Transduction Channels in Vertebrate Inner Ear Hair Cells. *Neuron* **2018**, *99*, 736–753.e6. [CrossRef] [PubMed]
29. Delpire, E.; Lu, J.; England, R.; Dull, C.; Thorne, T. Deafness and imbalance associated with inactivation of the secretory Na-K-2Cl co-transporter. *Nat. Genet.* **1999**, *22*, 192–195. [CrossRef]
30. Marcus, D.C.; Wu, T.; Wangemann, P.; Kofuji, P. KCNJ10 (Kir4.1) potassium channel knockout abolishes endocochlear potential. *Am. J. Physiol. Cell Physiol.* **2002**, *282*, C403–C407. [CrossRef]
31. Dallos, P. Cochlear amplification, outer hair cells and prestin. *Curr. Opin. Neurobiol.* **2008**, *18*, 370–376. [CrossRef]
32. Housley, G.D.; Ashmore, J.F. Ionic currents of outer hair cells isolated from the guinea-pig cochlea. *J. Physiol.* **1992**, *448*, 73–98. [CrossRef]
33. Dallos, P.; Zheng, J.; Cheatham, M.A. Prestin and the cochlear amplifier. *J. Physiol.* **2006**, *576*, 37–42. [CrossRef]
34. Marcotti, W.; Kros, C.J. Developmental expression of the potassium current $I_{K,n}$ contributes to maturation of mouse outer hair cells. *J. Physiol.* **1999**, *520*, 653–660. [CrossRef]
35. Winter, H.; Braig, C.; Zimmermann, U.; Geisler, H.-S.; Fränzer, J.-T.; Weber, T.; Ley, M.; Engel, J.; Knirsch, M.; Bauer, K.; et al. Thyroid hormone receptors TRα1 and TRβ differentially regulate gene expression of *Kcnq4* and prestin during final differentiation of outer hair cells. *J. Cell Sci.* **2006**, *119*, 2975–2984. [CrossRef]
36. Boettger, T.; Hübner, C.A.; Maier, H.; Rust, M.B.; Beck, F.X.; Jentsch, T.J. Deafness and renal tubular acidosis in mice lacking the K-Cl co-transporter Kcc4. *Nature* **2002**, *416*, 874–878. [CrossRef]

37. Kharkovets, T.; Hardelin, J.P.; Safieddine, S.; Schweizer, M.; El-Amraoui, A.; Petit, C.; Jentsch, T.J. KCNQ4, a K⁺ channel mutated in a form of dominant deafness, is expressed in the inner ear and the central auditory pathway. *Proc. Natl. Acad. Sci. USA* **2000**, *97*, 4333–4338. [CrossRef]
38. Mammano, F.; Ashmore, J.F. Differential expression of outer hair cell potassium currents in the isolated cochlea of the guinea-pig. *J. Physiol.* **1996**, *496*, 639–646. [CrossRef]
39. Beisel, K.W.; Nelson, N.C.; Delimont, D.C.; Fritzsch, B. Longitudinal gradients of KCNQ4 expression in spiral ganglion and cochlear hair cells correlate with progressive hearing loss in DFNA211Published on the World Wide Web on 13 September 2000. *Mol. Brain Res.* **2000**, *82*, 137–149. [CrossRef]
40. Oliver, D.; Knipper, M.; Derst, C.; Fakler, B. Resting potential and submembrane calcium concentration of inner hair cells in the isolated mouse cochlea are set by KCNQ-type potassium channels. *J. Neurosci. Off. J. Soc. Neurosci.* **2003**, *23*, 2141–2149. [CrossRef]
41. Beisel, K.W.; Rocha-Sanchez, S.M.; Morris, K.A.; Nie, L.; Feng, F.; Kachar, B.; Yamoah, E.N.; Fritzsch, B. Differential expression of KCNQ4 in inner hair cells and sensory neurons is the basis of progressive high-frequency hearing loss. *J. Neurosci. Off. J. Soc. Neurosci.* **2005**, *25*, 9285–9293. [CrossRef]
42. Kharkovets, T.; Dedek, K.; Maier, H.; Schweizer, M.; Khimich, D.; Nouvian, R.; Vardanyan, V.; Leuwer, R.; Moser, T.; Jentsch, T.J. Mice with altered KCNQ4 K⁺ channels implicate sensory outer hair cells in human progressive deafness. *EMBO J.* **2006**, *25*, 642–652. [CrossRef]
43. Carignano, C.; Barila, E.P.; Rías, E.I.; Dionisio, L.; Aztiria, E.; Spitzmaul, G. Inner Hair Cell and Neuron Degeneration Contribute to Hearing Loss in a DFNA2-Like Mouse Model. *Neuroscience* **2019**, *410*, 202–216. [CrossRef]
44. Rüttiger, L.; Sausbier, M.; Zimmermann, U.; Winter, H.; Braig, C.; Engel, J.; Knirsch, M.; Arntz, C.; Langer, P.; Hirt, B.; et al. Deletion of the Ca²⁺-activated potassium (BK) alpha-subunit but not the BKbeta1-subunit leads to progressive hearing loss. *Proc. Natl. Acad. Sci. USA* **2004**, *101*, 12922–12927. [CrossRef]
45. Selyanko, A.A.; Hadley, J.K.; Wood, I.C.; Abogadie, F.C.; Jentsch, T.J.; Brown, D.A. Inhibition of KCNQ1–4 potassium channels expressed in mammalian cells via M1 muscarinic acetylcholine receptors. *J. Physiol.* **2000**, *522 Pt 3*, 349–355. [CrossRef]
46. Alberti, P.W.; Symons, F.; Hyde, M.L. Occupational hearing loss. The significance of asymmetrical hearing thresholds. *Acta Otolaryngol.* **1979**, *87*, 255–263. [CrossRef]
47. World Health Organization. *Hearing Loss Due to Recreational Exposure to Loud Sounds: A Review*; World Health Organization: Geneva, Switzerland, 2015.
48. Konings, A.; Laer, L.V.; Camp, G.V. Genetic Studies on Noise-Induced Hearing Loss: A Review. *Ear Hear.* **2009**, *30*, 151–159. [CrossRef] [PubMed]
49. Pawelczyk, M.; van Laer, L.; Fransen, E.; Rajkowska, E.; Konings, A.; Carlsson, P.I.; Borg, E.; van Camp, G.; Sliwinska-Kowalska, M. Analysis of gene polymorphisms associated with K ion circulation in the inner ear of patients susceptible and resistant to noise-induced hearing loss. *Ann. Hum. Genet.* **2009**, *73 Pt 4*, 411–421. [CrossRef]
50. Sliwinska-Kowalska, M.; Pawelczyk, M. Contribution of genetic factors to noise-induced hearing loss: A human studies review. *Mutat. Res.* **2013**, *752*, 61–65. [CrossRef]
51. Guo, H.; Ding, E.; Sheng, R.; Cheng, J.; Cai, W.; Guo, J.; Wang, N.; Zhang, H.; Zhu, B. Genetic variation in KCNQ4 gene is associated with susceptibility to noise-induced hearing loss in a Chinese population. *Environ. Toxicol. Pharm.* **2018**, *63*, 55–59. [CrossRef] [PubMed]
52. Marchetta, P.; Möhrle, D.; Eckert, P.; Reimann, K.; Wolter, S.; Tolone, A.; Lang, I.; Wolters, M.; Feil, R.; Engel, J.; et al. Guanylyl Cyclase A/cGMP Signaling Slows Hidden, Age- and Acoustic Trauma-Induced Hearing Loss. *Front. Aging Neurosci.* **2020**, *12*, 83. [CrossRef] [PubMed]
53. Engel, J.; Braig, C.; Rüttiger, L.; Kuhn, S.; Zimmermann, U.; Blin, N.; Sausbier, M.; Kalbacher, H.; Münkner, S.; Rohbock, K.; et al. Two classes of outer hair cells along the tonotopic axis of the cochlea. *Neuroscience* **2006**, *143*, 837–849. [CrossRef]
54. Xiong, Q.; Gao, Z.; Wang, W.; Li, M. Activation of Kv7 (KCNQ) voltage-gated potassium channels by synthetic compounds. *Trends Pharmacol. Sci.* **2008**, *29*, 99–107. [CrossRef] [PubMed]
55. Rostock, A.; Tober, C.; Rundfeldt, C.; Bartsch, R.; Engel, J.; Polymeropoulos, E.E.; Kutscher, B.; Löscher, W.; Hönack, D.; White, H.S.; et al. D-23129: A new anticonvulsant with a broad spectrum activity in animal models of epileptic seizures. *Epilepsy Res.* **1996**, *23*, 211–223. [CrossRef]
56. Rundfeldt, C. The new anticonvulsant retigabine (D-23129) acts as an opener of K+ channels in neuronal cells. *Eur. J. Pharmacol.* **1997**, *336*, 243–249. [CrossRef]
57. Tober, C.; Rostock, A.; Rundfeldt, C.; Bartsch, R. D-23129: A potent anticonvulsant in the amygdala kindling model of complex partial seizures. *Eur. J. Pharmacol.* **1996**, *303*, 163–169. [CrossRef]
58. French, J.A.; Abou-Khalil, B.W.; Leroy, R.F.; Yacubian, E.M.T.; Shin, P.; Hall, S.; Mansbach, H.; Nohria, V. Randomized, double-blind, placebo-controlled trial of ezogabine (retigabine) in partial epilepsy. *Neurology* **2011**, *76*, 1555–1563. [CrossRef] [PubMed]
59. Gunthorpe, M.J.; Large, C.H.; Sankar, R. The mechanism of action of retigabine (ezogabine), a first-in-class K+ channel opener for the treatment of epilepsy. *Epilepsia* **2012**, *53*, 412–424. [CrossRef] [PubMed]
60. Tatulian, L.; Delmas, P.; Abogadie, F.C.; Brown, D.A. Activation of Expressed KCNQ Potassium Currents and Native Neuronal M-Type Potassium Currents by the Anti-Convulsant Drug Retigabine. *J. Neurosci.* **2001**, *21*, 5535–5545. [CrossRef] [PubMed]

61. Schenzer, A.; Friedrich, T.; Pusch, M.; Saftig, P.; Jentsch, T.J.; Grötzinger, J.; Schwake, M. Molecular Determinants of KCNQ (K_v7) K^+ Channel Sensitivity to the Anticonvulsant Retigabine. *J. Neurosci.* **2005**, *25*, 5051–5060. [CrossRef]
62. Friedman, A.K.; Juarez, B.; Ku, S.M.; Zhang, H.; Calizo, R.C.; Walsh, J.J.; Chaudhury, D.; Zhang, S.; Hawkins, A.; Dietz, D.M.; et al. KCNQ channel openers reverse depressive symptoms via an active resilience mechanism. *Nat. Commun.* **2016**, *7*, 11671. [CrossRef]
63. Fretwell, L.V.; Woolard, J. Cardiovascular responses to retigabine in conscious rats—Under normotensive and hypertensive conditions. *Br. J. Pharm.* **2013**, *169*, 1279–1289. [CrossRef] [PubMed]
64. Hayashi, H.; Iwata, M.; Tsuchimori, N.; Matsumoto, T. Activation of peripheral KCNQ channels attenuates inflammatory pain. *Mol. Pain* **2014**, *10*, 15. [CrossRef] [PubMed]
65. Korsgaard, M.P.G.; Hartz, B.P.; Brown, W.D.; Ahring, P.K.; Strøbæk, D.; Mirza, N.R. Anxiolytic Effects of Maxipost (BMS-204352) and Retigabine via Activation of Neuronal K_v7 Channels. *J. Pharmacol. Exp. Ther.* **2005**, *314*, 282–292. [CrossRef] [PubMed]
66. Redrobe, J.P.; Nielsen, A.N. Effects of neuronal Kv7 potassium channel activators on hyperactivity in a rodent model of mania. *Behav. Brain Res.* **2009**, *198*, 481–485. [CrossRef] [PubMed]
67. Brickel, N.; Gandhi, P.; VanLandingham, K.; Hammond, J.; DeRossett, S. The urinary safety profile and secondary renal effects of retigabine (ezogabine): A first-in-class antiepileptic drug that targets KCNQ (Kv7) potassium channels. *Epilepsia* **2012**, *53*, 606–612. [CrossRef]
68. Wainger, B.J.; Macklin, E.A.; Vucic, S.; McIlduff, C.E.; Paganoni, S.; Maragakis, N.J.; Bedlack, R.; Goyal, N.A.; Rutkove, S.B.; Lange, D.J.; et al. Effect of Ezogabine on Cortical and Spinal Motor Neuron Excitability in Amyotrophic Lateral Sclerosis: A Randomized Clinical Trial. *JAMA Neurol.* **2021**, *78*, 186–196. [CrossRef]
69. van Rijn, C.M.; van Bree, E.W. Synergy between retigabine and GABA in modulating the convulsant site of the GABAA receptor complex. *Eur. J. Pharm.* **2003**, *464*, 95–100. [CrossRef]
70. Schroder, R.L.; Jespersen, T.; Christophersen, P.; Strobaek, D.; Jensen, B.S.; Olesen, S.P. KCNQ4 channel activation by BMS-204352 and retigabine. *Neuropharmacology* **2001**, *40*, 888–898. [CrossRef]
71. Li, T.; Wu, K.; Yue, Z.; Wang, Y.; Zhang, F.; Shen, H. Structural Basis for the Modulation of Human KCNQ4 by Small-Molecule Drugs. *Mol. Cell* **2020**, *81*, 25–37. [CrossRef]
72. Wuttke, T.V.; Seebohm, G.; Bail, S.; Maljevic, S.; Lerche, H. The new anticonvulsant retigabine favors voltage-dependent opening of the Kv7.2 (KCNQ2) channel by binding to its activation gate. *Mol. Pharm.* **2005**, *67*, 1009–1017. [CrossRef] [PubMed]
73. Zhang, H.; Craciun, L.C.; Mirshahi, T.; Rohács, T.; Lopes, C.M.B.; Jin, T.; Logothetis, D.E. PIP2 Activates KCNQ Channels, and Its Hydrolysis Underlies Receptor-Mediated Inhibition of M Currents. *Neuron* **2003**, *37*, 963–975. [CrossRef]
74. Zaydman, M.A.; Silva, J.R.; Delaloye, K.; Li, Y.; Liang, H.; Larsson, H.P.; Shi, J.; Cui, J. Kv7.1 ion channels require a lipid to couple voltage sensing to pore opening. *Proc. Natl. Acad. Sci. USA* **2013**, *110*, 13180–13185. [CrossRef] [PubMed]
75. Sheppard, A.M.; Chen, G.-D.; Salvi, R. Potassium ion channel openers, Maxipost and Retigabine, protect against peripheral salicylate ototoxicity in rats. *Hear. Res.* **2015**, *327*, 1–8. [CrossRef]
76. Wang, L.; Qiao, G.-H.; Hu, H.-N.; Gao, Z.-B.; Nan, F.-J. Discovery of Novel Retigabine Derivatives as Potent KCNQ4 and KCNQ5 Channel Agonists with Improved Specificity. *ACS Med. Chem. Lett.* **2019**, *10*, 27–33. [CrossRef]
77. Liu, R.; Tzounopoulos, T.; Wipf, P. Synthesis and Optimization of Kv7 (KCNQ) Potassium Channel Agonists: The Role of Fluorines in Potency and Selectivity. *ACS Med. Chem. Lett.* **2019**, *10*, 929–935. [CrossRef] [PubMed]
78. Dalby-Brown, W.; Jessen, C.; Hougaard, C.; Jensen, M.L.; Jacobsen, T.A.; Nielsen, K.S.; Erichsen, H.K.; Grunnet, M.; Ahring, P.K.; Christophersen, P.; et al. Characterization of a novel high-potency positive modulator of Kv7 channels. *Eur. J. Pharmacol.* **2013**, *709*, 52–63. [CrossRef] [PubMed]
79. Jepps, T.A.; Bentzen, B.H.; Stott, J.B.; Povstyan, O.V.; Sivaloganathan, K.; Dalby-Brown, W.; Greenwood, I.A. Vasorelaxant effects of novel Kv 7.4 channel enhancers ML213 and NS15370. *Br. J. Pharmacol.* **2014**, *171*, 4413–4424. [CrossRef] [PubMed]
80. Marks, R.; Pearse, A.D.; Walker, A.P. The effects of a shampoo containing zinc pyrithione on the control of dandruff. *Br. J. Derm.* **1985**, *112*, 415–422. [CrossRef]
81. Xiong, Q.; Sun, H.; Li, M. Zinc pyrithione-mediated activation of voltage-gated KCNQ potassium channels rescues epileptogenic mutants. *Nat. Chem. Biol.* **2007**, *3*, 287–296. [CrossRef]
82. Xiong, Q.; Sun, H.; Zhang, Y.; Nan, F.; Li, M. Combinatorial augmentation of voltage-gated KCNQ potassium channels by chemical openers. *Proc. Natl. Acad. Sci. USA* **2008**, *105*, 3128–3133. [CrossRef] [PubMed]
83. Hewawasam, P.; Gribkoff, V.K.; Pendri, Y.; Dworetzky, S.I.; Meanwell, N.A.; Martinez, E.; Boissard, C.G.; Post-Munson, D.J.; Trojnacki, J.T.; Yeleswaram, K.; et al. The synthesis and characterization of BMS-204352 (MaxiPost™) and related 3-fluorooxindoles as openers of maxi-K potassium channels. *Bioorg. Med. Chem. Lett.* **2002**, *12*, 1023–1026. [CrossRef]
84. Lobarinas, E.; Dalby-Brown, W.; Stolzberg, D.; Mirza, N.R.; Allman, B.L.; Salvi, R. Effects of the potassium ion channel modulators BMS-204352 Maxipost and its R-enantiomer on salicylate-induced tinnitus in rats. *Physiol. Behav.* **2011**, *104*, 873–879. [CrossRef] [PubMed]
85. Bentzen, B.H.; Schmitt, N.; Calloe, K.; Dalby Brown, W.; Grunnet, M.; Olesen, S.P. The acrylamide (S)-1 differentially affects Kv7 (KCNQ) potassium channels. *Neuropharmacology* **2006**, *51*, 1068–1077. [CrossRef] [PubMed]
86. Wu, Y.J.; Boissard, C.G.; Greco, C.; Gribkoff, V.K.; Harden, D.G.; He, H.; L'Heureux, A.; Kang, S.H.; Kinney, G.G.; Knox, R.J.; et al. (S)-N-[1-(3-morpholin-4-ylphenyl)ethyl]-3-phenylacrylamide: An orally bioavailable KCNQ2 opener with significant activity in a cortical spreading depression model of migraine. *J. Med. Chem.* **2003**, *46*, 3197–3200. [CrossRef] [PubMed]

87. Blom, S.M.; Rottländer, M.; Kehler, J.; Bundgaard, C.; Schmitt, N.; Jensen, H.S. From pan-reactive KV7 channel opener to subtype selective opener/inhibitor by addition of a methyl group. *PLoS ONE* **2014**, *9*, e100209. [CrossRef]
88. Landoulsi, Z.; Miceli, F.; Palmese, A.; Amoresano, A.; Marino, G.; El Ayeb, M.; Taglialatela, M.; Benkhalifa, R. Subtype-Selective Activation of K_v7 Channels by AaTXK$\beta_{(2-64)}$, a Novel Toxin Variant from the *Androctonus australis* Scorpion Venom. *Mol. Pharmacol.* **2013**, *84*, 763–773. [CrossRef]
89. Zhang, X.; An, H.; Li, J.; Zhang, Y.; Liu, Y.; Jia, Z.; Zhang, W.; Chu, L.; Zhang, H. Selective activation of vascular Kv 7.4/Kv 7.5 K^+ channels by fasudil contributes to its vasorelaxant effect. *Br. J. Pharmacol.* **2016**, *173*, 3480–3491. [CrossRef]
90. Yu, H.; Wu, M.; Townsend, S.D.; Zou, B.; Long, S.; Daniels, J.S.; McManus, O.B.; Li, M.; Lindsley, C.W.; Hopkins, C.R. Discovery, Synthesis, and Structure–Activity Relationship of a Series of N-Aryl-bicyclo [2.2.1]heptane-2-carboxamides: Characterization of ML213 as a Novel KCNQ2 and KCNQ4 Potassium Channel Opener. *ACS Chem. Neurosci.* **2011**, *2*, 572–577. [CrossRef] [PubMed]

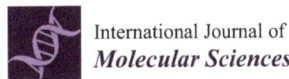
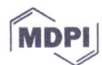

Review

Hyperbaric Oxygenation as Adjunctive Therapy in the Treatment of Sudden Sensorineural Hearing Loss

Dorota Olex-Zarychta

Institute of Sport Sciences, Academy of Physical Education in Katowice, 40-065 Katowice, Poland; d.olex@awf.katowice.pl

Received: 14 October 2020; Accepted: 11 November 2020; Published: 14 November 2020

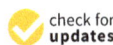

Abstract: Sudden sensorineural hearing loss seems to become a serious social health problem in modern societies. According to the World Health Organization (WHO) reports, adult-onset sensorineural hearing loss is found to be one of the leading diseases at the global level, especially in high-income countries, and is foreseen to move up from the 14th to 7th leading cause of the global burden of diseases by the year 2030. Although the direct mortality rate of this disease is very low, its influence on quality of life is huge; that is the reason why the implementation of the most effective and the safest therapies for the patient is crucial for minimizing the risk of complications and adverse reactions to treatment. The aim of this paper is to present hyperbaric oxygen therapy (HBOT) as a medical procedure useful in the treatment of sudden sensorineural hearing loss as adjunctive therapy of high efficacy. This paper focuses on the molecular mechanisms of action and clinical effectiveness of HBOT in the treatment of idiopathic sudden deafness, taking into consideration both the benefits and potential risks of its implementation.

Keywords: sensorineural hearing loss; hyperbaric oxygenation; adjunctive therapy

---

1. Introduction

Clinical hyperbaric oxygen therapy (HBOT) is defined as placing a patient's entire body in an increased pressure environment and having that patient inhale 100% oxygen for their specific diagnosis, for a defined period of time per treatment [1]. HBOT can be used as the leading or a complementary therapy to address several medical problems. HBOT is undertaken in Europe on the basis of the indications of the European Committee of Hyperbaric Medicine (ECHM). Actual indications for the medical use of HBOT in Europe were established during the ECHM Consensus Conference in 2016, taking into account three different types of recommendations for using HBOT as a medical procedure.

A Type I recommendation is where HBOT is strongly recommended, because this approach guarantees a positive treatment effect. Recommendations include decompression illness and CO poisoning, prevention and treatment of osteoradionecrosis (mandible), soft tissue radionecrosis (cystitis and proctitis), gas embolism, open fractures with a crush injury, anaerobic or mixed bacterial infections, and sudden sensorineural hearing loss (SSNHL). Recommendations and standards are supported by strong evidence of beneficial action based on at least two concordant, large, double-blind, randomized controlled trials, with no or only weak methodological bias.

A Type II recommendation is when HBOT is recommended because of its positive therapeutic effect. Recommendations include diabetic foot lesions, femoral head necrosis, compromised skin grafts and musculo-cutaneous flaps, a crush injury without a fracture, osteoradionecrosis (bones other than the mandible), radio-induced lesions of soft tissues (other than cystitis and proctitis), ischemic ulcers, refractory chronic osteomyelitis, and 2nd-degree burns over more than 20% of the body surface area. Recommendations or guidelines are supported by evidence of beneficial action based on double-blind, randomized controlled trials, but with some methodological bias, such as concerning only small samples or only a single study.

A Type III recommendation is when choosing HBOT may be optional, such as for radio-induced lesions, post-vascular procedure reperfusion syndrome and limb replantation, and selected non-healing wounds secondary to systemic processes. Recommendations are supported by weak evidence of beneficial action based only on uncontrolled studies-a historical control group, a cohort study, etc. [2].

Sensorineural hearing loss seems to become a serious social health problem in modern societies. According to the World Health Organization (WHO) reports, sensorineural hearing loss is one of the leading diseases at the global level, especially in high-income countries, and is foreseen to move up from the 14th to 7th leading cause of the global burden of diseases by the year 2030 [3]. Although the direct mortality rate of this disease is very low, its influence on quality of life is significant; that is, the reason why the implementation of the most effective and the safest therapies for the patient is crucial for minimizing the risk of complications and adverse reactions to treatment. The aim of this paper is to present HBOT as a medical procedure useful in the treatment of sudden sensorineural hearing loss (SSNHL) as an adjunctive therapy of high efficacy. This paper focuses on the mechanisms of action and clinical usefulness of HBOT in the treatment of idiopathic sudden deafness, taking into consideration both the benefits and potential risks of its implementation.

2. Physiology of Hyperbaric Oxygenation in Human

For oxygenation in hyperbaric conditions, pressure is expressed as multiples of the atmospheric pressure measured at sea level, which is 1 atmosphere absolute (1 ATA). In normobaric conditions at sea level, most of the oxygen in the blood is in a complex with the hemoglobin from the red blood cells (98%), with just a tiny amount of oxygen actually dissolved in the plasma (0.3 mL oxygen/100 mL). Assuming normal perfusion, tissues at rest extract about 6 mL of oxygen per 100 mL of blood. Breathing with pure oxygen in hyperbaric conditions leads to an increase in oxygen partial pressure in the lungs, and thus a significant increase in its concentration in the plasma on the basis of physical dissolution in amounts of up to 20 times higher than at ambient pressure. Hyperbaric oxygenation increases the oxidative capacity of the blood serum. Breathing 100% oxygen under hyperbaric conditions (f. ex. 2.5 ATA) leads to increased amounts of oxygen in blood serum to about 5 mL/100 mL. During HBOT, the pressure is raised to 3 ATA and the amount of oxygen delivered with the blood increases from 10 to 15 times above the norm, which gives a quantity sufficient for life support even in the case of absence of hemoglobin [4]. In hyperbaric conditions, the amount of oxygen that is dissolved in the blood plasma is sufficient to meet resting requirements. Administering 100% oxygen at 3 ATA, the dissolved oxygen content is approximately 6 mL per 100 mL, while in normobaric conditions breathing pure oxygen increases the amount of oxygen dissolved in the blood only from 0.3 to 1.5 mL per 100 mL. Breathing 100% oxygen in hyperbaric conditions above 1.4 ATA contributes to a significant increase in the diffusion radius of the oxygen from the capillaries to the surrounding tissues. At 3 ATA, its plasma pressure can be as high as 2000 mmHg, which increases the diffusion of oxygen to the tissues four times on the arterial side, and twice on the venous side of the capillary blood circulation [5]. Breathing 100% oxygen under normobaric conditions (1 ATA) is not qualified as HBOT, since it increases the amount of oxygen dissolved in the blood serum only about 2 mL/100 mL [6]. HBOT also causes an increase in the elasticity of erythrocytes and reduces the viscosity of blood, thus improving microcirculation [6,7]. Inhaling the oxygen at 3 ATA increases the partial pressure of the oxygen in the blood to 200 kPa and more, which leads to an increase in the oxygen concentration in arterial blood of about 6.6–6.8 mL oxygen/100 mL [4].

The influence of HBOT on organs and tissues is diverse. In conditions of high pressure and high partial concentrations, the oxygen becomes a drug exerting many important phenomena in a patient's body, the most important of which is metabolism [5]. Hyperbaric oxygen is proven to have a beneficial influence on local hypoxia in tissues. Proper oxygen tension is essential for angiogenesis because it is a prerequisite for the formation of the collagen matrix [8]. The use of HBOT decreases the ability of neutrophils to adhere to the vessel walls, thus reducing endothelial damage, and allowing vasoconstriction of vessels in areas with a normal oxygen concentration without changes in the circulation in areas with impaired flow, restoration of collagen production and fibroblast growth, stimulation of peroxide dismutase production, and storage of adenosine-triphosphate (ATP) in cell membranes. This has an influence on the reduction of edema in tissues, limitation of some forms of immune response, stimulation of osteoclasts activity, capillary proliferation, inhibition of production the surfactant in the lungs, and blockage of lipid peroxidation in carbon monoxide (CO) poisoning and its accelerated removal from hemoglobin [7]. In conditions caused by the formation of gas (f ex. in cases of decompression sickness), through increasing the pressure HBOT causes a reduction in the volume of the inert gas bubbles in the blood vessels and tissues. At 2.8 ATA, the bubble volume is reduced by almost two thirds. Treatment with HBOT serves to decrease the bubble size, thus reducing pain and restoring blood flow, while also correcting tissue hypoxia and inducing a large inert gas gradient to expedite washout. Hyperbaric oxygenation hastens additionally the dissolution of the gas bubbles by replacing the inert gas in the bubble with oxygen (metabolized rapidly by the tissues) and prevents the formation of new bubbles [9].

The administration of pure hyperbaric oxygen extends the leukocyte antibacterial activity. It increases the rate of killing of some common bacteria and phagocytes. HBOT is bactericidal for certain anaerobes, including *Clostridium perfringens*, and research showed that it is bacteriostatic for some species of *Escherichia* and *Pseudomonas* [10]. The action of HBOT on anaerobes is based on the production of free radicals, such as superoxide, dismutase, catalase, and peroxidase. Many different clostridial exotoxins have been identified so far, and the most prevalent is alphatoxine (phospholipase C), which is hemolytic and tissue necrotizing, as well as thetatoxine, which is responsible for vascular injury and in consequence for acceleration of tissue necrosis. HBOT blocks the production of alphatoxine and thetatoxine and acts as inhibitors of bacterial growth [11]. Hyperbaric oxygen is documented to reduce ischemia/reperfusion injury in a number of different experimental models. Mechanisms responsible for the beneficial effect of HBOT in the treatment of ischemia/reperfusion injury involve suppression of neutrophil–endothelial adhesion [12]. The effect of inhibiting leukocyte adhesion to the endothelium is present after HBOT, and it leads to improvement in microcirculation [13]. Huang and Obenaus [14] reported the neuroprotective effect of HBOT in an animal model. They observed anti-inflammatory effects and an improvement in tissue oxidation, as well as inhibition of mitochondria-associated apoptosis. There is little available data on the influence of HBOT on the motor control and neurocognitive functioning of humans; however, a positive effect of HBOT on sensorimotor functions in mammals was suggested in some previous research. A positive effect of HBOT on simple reaction time is showed in the research of Olex-Zarychta [15], where after 15 sessions at 2.5 ATA the reaction time of the patient visibly improved, and 3 weeks after the last session slightly decreased, but still exceeded the output level. Research of Kenneth and Stoller [16] presented the beneficial effects of HBOT on human psychomotor functions, but the effects of therapy were transient; maintaining the positive effect of HBOT required repeated administering. The potential mechanism that may underline the effectiveness of hyperbaric oxygenation on neurocognitive functions of humans is still not clear. It is supposed that HBOT leads to a higher amount of oxygen available to the brain and, therefore, it results in an increase in the cognitive processing of the human. Appropriate HBOT exposure results in an increase in the oxygen content of arterial blood. This increase in oxygen and the subsequent increase in the oxygen diffusion gradient between the blood and tissues has been termed the primary effect of HBOT therapy. A secondary effect of HBOT therapy is a reduction in the inflammatory response due to a vasoconstriction mediated by the oxygen [17]. Such therapy can indirectly result in an increased ability to repair blood vessels, improvement in the circulation in brain tissue, and may increase the ability of vascular endothelium toward axon regeneration or nitrogen synthesis [18].

3. The Use of Hyperbaric Oxygenation in Medicine

Hyperbaric oxygenation as a medical procedure involves a patient inhaling pure oxygen using a pressure of 2 to 3 ATA, which is provided by properly constructed pressure chambers. Breathing 100% oxygen at ambient pressure of 1 ATA, or displaying only parts of the body at 100% oxygen, should not be qualified as HBOT [6,7]. Current knowledge indicates that the pressure in a hyperbaric chamber during HBOT should be at least 1.4 ATA [4]. According to ECHM standards and guidelines, one typical session of HBOT in a multi-site chamber lasts about 90 min and consists of three main phases. The first phase lasts about 10 min and contains air compression to the pressure of 2.0–2.5 ATA (equivalent to the depth of 10–15 m under water) and lasts 70 min. During the second phase, the patient breathes pure oxygen through a mask three times for 20 min, taking two air breaks (5 min each) with the mask off. The last phase of the session is decompression [6]. The procedure for administering pure oxygen in an intermittent way is to avoid symptoms of oxygen toxicity. In almost all centers of hyperbaric medicine around the world, 100% oxygen is administered in hyperbaric conditions of 2–3 ATA in an intermittent way, in a time not exceeding 1 h.

Clinically, HBOT is highly efficacious in the treatment of several conditions spanning a broad pathological range [19]. Actual European indications for the medical use of HBOT were established during the ECHM Consensus Conference in 2016, taking into account three types of recommendations for using HBOT as a medical procedure—from strongly recommended to optional use, depending on the strength of the evidence of its beneficial action [2]. In the USA, such indications are prepared by the Undersea and Hyperbaric Medical Society (UHMS). Both the ECHM and UHMS create and update lists of indications for treatment with hyperbaric oxygen every few years. Differences between the actual lists include the lack of indications for SSNHL in UHMS recommendations (present on the ECHM list) and the lack of indications for a state of extremely high blood loss on the ECHM list (present on the UHMS list). HBOT is also used in treatment of diseases not included in the official lists of indications, although further studies need to confirm the efficacy of such an approach [5]. Some authors indicate the neurotherapeutic effects of hyperbaric oxygen in traumatic brain injuries, in the light of recent evidence for HBOT efficacy in brain repair [20]. Some observations and experiments indicated HBOT as a potent means of delivering to the brain sufficient oxygen needed for activation of neuroplasticity and restoration of impaired brain functions [21]. However, there is no strong evidence of the effectiveness of HBOT in neurodegenerative illnesses so far. The lack of a clear and confirmed clinical effect of HBOT is why in the 2016 recommendations it could not be used in autism spectrum disorders, placental insufficiency, multiple sclerosis, cerebral palsy, and acute phase of stroke [2]. Complete contraindications to HBOT are untreated pneumothorax and chemotherapy. Relative contraindications to oxygenation in hyperbaric conditions are upper respiratory tract infections, emphysema with CO_2 retention, asymptomatic air cysts or blebs in the lungs, high body temperature, pregnancy, claustrophobia, low seizure threshold, bleomycin therapy, and a history of thoracic or ear surgery [2,7].

4. HBOT in the Treatment of Sudden Sensorineural Hearing Loss

Sudden sensorineural hearing loss (SSNHL) is a deterioration of hearing greater than 30 dB occurring in at least three consecutive audiometric frequencies over a period of up to 72 h [22]. Idiopathic SSNHL affects 5 to 20 per 100,000 individuals with the probability of appearance increasing with age. This illness is considered to be a true otologic emergency [23]. For smaller losses, some patients regain their pre-loss hearing threshold without medical therapy due to the repair capacity of the cochlea, but in cases of profound hearing impairment the chance of complete recovery is limited [19]. The majority (about 90%) of SSNHL cases is idiopathic and several causes have been proposed to explain its etiopathogenesis (i.e., viral infection, otologic disease, trauma, vascular causes, and neoplastic disease, in order from the most frequent to rare [24]. Diagnosis and treatment should be preceded by a thorough medical history and physical examination of the patient. Adult-onset SSNHL typically affects women and men in the age between 43 and 53, with no significant gender differences. Patients typically present with tinnitus, vertigo, or ear fullness along with hearing loss. Tinnitus (a phantom auditory sensation without external sound, often described as a ringing, buzzing, or roaring in the ear) is the most frequent secondary symptom of idiopathic SSNHL; recent trials reported incidence rates as high as 73% to 84% [25]. The majority of sudden deafness cases are unilateral. Bilateral symptoms occur in less than 2% of all cases [26]. During the onset of SSNHL, the following variables are correlated with a worse prognosis: dizziness, profound hearing loss, impaired hearing in the contralateral ear, and delay to start treatment. Tinnitus at the onset of idiopathic SSNHL is reported to correlate with a better prognosis [27]. Idiopathic healing occurs in 32–65% of patients; the majority within the first 2 weeks after symptoms onset. Complete hearing recovery and full tinnitus remission were both reported about three times more frequent in mild–moderate hearing loss patients than in severe–profound cases [25].

The pathophysiology of SSNHL seems to be closely associated with the state of the inner ear. In the research of Gupta et al. [28], a low birth weight of infants (<5.5 lbs) was associated with higher risk of adult-onset hearing loss. The authors supposed that among the low birth-weight infants, exposure to malnutrition or stress may adversely affect cochlear development and influence the inner ear functioning in adult life. There is evidence suggesting that chronic inflammation may be involved in the development of idiopathic sensorineural deafness as a molecular basis of this illness [29–31]. It can lead to microvascular injury and atherogenesis and increase the risk of ischemia [32]. Inflammation can result in endothelial dysfunction, which can cause a thrombotic event that alters the blood supply to the inner ear [29]. The cochlea is an organ dependent on adequate oxygen levels in the blood [33]. However, because of the protected location of the cochlea in the temporal bone, blood supply to this organ is quite limited [34]. Blood is supplied to the cochlea mainly through a single terminal (labyrinthine) artery. Cochlear hair cells have a high oxygen consumption and poor tolerance of hypoxia, which is the reason why the inner ear is prone to changes in circulation. SSNHL appears to be characterized by hypoxia in the perilymph and, therefore, in the scala tympani and the organ of Corti. Thus, a mechanism playing a possible role in idiopathic SSNHL seems to be of vascular origin related to the lack of oxygen.

The prognosis in cases of isolated SSNHL is generally good, and an improvement within a matter of days is common. Patients in whom there is no change within 2 weeks are unlikely to show much recovery. However, the time between onset and treatment seems to be crucial in the prognosis. According to studies, 65% of patients with idiopathic SSNHL recovered their hearing irrespective of the type of treatment, with most recovering within 14 days [35].

Different therapeutic approaches are based on the supposed pathophysiological mechanisms responsible for inner ear dysfunction. Therapies of idiopathic SSNHL include corticosteroids, vasodilators, anticoagulants, antioxidants, plasma expanders and HBOT [36–38]. The first-line treatment for idiopathic SSNHL are oral or/and intratympanic corticosteroids to reduce the supposed inflammatory response. Steroids are one of the most used options among the therapeutic armamentarium without any strong recommendation to refer to. Oral steroids are usually proposed as a first-line treatment based on an evaluation of the ratio risk versus benefit [39]. The side effects expected from an acute therapy with oral steroids are mild [38]. However, trans-tympanic steroids are also recommended, because this mode of administration avoids the undesirable effects of systemic steroids. Trans-tympanic steroids in the treatment of SSNHL may be used as a primary therapy alone or in combination with systemic steroids, or as a salvage therapy after the failure of systemic steroids [38,39]. Research showed that intratympanic treatment was not inferior to oral corticosteroids treatment [38]. The success rate of the initial steroid therapy depends on many factors, such as the severity of the initial hearing loss and the time of the onset of treatment. In cases where the initial therapy of idiopathic SSNHL has no or an unsatisfactory result, adjunctive or salvage therapies are implemented. HBOT is mostly used as salvage therapy after the failure of the initial steroid therapy or as adjunctive therapy of idiopathic cases of sudden deafness treated with corticosteroids [2,22,37,39–41].

HBOT in the treatment of SSNHL is used to reverse the lack of oxygen in the inner ear. It increases the partial oxygen pressure to improve the blood oxygen profile and microcirculation. Oxygen supply is very important for hearing due to essential role of the endocochlear potential in auditory transduction in human. The cochlea mediates the transduction of sound waves into nerve impulses and this process depends on the endocochlear potential. Its magnitude is dependent on the oxygen supply. When the oxygen content of blood is increased, the magnitude of the endocochlear potential is elevated and auditory sensitivity is enhanced. The metabolic demand for the generation of endocochlear potential requires a dense capillary network for the delivery of the oxygen and removal of CO_2. The lack of oxygen causes the lack of endovascular potential and results in sensorineural hearing loss. In a state of low oxygen tension, the endocochlear potential was found to be more negative than in the oxygenated state [19]. It was found that perilymphatic oxygen tension decreased in patients with SSNHL, while under hyperbaric conditions, the oxygen tension in the perilymphatic fluid increased by 450% [37]. According to the results of actual research, HBOT improves hearing in SSNHL patients by suppressing the inflammatory response induced by Toll-like receptors, which play a critical role in the inflammatory response [30]. These shed light on the molecular mechanism of the therapeutic effects of HBOT on hearing loss. By increasing the oxygen delivery to the cochlea, HBOT influence the endocochlear potential. HBOT seems to decrease the expression of inflammation-related cytokines in peripheral blood, leading to an improvement in the hearing levels in SSNHL patients [30,31].

HBOT was first used for SSNHL in the late 1970s [42]. Today oxygenation in hyperbaric conditions is still the only known method of increasing the oxygen level in the liquids of the inner ear. The purpose of HBOT in the treatment of SSNHL is to increase the partial pressure of oxygen in the blood and then, via diffusion, to increase the partial pressure of oxygen in the inner ear fluids that nourish the sensory and neural elements of the cochlea [19,20,42]. Oxygenation in hyperbaric conditions has gained popularity as a treatment for SSNHL in combination with pharmacologic agents. Recent evidence suggests that HBOT confers a significant additional therapeutic benefit when used in combination with steroid therapy for idiopathic sudden deafness. Results of recent research showed that HBOT combined with oral or intratympanic corticosteroids increased hearing gain in SSNHL patients compared to steroids treatment alone. According to the results of current research, when combined with a large-dose steroid treatment, HBOT gives positive results in 59.7–86.67% of patients with a greater rate of improvement (defined as gain of hearing of at least 10 dB on pure tone average) in patients treated with adjunctive hyperbaric oxygen than in patients treated only with corticosteroids [30,42–48]. In the majority of available research, the overall hearing recovery rate was significantly higher for the patients treated with hyperbaric oxygen and systemic steroids than for those treated with systemic steroids alone or systemic steroids combined with intratympanic steroids (Table 1).

Table 1. The percentage of hearing gain and recovery in comparative studies of hyperbaric oxygen therapy (HBOT) and pharmacotherapy with corticosteroids (CS) in sudden sensorineural hearing loss (SSNHL).

Author	Year	Percentage of Hearing Gain, $p < 0.005$	
		CS	CS + HBOT
Satar et al. [48]	2006	76.4%	60.0% *
Fujimura et al. [42]	2007	39.7%	59.7%
Capuano et al. [49]	2015	68%	84%
Cho et al. [46]	2018	40.8%	65.7%
Krajcovicova et al. [45]	2018	28.6%	61.7%
Yücel and Özbuğday [50]	2020	60%	68.2% *
Liu et al. [30]	2020	66.67%	86.67%

* Result not significant.

There is only a small number of research that showed no significant differences between the steroid and steroid + HBOT groups in terms of hearing gain [48,50]; however, in some of these studies the treatment was implemented up to 30 days from the symptoms onset, which could influence the results of therapy.

The actual results present no significant differences in therapeutic effect of HBOT alone in the treatment of SSNHL. In the research of Sun et al., corticosteroids showed a much better improvement of tinnitus than HBOT [51]. It stays in concordance with the actual EHMS recommendation for not using HBOT in the treatment of tinnitus due to a lack of a clear and confirmed clinical effect [2].

4.1. Implementation of Treatment

In the available literature and guidelines regarding the treatment of SSNHL with the use of HBOT, special attention is paid to the time elapsed between the occurrence of symptoms and the commencement of treatment, with emphasis on the necessity of quick therapy implementation [2,19,40,41,47,49,52]. The effectiveness of HBOT is time-dependent and decreases with an increasing delay in administration. Generally, it is recommended to start with therapy as early as possible, preferably within 48 h [19]; however, there are discrepancies in the results of studies on the efficacy of HBOT treatment as a function of time. Research by Wang et al. [40] showed that the starting time of HBOT ≤ 7 days from disease onset was independently associated with hearing recovery. Capuano et al. found that recovery was significantly better when patients were treated with HBOT in the first 14 days after sudden deafness symptoms onset, compared to those treated after 14 days [49]. According to some reports, the rate of no recovery was significantly higher in patients who started treatment after 10 days of SSNHL onset [47]. Holy et al. found that patients who were treated with HBOT within 10days had significantly more improvement than those treated later than 10 days (66% vs. 39%). They describe treatment that started during the first 10 days following the onset of hearing loss as more effective than delayed treatment, even by only a few weeks [52]. Based on recent evidence, addition of HBOT to corticosteroids may be beneficial only when initiated early. The most favorable prognoses concern SSNHL patients with a medium or deep level of hearing loss (>41 dB), for whom HBOT was implemented within 14 days of the occurrence of the hearing loss [19,37,40–42,47–49,51–53]. According to the EHMS recommendation, it would be reasonable to use HBOT as an adjunct to corticosteroids in patients presenting after the first two weeks but not later than one month, particularly in patients with severe and profound hearing loss [2]. On the Consensus Conference on Hyperbaric Medicine in 2016, the EHMS recommended HBOT in the treatment of SSNHL as a Type 1 recommendation (therapy strongly recommended). However, the EHMS recommends HBOT combined with medical therapy only in patients with acute idiopathic SSNHL who present within two weeks from disease onset. According to EHMS, it would also be reasonable to use HBOT as an adjunct to corticosteroids in patients with severe or profound hearing loss (≥70 dB), but only in cases presented not later than one month after symptoms onset. There is no recommendation for HBOT in patients with SSNHL after six months of disease onset, due to the lack of randomized controlled clinical trials to confirm any positive effect of HBOT in such cases [2]. The guideline for clinical practice for idiopathic SSNHL, which was updated in 2019, states that HBOT can be administered as the initial therapy in combination with steroids within the first two weeks of symptoms onset, or as salvage therapy within the first month [54].

4.2. Severity of the Initial Hearing Loss

In the light of current research, the addition of HBOT to primary conventional therapy improves the results when started early after the onset of SSNHL. The results of the treatment are also related to the severity of the initial hearing loss. In the research of Ajduk et al., a significant difference in the hearing thresholds after HBOT, used as salvation therapy after the failure of steroid therapy, was found at all frequencies in patients with a hearing loss of >61 dB. The group of patients with a hearing threshold of ≤60 dB had a significant improvement only at 250 and 500 Hz [37]. Similar results are reported by Hara et al. [55], who hypothesized that HBOT improves hearing in idiopathic SSNHL patients at lower frequencies. Using early HBOT as adjunctive therapy to pharmacological treatment in many research studies showed the most promising therapeutic effects among patients with severe/profound (≥70 dB) and complete hearing loss [19,39,40,42,47,51,55–57]. Hosokawa et al. [44] found significantly better improvement rates in patients who were 60 years old or younger (74.8%) compared to patients older than 60 years (62.9%). Current research demonstrated also that a lower proportion of men was associated with a greater benefit of HBOT in comparison to women [56]. Early-stage combination therapy for patients in many research studies was associated with better audiometric results at higher frequencies and a better clinical outcome score [58].

4.3. HBOT Strategy

For HBOT to be properly effective in the treatment of SSNHL, the pressure in the hyperbaric chamber during HBOT should be at least 1.4 ATA. Only breathing 100% oxygen in hyperbaric conditions above 1.4 ATA contributes to a significant increase in the diffusion radius of the oxygen from the capillaries to the surrounding tissues [4–6]. Contemporary research show that increasing the maximal pressure during HBOT higher than 2.5 ATA did not provide any benefit for hearing recovery; so, an air pressure kept at 2.0 to 2.5 ATA is currently recommended for the treatment of SSNHL [56]. In terms of HBOT strategy, the optimal number of sessions in the treatment of sudden deafness should be determined individually for each case; however, there is no evidence in the literature for the effectiveness of HBOT longer than 10–20 sessions [59]. The lowest effective number of HBOT sessions should be implemented. Research reported a positive therapeutic effect of HBOT at 2.5 ATA in a 2-week protocol with a 90-min session per day, applied together with pharmacological treatment [41,55,56,59,60]. In a report of Olex-Zarychta [41], a full hearing recovery after 15 daily HBOT sessions was observed, with hearing gain reported by the patient after six sessions. In the research of Rhee et al. [56], complete hearing recovery was favored in SSNHL patients with a total HBOT duration of at least 1200 min. The authors recommended that 100% oxygen at 2.0 to 2.5 ATA should be administered for 10 to 20 days, with a 90-min session each day. Hara et al. [55] presented a protocol consisting of HBOT for 20 sessions, together with pharmacotherapy once a day for seven consecutive days, performed 3 h before the HBOT session. Generally, early implementation of a 10-day protocol with a 90-min session per day is recommended, or, alternatively, a 20-day protocol with a 60-min session per day to achieve a total HBOT duration of at least 1200 min. A medical consultation by a specialist in hyperbaric medicine before starting HBOT is recommended [41]. According to ECHM guidelines, a treatment series of HBOT in the treatment of SSNHL should consist of 15 daily 60-min exposures to 100% oxygen at 2.5 atmosphere ATA. All sessions should take place at the same time every day and at the same place (professional mono-place or multi-place hyperbaric chamber). According to official ECHM recommendations, each session of HBOT should last 90 min and should be divided into several phases: 10 min for air compression, 70 min of therapy (3 × 20 min of breathing pure oxygen through the mask with two 5-min breaks with the mask off), and about 10 min for decompression [2,41].

5. Adverse Reactions to HBOT

The use of oxygenation in hyperbaric conditions as a medical procedure is associated with the possibility of side effects and complications. HBOT remains among the safest therapies used today; however, some side effects are associated with this procedure [61–65]. HBOT side effects are primarily the result of increased pressure or hyperoxia. Possible complications during HBOT include barotraumatic lesions (middle ear, nasal sinuses, inner ear, lung, and teeth), oxygen toxicity (central nervous system, and lung), confinement anxiety (claustrophobia), and ocular effects (myopia and cataract growth) [2,6,7,61–65]. Undesirable reactions may occur during and after exposure to 100% oxygen, and its toxicity must always be taken into consideration before the implementation of HBOT in the treatment of SSNHL.

5.1. Effects of Pressure

The predominant complication is represented by pressure equalization problems within the middle ear that occur during the compression phase of the HBOT session. The most frequent complication of HBOT is barotrauma; it may affect the middle ear, but also the accessory sinuses of the nose and lungs. For example, 15–43% of patients experience symptoms of barotrauma in the middle ear during the compression phase of the HBOT procedure [2,7,61–64]. They have ear ache or problems with unblocking the hearing tube to relieve pressure. Recent publications indicated a vast majority (84%) of barotrauma complications being minor trauma (tympanic membrane injection or its slight hemorrhage) and no cases of tympanic membrane rupture. Risk factors that have been identified include a very slow or high rate of compression, intubation, acute upper respiratory infection, and a history of head and neck malignancy [64]. In order to prevent pressure injuries, pharmacologic agents are administered either orally or intranasally, and paracentesis can also be performed. In some cases, the procedure of compression must be interrupted, and the patient must leave the hyperbaric chamber. A pressure shock may occur on a one-off basis and often affects only one ear. To minimize the risk of pressure injuries, the compression and decompression phases of the HBOT protocol are recommended to be done very slowly [2,7]. Otherwise, edema in the middle ear may occur as well as retraction or even perforation of the tympanic membrane, which may lead to hearing deficits. In rare cases, pressure trauma to the middle ear can damage the inner ear and impair its function. There is a risk of rupture of the oval or round window membranes [61,63].

5.2. Pulmonary Oxygen Toxicity

Pulmonary oxygen toxicity is not expected from routine daily HBOT when used for typical elective indications, but it is a possible side effect of oxygenation in hyperbaric conditions [64]. Pulmonary toxicity from the oxygen is associated with long-term exposure of the body to 100% oxygen under both normal and elevated pressure conditions. An oxygen toxicity seizure is relatively rare at typical clinical treatment pressures (2–3 ATA). It is difficult to predict on an individual basis. It was traditionally reported at ~1 in 10,000 treatments [61]. Early symptoms of oxygen poisoning are irritation of the larynx and trachea, periodontal pain of the larynx, and swelling of the nasal mucosa. Such symptoms may appear after approx. 6 h of breathing with 100% oxygen at 2 ATA. Oxygen delivery by the intermittent method and a limited time of exposure (about 60–70 min) are practical ways to avoid symptoms of pulmonary oxygen toxicity under hyperbaric conditions.

5.3. Ocular Side Effects

Eye complications related to HBOT include short-sightedness (myopia) and cataracts. Myopia is a transient condition occurring in about 20–100% of patients undergoing oxygen therapy in hyperbaric chambers [61–63]. Progressive myopic changes to the eye may occur after repetitive HBOT. The cause of periodic visual impairment related to HBO intervention is not clear. The exact mechanism is not fully understood, but it is thought that oxygen toxicity causes changes to the crystalline lens, hardening the lens and increasing its refractive power. It is believed that temporary visual impairment can be inter alia because of changes in the curvature of the cornea caused by variations in pressure during the compression and/or decompression, metabolic changes in the cornea, or changes in the refractive lens [6]. Research also showed a possible increase in the risk of irreversible refractive changes if the number of therapies exceeds 100 [66]. Most of the myopic changes are reversible after cessation of the therapy. Many studies report this effect to last from days to months. Myopia is a reversible effect; in the majority of cases, the pre-therapy level of vision is reached within 6–8 weeks of HBOT completion [61,64]. However, in some reports the time for eyesight to normalize after HBOT was reported to be different. In a study by Olex-Zarychta, the reversal of myopia was rapid, within the first ten days after the last HBOT session. In this particular case the therapy included only 15 HBOT exposures [41]. However, reversal of myopia may progress more slowly over months up to a year from the date of completion of HBOT [6].

An excess of reactive oxygen species in tissues due to their cytotoxic properties and/or deficiencies in antioxidant activity may contribute to complications of HBOT, such as cataracts. The exact mechanism of cataractogenesis is not completely understood. The pathogenetic processes in the keratoconus seem to be contributing by deficiencies in antioxidant activities and reactive oxygen species. It is supposed that such an impact may be exacerbated during HBOT by exposure to additional reactive oxygen species [62]. The development of both nuclear cataracts and a reversible myopic shift in hyperbaric patients strongly suggests that oxidative damage to the lens proteins is responsible for these ocular complications of HBOT [66].

Limited exposure to HBOT (no more than 20–60 treatment sessions) does not seem to cause cataracts. According to reports, cataract formation may occur only in a long treatment series greatly exceeding 60 sessions. However, HBOT can lead to more rapid progression of existing cataracts [61,64,66,67]. In the literature, the role of the age of the patient is emphasized. Cataracts remain the leading cause of visual impairment and blindness worldwide and usually occurs after the age of 65 [61]. The senescent eye is supposed to be particularly prone to oxidative damage, exemplified by cataract and macular degeneration. The retina is particularly susceptible to oxidative stress, because of its high consumption of the oxygen. Age-related macular degeneration involves oxidative stress and death of the retinal pigment epithelial cells. HBOT may exacerbate these processes. That is the reason why cataracts as well as age-related macular degeneration and keratoconus may be contraindications to HBOT and exposure to the therapy-related oxidative stress. In the study by Palmquist et al. [66], over 40% of patients with no evidence of a cataract before therapy developed nuclear cataracts, with the first evidence appearing after 150 HBOT sessions. Long-term exposure to hyperbaric oxygenation, resulting in oxidative damage to the lens proteins, seems to play a critical role in this ocular complication of HBOT [61,66,67]. It should be underlined that ocular changes are not fully reversible after cessation of prolonged HBOT. Careful pre-examination and evaluation of the potential risks and benefits from HBOT should be warranted to the patient. Delivery of HBOT may need to be modified or it may even be contraindicated in some cases [61,62,67]. Patients who undergo multiple HBOT treatments and complain of visual changes persisting for more than two to three months after completion of the HBOT course should be seen by an ophthalmologist to assess their vision and obtain a diagnosis of the cause of any impairment [67].

5.4. Central Nervous System Oxygen Toxicity

The effects of HBOT on neural elements remain poorly understood [65]. The toxic effect of oxygen on the central nervous system (CNS) can manifest itself after even a short breathing time of 100% oxygen at an elevated pressure (at least 2 ATA). The recognized presentation of CNS oxygen toxicity during clinical hyperbaric oxygen treatment is an oxygen toxicity seizure. Recent evidence over the past 15 years puts the incidence at ~1 in 2000–10,000 treatments [61,66]. HBOT-induced seizures are defined as brief, oxygen-related, generalized tonic–clonic convulsions usually occurring toward the end of the treatment [68]. The higher the compression pressure, the faster the clinical symptoms of the toxic effects of oxygen on the CNS may appear [63]. The most characteristic symptom of CNS oxygen toxicity is generalized grand mal convulsions. The seizure may be preceded by muscular tremors around the mouth, eyes, and by trembling hands [6,7,61,65]. HBOT seems to be a safe method for patients with neurological disorders, excluding those who suffer from uncontrolled epilepsy [68]. Cerebral toxicity of the oxygen may be avoided by strict adherence to medical procedures for HBO treatment, including intermittent and controlled oxygen administration in hyperbaric chambers. The reason for the increased incidence for CNS oxygen toxicity during HBOT appears to be related to patient selection and changes in hyperbaric oxygen treatment protocols [61,68].

6. Conclusions

SSNHL appears to be characterized by hypoxia in the perilymph in the scala tympani and the organ of Corti. It is supposed that a possible mechanism of idiopathic SSNHL is of vascular origin and related to the lack of oxygen. HBOT is still the only known method of increasing the oxygen level in the liquids of the inner ear. Due to limited adverse reactions and compelling positive outcomes stemming from HBOT in the literature, this procedure is recommended clinically as adjunctive therapy for the treatment of SSNHL. Hyperbaric oxygen therapy remains an option, but only when combined with steroid therapy for either initial treatment or salvage therapy after the failure of pharmacological treatment. The high effectiveness of early HBOT implementation together with standard pharmacological treatment has been proven clinically and from 2016 is strongly recommended by EHMS for patients with acute idiopathic sudden deafness who present within two weeks of disease onset, or as a salvage therapy implemented within 1 month of onset of sensorineural hearing loss. The optimal number of HBOT sessions in the treatment of SSNHL depends on the severity and duration of the symptoms and on the response to the treatment. Standard treatment includes on average 10/20 daily sessions making a total HBOT duration of at least 1200 min. The typical time of one HBOT session recommended by EHMS is 90 min divided into three main phases; the time of breathing pure oxygen in the main phase of the session is about 60 min. Delivery of hyperbaric oxygenation may need to be modified or contraindicated in individual cases due to possible complications. Patients scheduled for HBOT need a careful pre-examination and monitoring. If safety guidelines are strictly followed, HBOT is a treatment method with a relatively low rate of adverse reactions.

Funding: This research received no external funding.

Conflicts of Interest: The author has no conflict of interest to disclose.

Abbreviations

ATA	atmosphere absolute
ATP	adenosine-triphosphate
CNS	central nervous system
CO	carbon monoxide
CO_2	carbon dioxide
ECHM	European Committee of Hyperbaric Medicine
HBOT	hyperbaric oxygen therapy
NO	nitric oxide
SSNHL	sudden sensorineural hearing loss
UHMS	Undersea and Hyperbaric Medical Society
WHO	World Health Organization

References

1. Kirby, J.P.; Snyder, J.; Schuerer, D.J.; Peters, J.S.; Bochicchio, G.V. Essentials of Hyperbaric Oxygen Therapy: 2019 Review. *Mol. Med.* **2019**, *116*, 176–179.
2. Mathieu, D.; Marroni, A.; Kot, J. Tenth European Consensus Conference on Hyperbaric Medicine: Recommendations for accepted and non-accepted clinical indications and practice of hyperbaric oxygen treatment. *SPUMS J.* **2017**, *47*, 24–32.
3. World Health Organization. The Global Burden of Disease 2004 Update. 2008. Available online: http://www.who.int/healthinfo/global_burden_disease/GBD_report_2004update_full.pdf (accessed on 8 September 2020).
4. Kujawski, S.; Kujawska, A.; Kozakiewicz, M.; Olszanski, R.; Siermontowski, P.; Zalewski, P. The effect of hyperbaric oxygen therapy on the nervous system. Systematic review. *Pol. Hyp. Res.* **2015**, *4*, 19–27. [CrossRef]
5. Kawecki, M.; Knefel, G.; Szymańska, B.; Nowak, M.; Sieroń, A. present indications and capabilities of HBO applying. *Acta Balneol.* **2006**, *4*, 202–206.
6. Mathieu, D. *Handbook on Hyperbaric Medicine*; Springer: Dordecht, Germany, 2006.
7. Jain, K. *Textbook of Hyperbaric Medicine, 4th Revised and Expanded Edition*; Hogrefe & Huber Publishers: Göttingen, Germany, 2004.
8. Marx, R.E.; Ehler, W.J.; Tayapongsak, P.; Pierce, L.W. Relationship of oxygen dose to angiogenesis induction in irradiated tissue. *Am. J. Surg.* **1990**, *160*, 519–524. [CrossRef]
9. Ciarlone, G.E.; Hinojo, C.M.; Stavitzski, N.M.; Dean, J.B. CNS function and dysfunction during exposure to hyperbaric oxygen in operationa land clinical settings. *Redox Biol.* **2019**, *27*, 101159. [CrossRef]

10. Park, M.K.; Muhvich, K.H.; Myers, R.M.; Marzella, L. Hyperoxia prolongs the aminoglycoside-induced post antibiotic effect in Pseudomonas aeruginosa. *Antimicrob. Agents Chemother.* **1991**, *35*, 691–695. [CrossRef]
11. Barata, P.; Cervaens, M.; Resende, R.; Camacho, Ó.; Marques, F. Hyperbaric oxygen effects on sport injuries. *Ther. Adv. Musculoskelet. Dis.* **2011**, *3*, 111–121. [CrossRef]
12. Buras, J.F.; Reenstra, W.R. Endothelial–neutrophil interactions during ischemia and reperfusion injury: Basic mechanisms of hyperbaric oxygen. *Neurol. Res.* **2007**, *29*, 127–131. [CrossRef]
13. Mortensen, C. Hyperbaric oxygen therapy. *Curr. Anaesth. Crit. Care* **2008**, *19*, 333–337. [CrossRef]
14. Huang, L.; Obenaus, A. Hyperbaric oxygen therapy for traumatic brain injury. *Med. Gas. Res.* **2011**, *1*, 21. [CrossRef] [PubMed]
15. Olex-Zarychta, D. Improvement of human reaction time with hyperbaric oxygen therapy. *J. Case Rep. Med. Sci.* **2017**, *3*, 26–28.
16. Kenneth, P.; Stoller, K.P. Quantification of neurocognitive changes before, during, and after hyperbaric oxygen therapy in a case of fetal alcohol syndrome. *Pediatrics* **2005**, *116*, 586–591.
17. Harrison, B.; Robinson, D.; Davison, B.J.; Foley, B.; Seda, E.; Byrnes, W.C. Treatment of exercise-induced muscle injury via hyperbaric oxygen therapy. *Med. Sci. Sports Exerc.* **2001**, *33*, 36–42. [CrossRef]
18. Günther, A.; Küppers-Tiedt, L.; Schneider, P.M.; Kunert, I.; Berrouschot, J.; Schneider, D.; Rossner, S. Reduced infarct volume and differential effects on glial cell activation after hyperbaric oxygen treatment in rat permanent focal cerebral ischaemia. *Eur. J. Neurosci.* **2005**, *21*, 3189–3194. [CrossRef]
19. Bayoumy, A.B.; DeRu, J.A. The use of hyperbaric oxygen therapy in acute hearing loss: A narrative review. *Eur. Arch. Otorhinolaryngol.* **2019**, *276*, 1859–1880. [CrossRef]
20. Efrati, S.; Ben-Jacob, E. Reflections on the neurotherapeutic effects of hyperbaric oxygen. *Expert Rev. Neurother.* **2014**, *14*, 233–236. [CrossRef]
21. Efrati, S.; Fishlev, G.; Bechor Volkov, O.; Bergan, J.; Kliakhandler, K.; Kamiager, I.; Gal, N.; Friedman, N.; Ben-Jacob, E.; Golan, H. Hyperbaric oxygen induce slate neuroplasticity in post stroke patients–randomized, prospective trial. *PLoS ONE* **2013**, *8*, e53716. [CrossRef]
22. Imsuwansri, T.; Poonsap, P.; Snidvongs, K. Hyperbaric oxygen therapy for sudden sensorineural hearing loss after failure from oral and intratympanic corticosteroid. *Clin. Exp. Otorhinolaryngol.* **2012**, *5* (Suppl. 1), 99–102. [CrossRef]
23. Cvorovic, L.; Jovanovic, M.B.; Milutinovic, Z.; Arsovic, N.; Djeric, D. Randomized prospective trail of hyperbaric oxygen therapy and intratympanic steroid injection as salvage treatment of sudden sensorineural hearing loss. *Otol. Neurotol.* **2013**, *34*, 1021–1026. [CrossRef]
24. Quaranta, N.; De Ceglie, V.; D'Elia, A. Endothelia dysfunction in idiopathic sudden sensorineural hearing loss: A review. *Audiol. Res.* **2016**, *6*, 151. [CrossRef]
25. Mühlmeier, G.; Baguley, D.; Cox, T.; Suckfüll, M.; Meyer, T. Characteristics and spontaneous recovery of tinnitus related to idiopathic sudden sensorineural hearing loss. *Otol. Neurotol.* **2016**, *37*, 634–641. [CrossRef] [PubMed]
26. Khamvongsa, P.; Patel, N.; Aziz Ali, A.; Bodoukhin, N.; Carreno, O. Using corticosteroids to treat sudden sensorineural hearing loss in pregnancy: A case report and literature review. *Case Rep. Woman's Health* **2020**, *27*, e00201. [CrossRef] [PubMed]
27. Bogaz, E.A.; Maranhão, A.S.; Inoue, D.P.; Suzuki, F.A.; Penido, N.d.O. Variables with prognostic value in the onset of idiopathic sudden sensorineural hearing loss. *Braz. J. Otorhinolaryngol.* **2015**, *81*, 520–526. [CrossRef] [PubMed]
28. Gupta, S.; Wang, M.; Hong, B.; Curhan, S.G.; Curhan, G.C. Birth weight and adult-onset hearing loss. *Ear Hear.* **2020**, *41*, 1208–1214. [CrossRef] [PubMed]
29. Chen, L.N.; Zhang, G.; Zhang, Z.; Wang, Y.; Hu, L.; Wu, J. Neutrophil-tolymphocyte ratio predictsdiagnosis and prognosis of idiopathic sudden sensorineural hearing loss: A systematic review and meta-analysis. *Medicine* **2018**, *97*, e12492. [CrossRef]
30. Liu, X.H.; Liang, F.; Jia, X.Y.; Zhao, L.; Zhou, Y.; Yang, J. Hyperbaric oxygen treatment improves hearing level via attenuating TLR4/NF-κB mediated inflammation in sudden sensorineural hearing loss patients. *Biomed. Environ. Sci.* **2020**, *33*, 331–337.
31. Yang, C.H.; Hwang, C.F.; Yang, M.Y.; Lin, P.M.; Chuang, J.H. Expression of toll-like receptor genes in leukocytes of patients with sudden sensorineural hearing loss. *Laryngoscope* **2015**, *125*, 382–387. [CrossRef]

32. Chang, S.L.; Hsieh, C.C.; Tseng, K.S.; Weng, S.F.; Lin, Y.S. Hypercholesterolemia is correlated with an increased risk of idiopathic sudden sensorineural hearing loss: A historical prospective cohort study. *Ear Hear.* **2014**, *35*, 256–261. [CrossRef]
33. Tabuchi, K.; Nishimura, B.; Tanaka, S.; Hayashi, K.; Hirose, Y.; Hara, A. Ischemia-reperfusion injury of the cochlea: Pharmacological strategies for cochlear protection and implications of glutamate and reactive oxygen species. *Curr. Neuropharmacol.* **2010**, *8*, 128–134. [CrossRef]
34. Shi, X. Physiopathology of the cochlear microcirculation. *Hear. Res.* **2011**, *282*, 10–24. [CrossRef] [PubMed]
35. Schreiber, E.B.; Agrup, C.; Haskard, D.O.; Luxon, L.M. Sudden sensorineural hearing loss. *Lancet* **2010**, *375*, 1203–1211. [CrossRef]
36. Ganesan, P.; Kothandaraman, P.P.; Swapna, S.; Manchaiah, V. A retrospective study of the clinical characteristics and post-treatment hearing outcome in idiopathic sudden sensorineural hearing loss. *Audiol. Res.* **2017**, *7*, 168. [CrossRef] [PubMed]
37. Ajduk, J.; Ries, M.; Trotic, R.; Marinac, I.; Vlatka, K.; Bedekovic, V. Hyperbaric oxygen therapy as salvage therapy for sudden sensorineural hearing loss. *J. Int. Adv. Otol.* **2017**, *13*, 61–64. [CrossRef] [PubMed]
38. Rauch, S.D.; Halpin, C.F.; Antonelli, P.J.; Babu, S.; Carey, J.P.; Gantz, B.J.; Goebel, J.A.; Hammerschlag, P.E.; Jeffrey, P.; Harris, J.P.; et al. Oral vs intratympanic corticosteroid therapy for idiopathic sudden sensorineural hearing loss. A randomized trial. *JAMA Otolaryngol. Head Neck Surg.* **2011**, *305*, 2071–2079.
39. Marx, M.; Younes, E.; Chandrasekhar, S.S.; Ito, J.; Plontke, S.; O'Leary, S.; Sterkers, O. International consensus (ICON) on treatment of sudden sensorineural hearing loss. *Eur. Ann. Otorhinolaryngol. Head Neck Dis.* **2018**, *135*, 23–28. [CrossRef] [PubMed]
40. Wang, Y.; Gao, Y.; Wang, B.; Chen, L.; Zhang, X. Efficacy and prognostic factors of combined hyperbaric oxygen therapy in patients with idiopathic sudden sensorineural hearing loss. *Am. J. Audiol.* **2019**, *28*, 95–100. [CrossRef]
41. Olex-Zarychta, D. Successful treatment of sudden sensorineural hearing loss by means of pharmacotherapy combined with early hyperbaric oxygen therapy. *Medicine* **2017**, *96*, e9397. [CrossRef]
42. Fujimura, T.; Suzuki, H.; Shiomori, T.; Udaka, T.; Mori, T. Hyperbaric oxygen and steroid therapy for idiopathic sudden sensorineural hearing loss. *Eur. Arch. Otorhinolaryngol.* **2007**, *264*, 861–866. [CrossRef]
43. Hosokawa, S.; Hosokawa, K.; Takahashi, G.; Sugiyama, K.; Nakanishi, H.; Takebayashi, S.; Mineta, H. Hyperbaric oxygen therapy as concurrent treatment with systemic steroids for idiopathic sudden sensorineural hearing loss: A comparison of three different steroid treatments. *Audiol. Neurootol.* **2018**, *23*, 145–151. [CrossRef]
44. Hosokawa, S.; Sugiyama, K.; Takahashi, G.; Takebayashi, S.; Mineta, H. Prognostic factors for idiopathic suddensen sorineural hearing loss treated with hyperbaric oxygen therapy and intravenous steroids. *J. Laryngol. Otol.* **2017**, *131*, 77–82. [CrossRef] [PubMed]
45. Krajcovicova, Z.; Melus, V.; Zigo, R.; Matisakova, I.; Vecera, J.; Kaslikova, K. Efficacy of hyperbaric oxygen therapy as a supplementary therapy of sudden hearing loss in the Slovak Republic. *Undersea Hyperb. Med.* **2018**, *45*, 363–370. [PubMed]
46. Cho, I.; Lee, H.-M.; Choi, S.-W.; Kong, S.-K.; Lee, I.-W.; Goh, E.-K.; Oh, S.-J. Comparison of two diferent treatment protocols using systemic and intratympanic steroids with and without hyperbaric oxygen therapy in patients with severe to profound idiopathic sudden sensorineural hearing loss: A randomized controlled trial. *Audiol. Neurootol.* **2018**, *23*, 199–207. [CrossRef] [PubMed]
47. Eryigit, B.; Ziylan, F.; Yaz, F.; Thomeer, H. The efectiveness of hyperbaric oxygen in patients with idiopathic sudden sensorineural hearing loss: A systematic review. *Eur. Arch. Otorhinolaryngol.* **2018**, *275*, 2893–2904. [CrossRef]
48. Satar, B.; Hidir, Y.; Yetiser, S. Efectiveness of hyperbaric oxygen therapy in idiopathic sudden hearing loss. *J. Laryngol Otol.* **2006**, *120*, 665–669. [CrossRef]
49. Capuano, L.; Cavaliere, M.; Parente, G.; Damiano, A.; Pezzuti, G.; Lopardo, D.; Iemma, M. Hyperbaric oxygen for idiopathic sudden hearing loss: Is the routine application helpful? *Acta Otolaryngol.* **2015**, *135*, 692–697. [CrossRef]
50. Yücel, A.; Özbuğday, Y. Comparison of steroid treatment with and without hyperbaric oxygen therapy for idiopathic sudden sensorineural hearing loss. *J. Audiol. Otol.* **2020**, *24*, 127–132. [CrossRef]

51. Sun, H.; Qiu, X.; Hu, J.; Ma, Z. Comparison of intratympanic dexamethasone therapy and hyperbaric oxygen therapy for the salvage treatment of refractory high-frequency sudden sensorineural hearing loss. *Am. J. Otolaryngol.* **2018**, *39*, 531–535. [CrossRef]
52. Holy, R.; Navara, M.; Dosel, P.; Fundova, P.; Prazenica, P.; Hahn, A. Hyperbaric oxygen therapy in idiopathic sudden sensorineural hearing loss (ISSNHL) in association with combined treatment. *Undersea Hyperb. Med.* **2011**, *38*, 137–142.
53. Goodrich, E.; Goodrich, R.P.; Reese, C.A. Sensorineural hearing loss after spine surgery treated with hyperbaric oxygen therapy: Two case reports. *Undersea Hyperb. Med.* **2018**, *45*, 217–224. [CrossRef]
54. Chandrasekhar, S.S.; Tsai Do, B.S.; Schwartz, S.R.; Bontempo, L.J.; Faucett, E.A.; Finestone, S.A.; Hollingsworth, D.B.; Kelley, D.M.; Kmucha, S.T.; Moonis, G.; et al. Clinical practice guideline: Sudden hearing loss (Update). *Otolaryngol. Head Neck Surg.* **2019**, *161* (Suppl. 1), 1–45. [CrossRef] [PubMed]
55. Hara, S.; Kusunoki, T.; Honma, H.; Kidokoro, Y.; Ikeda, K. Efficacy of the additional effect of hyperbaric oxygen therapy in combination of systemic steroid and prostaglandin E_1 for idiopathic sudden sensorineural hearing loss. *Am. J. Otolaryngol.* **2020**, *41*, 102363. [CrossRef] [PubMed]
56. Rhee, T.M.; Hwang, D.; Lee, J.S.; Park, J.; Lee, J.M. Addition of hyperbaric oxygen therapy vs medical therapy alone for idiopathic sudden sensorineural hearing loss: A systematic review and meta-analysis. *JAMA Otolaryngol. Head Neck Surg.* **2018**, *144*, 1153–1161. [CrossRef] [PubMed]
57. Sevil, E.; Bercin, S.; Muderris, T.; Gul, F.; Kiris, M. Comparison of two different steroid treatments with hyperbaric oxygen for idiopathic sudden sensorineural hearing loss. *Eur. Arch. Otorhinolaryngol.* **2016**, *273*, 2419–2426. [CrossRef]
58. Bayoumy, A.B.; van der Veen, E.L.; van Ooij, P.-J.A.M.; Besseling-Hansen, F.S.; Koch, D.A.; Stegeman, I.; de Ru, J.A. Effect of hyperbaric oxygen therapy and corticosteroid therapy in military personnel with acute acoustic trauma. *BMJ Mil. Health.* **2020**, *166*, 243–248. [CrossRef]
59. Murphy-Lavoie, H.; Piper, S.; Moon, R.E.; Legros, T. Hyperbaric oxygen therapy for idiopathic sudden sensorineural hearing loss. *Undersea Hyperb. Med.* **2012**, *39*, 777–792.
60. Taşdöven, G.E.; Derin, A.T.; Yaprak, N.; Özçağlar, H.Ü. The place of hyperbaric oxygen therapy and ozone therapy in sudden hearing loss. *Braz. J. Otorhinolaryngol.* **2017**, *83*, 457–463. [CrossRef]
61. Heyboer, M., III; Sharma, D.; Santiago, W.; McCulloch, N. Hyperbaric oxygen therapy: Side effect defined and quantified. *Adv. Wound Care* **2017**, *6*, 210–224. [CrossRef]
62. McMonnies, C.W. Hyperbaric oxygen therapy and the possibility of ocular complications or contraindications. *Clin. Exp. Optom.* **2015**, *98*, 122–125. [CrossRef]
63. Plafki, C.; Peters, P.; Almeling, M.; Welslau, W.; Busch, R. Complications and side effects of hyperbaric oxygen therapy. *Aviat Space Environ. Med.* **2000**, *71*, 119–124.
64. Heyboer, M., 3rd. Hyperbaric Oxygen Therapy Side Effects-Where Do We Stand? *J. Am. Coll. Clin. Wound Spec.* **2018**, *8*, 2–3. [CrossRef] [PubMed]
65. Bitterman, N. CNS oxygen toxicity. *Undersea Hyperb. Med.* **2004**, *31*, 63–72. [PubMed]
66. Palmquist, B.M.; Philipson, B.; Barr, P.O. Nuclear cataract and myopia during hyperbaric oxygen therapy. *Br. J. Ophthalmol.* **1984**, *68*, 13–17. [CrossRef] [PubMed]
67. Bennett, M.H.; Cooper, J.S. *Hyperbaric Cataracts*; Stat Pearls Publishing: Treasure Island, FL, USA, 2020.
68. Hadanny, A.; Meir, O.; Bechor, Y.; Fishlev, G.; Bergan, J.; Efrati, S. Seizures during hyperbaric oxygen therapy: Retrospective analysis of 62,614 treatment sessions. *Undersea Hyperb Med.* **2016**, *43*, 21–28.

Publisher's Note: MDPI stays neutral with regard to jurisdictional claims in published maps and institutional affiliations.

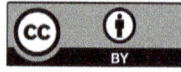

© 2020 by the author. Licensee MDPI, Basel, Switzerland. This article is an open access article distributed under the terms and conditions of the Creative Commons Attribution (CC BY) license (http://creativecommons.org/licenses/by/4.0/).

MDPI
St. Alban-Anlage 66
4052 Basel
Switzerland
Tel. +41 61 683 77 34
Fax +41 61 302 89 18
www.mdpi.com

International Journal of Molecular Sciences Editorial Office
E-mail: ijms@mdpi.com
www.mdpi.com/journal/ijms

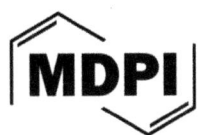